DRUGS LOOKING FOR DISEASES

Developments in Cardiovascular Medicine

VOLUME 120

DRUGS LOOKING FOR DISEASES

*Innovative Drug Research and the Development
of the Beta Blockers and the Calcium Antagonists*

by

REIN VOS

*Department of Pharmacology and Pharmacotherapeutics,
University Centre for Pharmacy,
University of Groningen,
Groningen, The Netherlands*

SPRINGER SCIENCE+BUSINESS MEDIA, B.V.

Library of Congress Cataloging-in-Publication Data

Vos, Rein, 1955-
    Drugs looking for diseases : innovative drug research and the
development of the beta blockers and the calcium antagonists / by
Rein Vos.
        p.   cm. -- (Developments in cardiovascular medicine ; v. 120)
    Includes bibliographical references.
    Includes index.
    ISBN 978-0-7923-0968-0   ISBN 978-94-011-3796-6 (eBook)
    DOI 10.1007/978-94-011-3796-6
    1. Drugs--Research. 2. Drugs--Design. 3. Adrenergic beta
blockers--Research--History. 4. Calcium--Antagonists--Research-
-History.   I. Title. II. Series.
    [DNLM: 1. Adrenergic Beta Receptor Blockaders--history.
2. Calcium Channel Blockers--history. 3. Drug Therapy. 4. Drugs.
5. Heart Disease--history. 6. Research. 7. Sociology, Medical.
W1 DE997VME v. 120 / QV 20.5 V959d]
RM301.25.V67   1991
615'.19--dc20
DNLM/DLC
for Library of Congress   90-5359

ISBN 978-0-7923-0968-0

Printed on acid-free paper

FOREWORD

We all know how much time, effort and money it takes to develop a new drug. Hundreds of chemical compounds have to be synthesized and thousands of different activities in biology, physiology, pharmacology, clinical investigation, management and marketing have to be initiated and coordinated. Each new drug starts a voyage of discovery through an unmapped terrain which is shrouded in mist and beset by pitfalls, as Dr. Rein Vos puts it in his absorbing inside story of the development of the beta-adrenoceptor blocking agents and the calcium antagonists.

Indeed we know, for example, how long it took before the theory of Ahlquist of the alpha and beta adrenergic receptors was widely accepted. Similarly, it suffices to memorize shortly the difficulty of expanding the new concept of calcium antagonism through the national German boundaries into the world. This shows how laborious and complex pharmaceutical progress is, and we all will benefit from a deeper understanding of the process of innovative drug research.

Dr. Vos provides an absorbing account of the origin of the pharmacodynamic concepts of beta blockade and calcium antagonism, and of the further development of these concepts as a new therapeutic rationale in cardiovascular medicine. The book is extremely interesting since it depicts the dominant trends in Anglo-American and German coronary therapy and the underlying theoretical concepts. I have never seen such a thorough study of cultural differences of medical thinking and their relevancy for progress in cardiovascular medicine. In this respect it is also really surprising how diligently my own work on calcium antagonism has been investigated in every detail. Such a scrutinizing study has never been made before, and I am sure that the colleagues in the various fields of cardiovascular and pharmaceutical research will have the same experience with respect to the subjects of their own expertise which are described in this book. Further, Dr. Vos' treatise of the interactions between industrial laboratory work, academic research and clinical investigation sheds light on the way of thinking by medicinal chemists, pharmacologists and physiologists, and clinical investigators and clinicians.

However, the most important prospect, as outlined in the book, seem to arise from the author's viewpoint that the drug discovery process can be studied and modeled. Throughout the book the view is developed that medical-pharmaceutical practice is an indispensable source of feedback to the discovery process. In this way Dr. Vos counteracts current views of drug research, yet simultaneously provides us with a new perspective on the shaping of new medicines.

Prof. Dr. A. Fleckenstein

Freiburg, West Germany
November 1990

CONTENTS

Chapter 4. Industrial research and beta blockade

Chapter 5. Verapamil: dying drug or sleeping beauty?

Chapter 6. Metamorphosis of a disease - Profiles of angina pectoris in Anglo-American medicine

Chapter 7. Targeting in drug research and the medical scene
The beta blocker project at Boehringer against the background of different views in German and Anglo-American medicine

Part 1. The medical scene - different views in German and Anglo-American medicine

Chapter 9. The enigma of drug discovery

PREFACE

The theme of this book is the role of medical-pharmaceutical practice as an indispensable source of feedback to the drug discovery process. The origin of medicines lies in the interface of development in the laboratory and the application of therapy in daily medical practice. This will be demonstrated with the help of the fascinating history of the beta adrenoceptor blocking agents and the calcium antogonists.

The search for the essentials of the drug discovery process delves into questions concerning the cognitive structures and types of knowledge representations in drug research. The view is developed that therapeutic change can be regarded as as the movement of patterns between profiles of drugs and diseases. Accordingly, the concept of profile, which forms a central part of communicating knowledge in the pharmaceutical and biomedical sciences, involves the kernel of this author's analysis.

Throughout, this analysis is interfered with the translation of the concept of profile into a set-theoretical model. Readers, primarily interested in the historical developments can easily skip the formal sections on the logic of drug and disease profiles, i.e. sections 2.6, 2.7, 5.7, and 7.4. These sections are intended, on the one hand, as a legitimation of the use of cognitive (and social) maps of medical knowledge in subsequent chapters and the application of the model to the collected historical material; on the other, as a way of first-order exploring of the computational foundations of the drug discovery process.

The study of these cognitive patterns not only contributes to theory development in cognitive science and science studies but offers also perspectives towards the modelling and improvement of the search processes in pharmaceutical research. This is of great importance considering the high costs and long development time in drug research, particulary in the context of the policy debate about the regulation of 'high tech' products from the research fronts in biotechnology and molecular biology.

The book attempts to set the foundation for a deeper understanding of how 'practice' contributes to the shaping of new medicines, that is it seeks to integrate the relevant aspects related to the construction of medical knowledge; classification of drugs and diseases; cultural differences in medical practice; drug regulatory affairs; the organization and development of clinical research programs; post-marketing-surveillance; drug utilization studies and pharmaco-epidemiology; and the history of drug research. These topics will become increasingly important to the medical profession and the pharmaceutical industry.

It is hoped that this book will provide the pharmaceutical industry, academia, government, clinical investigators, pharmacists, physicians, and research workers in the life sciences with a comprehensive view of drug discovery. Further, the concepts and views developed in this study might be interesting for scientists in the field of cognitive science and science studies, and philosophers and historians of science, technology and medicine.

The book has evolved over many years, and clearly it is impossible to thank all of the many people who have contributed to this project. The first exception is that I wish to express my special gratitude to Dr. Henk Bodewitz who introduced me to the field of drug innovation and regulation and to Prof. Dr. D.K.F. Meijer, Prof. Dr. A.J. Dunning and Prof. Dr. T.A.F. Kuipers who were promoters of the project leading to my Ph.D. in late 1989. Prof. Kuipers creatively contributed to the "Logic of profiles" and the set-theoretical model of drug discovery.

Secondly, I must record by gratitude to all participants in the field for being willing to invest so much and effort in the interviews in spite of their own busy schedules as well as for their invaluable comments on the draft-chapters of this book. Lack of space prevents me to thank to all of them separately – for this reason I have compiled a list of participants - but some of them I would like to name personally for making relevant contacts, for the thorough comments, or the provision of additional but indispensable information: Prof.Dr. B. Ablad, Prof.Dr. A.M. Barrett, Dr. J.D. Fitzgerald, Prof.Dr. A. Fleckenstein, Dr. R. Howe, Prof.Dr. G. Johnsson, Dr. I. Östholm, Dr. G. Pfennigsdorf, Prof.Dr. B.F. Robinson, and Prof.Dr. E.M. Vaughan Williams. A very special thank you goes to Prof.Dr. E. Kutter for allowing me to use the reports and the other material of the beta blocker project at Boehringer. This is also true for Dr. H.G. Köppe who has patiently endured my curiosity and has helped me to search for the relevant material.

Furthermore I am grateful to many people from whom I have received encouragement, criticism and support: Dr. Henk Buurma, Prof. Dr. M.N.G. Dukes, Dr. Johan Hoek, the late Prof. Dr. A.S. Horn, Dr. Reidar Lie, Dr. Annemarie Mol, Dr. Nico Punt, Dr. René Remie, Prof. Dr. W. van Rossum, Prof. Dr. Jochen Schaefer, Dr. Fred Steward, Dr. Dick Willems, Prof. Dr. J. Zaagsma and the colleagues of the Science Studies Unit, the International Institute for Theoretical Cardiology, the "Munga" group, and the Department of Pharmacology and Pharmacotherapeutics.

A special acknowledgment goes to my colleagues Petra Denig, Floor Haaijer, Lolkje de Jong, Anke van Trigt and Nicolien Wieringa. I appreciate the many discussions about drug utilization, pharmacoepidemiology and post-marketing-surveillance which I could participate in, and which, directly or indirectly, have influenced the ideas set forth in this thesis.

I greatly appreciate the patience and the skills of Nynke Bakker, Greet Popken, and Koos Jansen, the latter also for his help with the computerized search in MEDLARS database. For preparing the photographical part I owe much to Jacques Duitsch, Jacob Pleiter and Siep Noorman.

What are ideas without being able to communicate? This is particularly so because my lack of understanding of the English language diluted the impact of the story that I wished to convey clearly. If the story about the beta blockers and the calcium antagonists, and the philosophical view unfolding in this study, has been made transparent in its bare bones, then this is a tribute to the skills and understanding of Mrs. Biddy Schilizzi. Similarly, I would like to thank Dr. Fulco Teunissen for his excellent translation of the German quotations.

Rein Vos
Groningen, November 1990.

Acknowledgments

Chapter 3 is a (slightly) edited version of: Rein Vos and Henk Bodewitz, Experimental and therapeutic profiling in drug innovation - The early history of the beta blockers. Perspectives in Biology and Medicine 1988; 31: 469-479.

Permission of the publishing-firms for reproducing the figures/tables in this thesis - listed below - is gratefully acknowledged:

Figure 1.1
Fletcher SW, Fletcher RH, Greganti MA. Clinical research trends in general medical journals, 1946 - 1976. In: Roberts E, et al., eds. Biomedical innovation. Massachuchets: The MIT Press, 1980: 284-300.

Figure 1.3
Oates JA. Clinical investigation: a pathway to discovery [presidential address]. Trans Ass Am Phys 1982; 95:lxxviii-xc.

Figure 1.4
Oates JA [discussion]. In: Helms RB, ed. Drug development and marketing. Washington DC: American Enterprise Institute for Public Policy Research, 1975.

Table 1.1
Fletcher SW, Fletcher RH, Greganti MA. Clinical research trends in general medical journals, 1946 - 1976. In: Roberts E, et al., eds. Biomedical innovation. Massachuchets: The MIT Press, 1980: 284-300.

Figure 2.1
Figure 2.2
Maxwell RA. The state of the art of the science of drug discovery - an opinion. Drug Dev Res 1984; 4:375-389.

Table 2.1
Langley P, Simon HA, Bradshaw GL, Zytkow JM. Scientific discovery. Computational explorations of the creative processes. Cambridge [etc.]: The MIT Press, 1987.

Table 2.2
Table 2.4
Zsotér TT, Church JG. Calcium antagonists. Pharmacodynamic effects and mechanism of action. Drugs 1983; 25:93-112.

Table 2.5
Anderson JL. Pharmacologic interventions in acute myocardial infarction. In: Maronde RF. Topics in Clinical Pharmacology & Pharmacotherapeutics. New York [etc.]: Springer-Verlag, 1986: 108-134.

Figure 2.3
Wartak J, Fenna D, Callaghan JC. Numerical approach to classification of angina. Am Heart J 1984; 107:402-404.

Table 4.2
Barrett AM, Crowther AF, Dunlop D, Shanks RG, Smith LH. Cardio-selective ß-blockade [Short communications/Kurzreferate, Teil 2]. N-S Arch Ph 1967/1968; 259:152-153.

Table 4.3
Lands AM, Arnold A, McAuliff JP, Luduena FP, Brown, Jr., TG. Differentiation of receptor systems activated by sympathomimetic amines. Nature 1967; 214:597-598.

Table 4.4
Larsen AA, Lish PM. A new bio-isostere: alkylsulphonamidophenethanolamines. Nature 1964; 203:1283-1284.

Figure 4.5
Astra Chemical & Pharmaceuticals NV. Proceedings Swedish conference with Dutch specialists on hypertension. Gothenburg, May 17th-19th, 1972, Rijswijk: Astra, 1972: 15-24.

Figure 4.6
Forsberg S-A, Johnsson G. Hemodynamic effects of propranolol and H56/28 in man - a comparative study of two ß-adrenergic receptor antagonists. Life Sci 1967; 6:1147-1154.

Figure 5.1
Fleckenstein A, Döring HJ, Kammermeier H, Grün G. Influence of prenylamine on the utilization of high energy phosphates in cardiac muscle. Biochimica applicata 1968; 14 (S1):323-344.

Table 6.1
Prinzmetal M, Ekmeckci A, Kennamer R. Kwoczynski JK, Shubin H, Toyoshima H. Variant form of angina pectoris. Previously undelineated syndrome. JAMA 1960; 174:1794-1800.

Figure 6.8
Kübler W, Tillmans H. Management of coronary vasometric angina. Eur Heart J 1985; 6 (Suppl F):27-31.

Figure 7.5
Holzmann M. Differenzierungsmöglichkeiten bei der Angina Pectoris, Deut Med Wo 1954; 79:1109-1115.

Figure 7.6
Keller CH. Leitsymptom: "Herzschmerzen" und ihre Deutung. Münch med Wschr 1960; 30:1409-1415.

Figure 7.8
Figure 7.9
Köppe HG. Recent chemical developments in the field of beta adrenoceptor blocking drugs. Progr Clin Biochem Med 1986; 3:31-72.

Figure 8.2
Austel V, Kutter E. Practical procedures in drug design. In: Ariens EJ, ed. Drug Design. Medicinal Chemistry. A series of monographs, Vol X. New York [etc.]: Academic Press, 1980: 1-69.

Figure 9.1
Zandvoort H. Milieukunde en interdisciplinariteit. Kennis & Methode 1986; 10 (3):230-251.

Financial support by:

AB Hässle subsidiary of Astra, Mölndal, Sweden

Dutch Foundation for the Promotion of Medical - Pharmaceutical Research, Utrecht, The Netherlands

Knoll AG, Ludwigshafen, West-Germany

The Netherlands Heart Foundation, The Hague, The Netherlands

for the publication of this thesis is gratefully acknowledged.

List of Interviewed Participants

B. Ablad, Department of Pharmacology, AB Hässle Mölndal, Sweden.

A.M. Barrett, University of Buckingham, United Kingdom.

F. Bender, Kardiologie, Medizinische Klinik und Poliklinik der Westfalische Wilhelms-Universität Münster, Federal Republic Germany.

A. Berntsson, AB Hässle Mölndal, Sweden.

J.W. Black, The Rayne Institute, Analytical Pharmacology, King's College School of Medicine and Dentistry of King's College London, United Kingdom.

B. Brisse, Kardiologie, Medizinische Klinik und Poliklinik der Westfalische Wilhelms-Universität Münster, Federal Republic Germany.

R.T. Brittain, Glaxo Research Group Limited, Ware Hertfordshire, United Kingdom.

H. Brunner, Therwil, Switzerland.

D.M. Burley, Centre for Pharmaceutical Development/International Liaison, Pharmaceuticals Division Ciba-Geigy, Horsham, United Kingdom.

A. Carlsson, Department of Pharmacology, University of Göteborg, Sweden.

D.A. Chamberlain, Cardiac Care Unit, Royal Sussex County Hospital Brighton, United Kingdom.

D.J. Le Count, Imperial Chemical Industries Limited, Macclesfield, United Kingdom.

R.H. Davies, The Welsh School of Pharmacy Cardiff, United Kingdom.

C.T. Dollery, Royal Postgraduate Medical School, Hammersmith Hospital London, United Kingdom.

A.C. Dornhorst, Department of Medicine, Middlesex Hospital London, United Kingdom.

A. Engelhardt, Boehringer Ingelheim, Federal Republic Germany.

J.D. Fitzgerald, Materia Medica, Mere Cheshire, United Kingdom.

A. Fleckenstein, Physiologisches Institut, Albert Ludwigs Universität Freiburg, Federal Republic of Germany.

B. Folkow, Department of Physiology, University of Göteborg, Sweden.

H. Gülker, Kardiologie, Medizinische Klinik und Poliklinik der Westfalische Wilhelms-Universität Münster, Federal Republic Germany.

H. Haas, Bad Herrenalb, Federal Republic Germany.

F. Hagemeijer, Cardiologie, Sint Franciscus Gasthuis Rotterdam, The Netherlands.

R. Howe, Chemistry II Department, Imperial Chemical Industries Macclesfield, United Kingdom.

H. Huijbers, Marketing Manager Knoll BV Almere, The Netherlands.

D. Jack, Glaxo Holdings Greenford, Middlesex London, United Kingdom.

G.J. Johnsson, Cardiovascular Research & Development, AB Hässle Mölndal, Sweden.

M. Kaltenbach, Zentrum der Innere Medizin, Abteilung für Kardiologie, Klinikum der Johann Wolfgang Goethe Universität Frankfurt, Federal Republic Germany.

G. Kan, Cardiologie, Elisabeth Gasthuis Haarlem, The Netherlands.

H.G. Köppe, Chemistry Department Boehringer Ingelheim, Federal Republic Germany.

A. Lichterfeldt, Ockenheim, Federal Republic Germany.

B.J. Main, Chemistry II Department, Imperial Chemical Industries Macclesfield, United Kingdom.

M. Maier, Cardiovascular Research, Ciba-Geigy, Basle Switzerland.

F.A. Nelemans, Paasloo , The Netherlands.

I. Östholm, AB Hässle Mölndal, Sweden.

F. Ostermayer, Cardiovascular Research, Ciba-Geigy, Basle Switzerland.

G. Pfennigsdorf, Medizinisch-Wissenschaftliche Abteilung, Knoll AG Ludwigshafen, Federal Republic of Germany.

B.N.C. Prichard, Department of Clinical Pharmacology, University College Medical School, The Rayne Institute London, United Kingdom.

B.F. Robinson, Department of Pharmacology and Clinical Pharmacology, St. George's Hospital Medical School, University of London, United Kingdom.

R. Sannerstedt, Cardiology Sahlgren's Hospital, University of Göteborg, Sweden.

R.G. Shanks, Department of Therapeutics and Pharmacology, The Queen's University of Belfast, United Kingdom.

B. Silke, Department of Medical cardiology, The General Infirmary Leeds, United Kingdom.

L.H. Smith, Macclesfield, United Kingdom.

J. Thale, Kardiologie, Medizinische Klinik und Poliklinik der Westfalische Wilhelms-Universität Münster, Federal Republic Germany.

Th.A. Thien, Interne Geneeskunde, Sint Radboud Ziekenhuis Nijmegen, The Netherlands.

H. Tucker, Chemistry II Department, Imperial Chemical Industries Macclesfield, United Kingdom.

E.M. Vaughan Williams, University Department of Pharmacology, Oxford, United Kingdom.

L. Werkö, Stockholm, Sweden.

Introduction

Aim of the study

In the past it may have been possible for one person to generate most of the knowledge needed for innovating medical therapy. Comroe has pointed out that when Withering discovered and used digitalis in 1785, he *"needed little help from those in other branches of science because he himself was a botanist, clinician, mineralogist, and chemist. The interfaces in his discovery were between his own brain cells that stored information in botany, chemistry, and medicine, and these neural connections quickly enabled him to identify the foxglove as the only ingredient of a Shropsire potpourri that was likely to have potent biological activity"*. [1] Since Withering, the foxglove (digitalis) has become a successful therapy for heart disease for more than a hundred years.

Nowadays scientists have to search through a vast space of theories, facts, numerous drugs and techniques, for novel phenomena in order to create new drugs. The search for new drugs takes place in large industrial laboratories and the development of one drug frequently takes more than ten years and can cost over $ 100,- million dollars.

This process of drug discovery is the subject of this study the aim of which is threefold. The **first aim** is a plea to re-value the role of medical practice for its contribution to the discovery process. With the move of drug research to the laboratory in this century, views on drug discovery are increasingly neglecting medical practice as a source for new drugs. However, through the use of medicines in different conditions, novel aspects of therapy and disease are continuously discovered which form targets for new developments in the pharmaceutical and biological sciences. The thesis to be elaborated here is that the origin of new medicines lies in the interface of development in the laboratory and the application of therapy in daily medical practice. This implies that no particular area in medicine is an exclusive source for drug discovery but that the exchange of information is the crucial factor. This emphasis on communication is embodied by pharmacological therapy. Probably more than any other product of technology, drugs form highly sensitive tools at the frontiers of modern bio-molecular research, yet simultaneously they pervade the daily life of people. This is commonly neglected, partly because of the apparent simplicity of drugs themselves: they are in a little bottle, they are touchable, green, red or blue, and every human being can swallow them.

The **second aim** of this study is to develop a theory in order to describe the drug discovery process. The assumption is that improvement of pharmacological therapy consists of a bi-directional process of innovating knowledge about drugs or about diseases. Either new medicines evolve when new principles of drug action are revealed or when new knowledge about the nature of the disease process emerges. In this sense, drugs and diseases are natural partners engaged in an intimate dance. One partner makes the first move and the other follows, sometimes one of the partners makes a side-step and the other unfortunately is too late to react adequately. In taking this dance-metaphor a step further, drugs are too often considered the leading party, while diseases have a passive role. Presumably diseases are just as frequently important in the innovation of therapies, just as drugs can be invented which reveal new aspects of a disease. Indeed, a dance encompasses two partners and the pattern of movements makes up the dance. Needless to say how complex this becomes when the ball-room appears to be filled with many dancing couples and also an exchange of partners is allowed.

If the metaphor stands, drug discovery consists of patterns of movement during which drugs and diseases meet and separate. In fact, the description of the partners involved is not entirely adequate since not the "drugs" and "diseases" themselves are the partners but rather the knowledge concerning the two aspects involved. Therefore **knowledge patterns**, i.e. profiles of drugs and diseases are the starting point of the model. The drug discovery process will therefore be conceived as a process of **rapprochement** between profiles of drugs on the one hand and profiles of diseases on the other.

The **third aim** of this study is the historical description of the development of the beta blockers and the calcium antagonists, two classes of cardiovascular drugs that were developed in the 1960s and 1970s respectively and which have improved cardiovascular therapy significantly. Moreover both types of drugs exemplify what has been said: while used and being used by millions of patients in variable conditions these medicines continue to help scientists at the frontiers of medicine in the clarification of bio-molecular processes.

Nature and scope of the study

The essence of this study lies in the combination of philosophy and history. From the viewpoint of both disciplines, therapeutics is a rather uncommon subject of analysis. *"Historians"*, as Rosenberg wrote a decade ago, *"have always found therapeutics an awkward piece of business. On the whole, they have responded by ignoring it"*. [2] The same applies to philosophers. Philosophy only seems to be relevant in discussing long-term consequences of therapeutic innovation, i.e. its impact on human life, norms and values, health care, in addition to basic issues concerning human and animal experimentation. To attribute philosophy a central place in the therapeutic enterprise will tend to evoke bland smiles and compassionate looks. One reason for this is that traditional philosophy of science is usually abstract and remote from scientific reality. Through the upsurge of interest in social studies of science, focussing on actual developments in scientific and technological practices, a discipline of cognitive studies of science is developing. This forms an area of interest at the Science Studies Unit in Groningen and has been called by Kuipers an "empirical meta-science", that is, a descriptive science of science.[3] In the philosophy of medicine this has been termed "empirical"[4] or "experimental"[5] philosophy.[6] The chosen method leaves room for normative problems and goals and is aiming at the extrapolation of patterns of successful or unsuccessful cases to problematic cases in science and technology.

From this follows an important approach, that is, not to start from general philosophical problems but from medical reality aiming at the conceptual clarification of cognitive processes. This will also yield new philosophical questions. Therefore attention is given to the language of biological scientists and physicians through which they attempt to grasp the essentials of knowledge development. In part, sets of terms are used which stem from the positivist philosophy of science such as theory, law, hypothesis and observation but which are insufficient in fully describing therapeutic developments. The development of drugs embodies numerous strands of knowledge. Since theories and laws are powerful but specialized devices for using knowledge, other means of defining regular structures and storing knowledge have to be used in drug research. This is reflected in sets of terms which are outside the realm of philosophers but which reveal an epistemological structure.

In this study the **concept of profiles** is the subject of analysis. This concept forms a central part of daily communication both in the pharmaceutical sciences and in medicine. A profile is a pattern and enables one to recognize the specific features of an object and to set it apart from other items. The epistemology underlying this concept is taxonomy which is considered by many philosophers as a primitive mechanism of gathering and storing information. However, taxonomy as this study claims is a powerful device for representing and using knowledge gathered from different sources. The model of drug discovery which is developed in this study, will be largely based on the concept of profile. Next to an epistemological analysis the idea will be proposed that the concept of profile can be translated into the language of set theory.

The scope of this study is therefore threefold:
a) A model will be developed as a contribution to structuring the history of drugs. In particular the purpose is to clarify the intricate relationships between knowledge about drugs and diseases. On the one hand this model generates problems for historical research, on the other, the historical material collected challenges the model.
b) The model proposed is an instrument to investigate cognitive structures underlying the drug discovery process. It is not a normative theory of discovery but rather the description of the process is the target.
c) By paying attention to the concept of profiles, cognitive structures in experimental sciences and medicine are clarified. The exploration of these issues will hopefully contribute to the philosophy of science, the philosophy of medicine and cognitive science.

Methodological issues

Combining philosophy with history is a delicate affair. Either history serves to illustrate the philosopher's view and the full richness of the historical developments is undermined; or the richness of history is kept but no room is left for philosophy. From both disciplinary viewpoints some methodological issues have to be discussed.

The historical section describes the development of the beta blockers and calcium antagonists. This description focusses on developments in the field of angina pectoris and covers the period 1950 - 1975. Because of the importance of both classes of drugs in medicine, the long period of use of these medicines as well as their impact on the recent progress in basic science, the history of these drugs will reveal essential features of the drug discovery process. All the ingredients are available: basic science (receptor theory, biochemistry and physiology of the circulatory system), chemical synthesis, clinical experience and accidental observations, etc. This is not to claim that the patterns of development shown in these cases can be simply extrapolated to other areas in the pharmaceutical sciences. However, the components of the developmental processes described can be used to model various routes of drug discovery.

Various industrial research projects are examined against the background of developing views on angina pectoris, heart failure and other cardiovascular disorders. The basic approach consists of a comparative analysis of developments in the Anglo-American and German speaking medical world. It seems somewhat awkward in treating British and American medicine as a single unit. However, the similarities are greater than the contrasts when compared with the developments in German medicine. National differences, however, between the United States and the United Kingdom should not be forgotten nor the regional differences in both countries. No doubt the same applies to German medicine. The differences described in this respect were very helpful in the unravelling of the processes relevant to therapeutic progress.

The methods used in this thesis are interviews with participants, literature-analysis and scientometric methods. Scientometric methods encompass citation analysis techniques based on bibliometric studies including (computerized) search of the Science Citation Index (SCI). These are used in particular, to illustrate developments revealed by the other methods. The specific methods are explained in notes to match and the appendices II and III.

The major medical journals in both medical settings as well as cardiovascular journals have been screened systematically. The respective names of the disorders involved, such as "angina pectoris", "heart failure", "(ischemic/coronary) heart disease", in addition to the categories of drugs and their individual components, were used as the key-words.

The interviews were open and unstructured but a check-list was used and for each interview separately prepared; this list grew with time. The interviews lasted from about an hour to more commonly about three hours. In some cases a round-table conversation with participants took place; in other cases interviews were repeated to yield additional information. All participants were given the opportunity to read the text with the relevant passages in which the material taken from the recorder was used; in various cases additional information was provided by the participants. With respect to representing developments in various disciplines and social settings, a variety of participants were asked to co-operate. In addition interviews were held with scientists and clinicians in the Netherlands to represent "outsider" views.

Taking the hypothesis that medical-pharmaceutical practice is an important source of feedback to the drug discovery process as the starting point, the term practice has to be defined. Current views distinguish between clinical medicine and general practice. The former represents the scientific side of medicine and is often characterized by the use of sophisticated techniques. Medical practice in contrast takes care of individual patients and is responsible for the careful and rational application of knowledge and techniques. Thus clinical medicine is considered as the forward-line of basic sciences. Alternatively clinical medicine is distinguished from the pre-clinical sciences and is in line with general practice. Both ways of looking at clinical medicine declare themselves in the debated "double-position" of the clinician: being a scientist as well as a practitioner. Moreover the intricate relationship between biomedical science and clinical medicine is the subject of a long-lasting discussion.

This shows that the term practice requires clarification. Various definitions are proposed. Thus, the institutional setting in which physicians perform their tasks can be taken as starting point, e.g. the distinction between single- and group practice versus the complex organizational structure of hospitals. In addition, the nature of medical work, e.g. research versus patient care, or the disciplinary origin of medical professionals can be used to define practice. In medical sociology the term practice denotes the centre of defining the labels "health", "disease", "deviance" or "handicap" which mediate societal processes. In the philosophy of medicine attempts are made to define prac‿e in terms of therapeutic action, the intrinsic relationship of diagnosis and treatment with societal values, and the physician-patient interaction. However, no consensus exists on this issue which is considered an important mission in the philosophy of medicine. Heterogeneous terminology is the result, e.g. "science of actions", "practical science", "science of individuals", "science of practice" and "praxiology".[7]

In this study the term practice is used as in the main stream philosophy of medicine, i.e. that therapeutic intervention is essential to medicine. In this respect, emphasis lies on a particular source of medical knowledge: casual experience (or casuistry or knowledge of particulars). The various methods of gathering knowledge about pharmacotherapy will be revealed in this study. As far as clinical medicine uses casual experience it may be considered as practice.

Outline of the argumentation in this thesis

Present views of drug discovery seem to be based too much on the simple model of the application of knowledge. Medical science develops theories, and as a result techniques used by physicians to establish the diagnosis, to estimate the prognosis and to prescribe therapy. This model is inadequate to grasp the multi-faceted aspects of therapeutic development.

In this thesis the model of the body of knowledge is used to shed light on the role of medical practice in the drug discovery process. This body of knowledge is as complex as the human body. It is composed of mechanisms for information storage, retrieval and usage in order to maintain its homeostasis and to perform its functions. Various sources are continuously shaping and reshaping the body of medical knowledge. Therefore the juxtaposition of different methods of obtaining medical knowledge will form a continuous thread through this thesis.

In **chapter 1** this issue is taken up by discussing the conflict between the controlled clinical trial and casual experience. The clinical trial is generally considered as the crucial step in transferring knowledge from laboratory to practice. Viewed in the light of the generation of knowledge instead of the validation of knowledge, the clinical trial must be regarded as a poor instrument. Other sources of obtaining medical knowledge, amongst which casual experience, are more powerful devices in generating new knowledge. It will be shown how various ways of gathering knowledge interact, thus addressing a wide range of medical topics and continuously reshaping the body of knowledge.

This issue is pursued in **chapter 2** in which the basic features of the drug discovery process are discussed. The analysis of two sets of philosophical terms in the pharmaceutical sector, i.e. basic-applied and rational-empirical (including art-serendipity), reveals that scientists recognize the various sources of knowledge which range from theory through experimental skills and craftsmanship to sharp-sighted observation. Nevertheless, through these sets of terms they are selectively focussing on specific features of the discovery process. The term selectively focussing is particularly apt because scientific development is viewed from the formation of scientific theories, thus excluding other aspects of the creative process.

For this reason, attention is paid to the renewed interest of philosophers in the role of the experiment in science. Philosophers like Hacking who shape this "new philosophy of the experiment" criticize present positivist philosophy for splitting up scientific activity into theory and observation, experiments merely serving the purpose of providing the evidence for the theories to be developed. Instead it is argued that theory and experiment both have variable shapes and a life of their own. Hence, several types of relationships between theory, experiment, invention and techniques have to be discerned.

Thus, starting from the conflict between the controlled clinical trials as the prototype of general scientific knowledge and casual experience as the prototype of particular knowledge gathered in medical practice, a landscape of the various sources of invention is drawn. This sketch substantiates the point of departure of this thesis, i.e. that no area in medicine is an exclusive source for drug discovery but that the coordination of the different kinds of activities in medicine is decisive. Hence, the choice of the case studies can be justified in the sense that they reveal the components of the discovery process which can be used to model the various pathways of drug development.

At this point the tension between the different ways of gaining knowledge will not be pursued but will reappear in the last two chapters.

From this point, the body of knowledge becomes the subject of the analysis. This analysis starts with a short overview of the state of affairs in cognitive science, in particular as seen through the eyes of Langley, Simon and colleagues. This overview generates the useful distinctions between descriptive and normative theory of discovery, theory and data driven discovery, and the representation and usage of knowledge. It also provides the author with the important concept of viewing the scientific process as the transition of one state into another. Searching through the vast space of scientific knowledge, scientists proceed from the initial state to a goal-state, hereby continuously evaluating the success of intermediate states. In this way the model of the body of knowledge is transformed into the image of a universe of goal-states and realized states which scientists attempt to match.

This image of goal-states and realized states is developed further by analyzing the concept of profile which is used in the pharmaceutical sector and in medicine to represent the state of knowledge about drugs and diseases. This concept of profile is chosen as the instrument for characterizing the states in the aforementioned universe of knowledge. The epistemological analysis is followed by the development of a **set-theoretical model** of the **concept of profile**. Subsequently, the drug discovery process seen as a process of rapprochement of drugs and diseases is described as the **interaction between profiles** within and between separate domains of knowledge about drugs and diseases.

Apart from providing a historical picture of the development of the beta blockers and the calcium antagonists, **chapters 3 to 7** attempt to substantiate the thesis that the developed model is useful in structuring therapeutic developments. But simultaneously, the question about the role of medical practice in therapeutic development is intertwined with the historical analysis in four ways.

Firstly, attention is paid permanently to show how emanating profiles in clinical medicine and general practice yield therapeutic objectives. These objectives are the targets of industrial researchers for profiling the desired drugs by means of experiments. This is shown in the descriptions of the industrial projects of ICI and AB Hässle (chapter 4), and the project of Boehringer (chapter 7).

Secondly, the contribution of clinical issues in the development of scientific concepts is analyzed. This applies to Ahlquist's theory (chapter 3), Land's theory and the concept of intrinsic activity (chapter 4), and biochemical and physiological concepts of the cardiovascular system (chapters 4,5 and 7). In particular, this is the case when describing the concept of calcium antagonism developed by Fleckenstein (chapter 5). But in this part the importance of creatively filling drug profiles with its spin off both to the basic sciences and medical therapy receives considerable attention.

Thirdly, the description of the changing views of diseases and therapeutic interventions (chapter 6 and 7) also reveals the important role of clinical medicine and general practice in therapeutic developments. Fourthly and finally, the cultural differences between Anglo-Saxon and German medicine revealed by the comparative method in the historical analysis (chapter 6 and 7) makes the role of medical practice much clearer.

In **chapter 8** the philosophical analysis is taken up again. The critical limits of the developed model will be discussed by analyzing the search process in drug research, the epistemological status of the concept of profile, and the question raised by Collins about the possibility of explicating knowledge as presupposed in artificial intelligence research.

After this critical outline of the model, the issue of different ways of gaining medical knowledge receives renewed attention. Firstly, by introducing the epistemological map as developed by Toulmin, the concepts such as general, particular, theoretical and practical knowledge are clarified further. Moreover, the conflict between the controlled clinical trial and casual experience is analyzed anew. This analysis culminates into the unraveling of the mechanisms through which medical practice contributes to the scope of medical knowledge about drugs.

In the final **chapter 9**, the role of medical practice is discussed by starting from the evolving trend in the pharmaceutical sector, i.e. the view that the understanding of the biological processes at the bio-molecular level allows the drug designer and the biologist to develop powerful and selectively acting drugs. This view is gaining increasing popularity and does not seem to leave much room for medical practice.

This view will be criticized because it endangers the creation of new therapies. Consequently, the concept of communication in medicine will be elaborated by showing that whatever extremes are chosen, e.g. theoretical and applied knowledge, general and particular knowledge, or reductionist and holistic knowledge, there is a step-wise system of knowledge formation which is spread out between these extremes. In this step-wise system, scientists are involved in an iterate process in which information collected at one step is sent through to the generation of knowledge at another step, and back again. In this to and fro process of gathering knowledge, the medical practice is indispensable, and the mechanisms are clarified through which it contributes to the drug discovery processes.

It is much easier to write
upon a disease
than upon a remedy.

The former is in the hands of Nature
and a faithful observer with
an eye of tolerable judgment
cannot fail to delineate a likeness.

The latter will ever be subject
to the whim,
the inaccuracies and
the blunder
of mankind.

William Withering, 1741-1799[1]

Chapter 1. The controlled clinical trial - A model for the intricate relationships between clinical medicine and drug research

1.1. Introduction

Over the past 30 years the controlled clinical trial has become the norm in clinical medicine and the pharmaceutical sector. Through a comparative analysis of treatment effects in two groups of patients - one group receiving the new remedy, the other group standard therapy or placebo - the effectiveness of the new therapy can be assessed.[2] A great deal of the fascination clinicians have in the performance of the controlled clinical trial derives from its rational nature and clearly defined outcome. Moreover, the controlled clinical trial is demanded today by authorities and policy makers in the health field. The regulatory systems that rapidly developed after the thalidomide disaster around 1960, took the controlled clinical trial as the basis for licensing new drugs. It was to form a barrier for the stream of chemical compounds coming out of industrial laboratories, and sift the good from the bad. The controlled trial has structured the way clinical medicine, both in theory and practice, became involved in the drug discovery process.
In this chapter the controlled clinical trial is discussed as the model for the intricate relationships between clinical medicine and drug research. The aim is twofold. On the one hand a linear view on the role of clinical medicine in the drug discovery process will be revealed. On the other some epistemological issues are elucidated which form the subject of subsequent chapters. The evolution of the controlled clinical trial will be briefly reviewed (1.2.) and the

way the controlled clinical trial has been implemented in drug research will be discussed
(1.3.). Finally, both historical sections culminate in a critique of the classic view of clinical
medicine in drug discovery (1.4.).

1.2. The evolution of the controlled clinical trial (CCT)

Proponents have emphasized the value of the CCT in forceful language on two fronts.
The first was formed by the campaign against empiricism and casual experience in medical
practice which were considered as sources of self-validating pronouncements in therapeutics. Lasagna, an influential proponent of the controlled clinical trial, pointed out *"that in
the day-to-day clinical evaluation of possible new drugs we can do better than merely capitalize on
unplanned accidents or to observe more or less naturally occurring phenomena"*. [3] Antagonists of the
clinical trial are criticized by Lasagna for taking *"refuge in the sanctity of 'clinical experience', both
their own and that of other physicians"*. [4] The inadequacy of casual experience concerned the
"post hoc propter hoc" dilemma: when patients, or at least some of them, recover, is the result
due to the remedy or to the healing power of Nature - "vis medicatrix naturae"? In addition,
the beneficial effects of medical therapy might be due to a placebo effect, not to its claimed
therapeutic activity. When prescribing a new remedy to patients, physicians, consciously or
unconsciously, display enthusiasm or scepticism. Thus, the physician's (and patient's) bias
disturbs the proper evaluation of medical therapy. Casual experience in medical practice is
unable to separate the three sources of recovery, e.g. placebo-effect, spontaneous recovery
and treatment effect; nor can it avoid bias.
The second front consisted of the desire to keep clinical medicine in pace with the rapidly
developing laboratory sciences. The intellectual procedures of valid evidence, logical analysis
and demonstrable proofs of these sciences are in painful contrast with the hazy bedside
procedures of the clinician. [5]
Both fronts amalgamated into the controlled clinical trial. During the 1920s and 1930s the
Medical Research Council (MRC) in Britain institutionalized the testing of the efficacy of
new drugs under "controlled conditions". In 1931, for example, the Council created the
Therapeutics Trial Committee. During the 1930s various controlled clinical trials were set
up to test therapies, mainly in the field of infectious and nutritional diseases. These activities
merged into the famous Streptomycin Trial, initiated in 1946 under the auspices of the MRC
to test streptomycin - developed in 1944 - in the treatment of pulmonary tuberculosis.
Awareness had grown about the inadequacies of casual clinical experience and as remarked
by the Medical Research Council: *"The natural course of pulmonary tuberculosis is in fact so
variable and unpredictable that evidence of improvement or cure following the use of a new drug in
a few cases cannot be accepted as proof of the effect of that drug. The history of chemotherapeutic trials
in tuberculosis is filled with errors due to empirical evaluation of drugs; the exaggerated claims made
for gold treatment, persisting over 15 years, provide a spectacular example"*. [6] The streptomycin trial
set the standards for future clinical trials.[7] Soon thereafter, the MRC conducted new
controlled clinical trials on anti-tuberculosis chemotherapy.[8]
The controlled clinical trial concept started to make inroads into clinical medicine. More-

over, it expressed how clinical medicine could contribute to pharmaceutical development in this "Golden Age of Drug Discovery" of the 1940s and 1950s.

Growth and impact of the controlled clinical trial

Most authors describe the development of the controlled clinical trial (CCT) - also often called the randomized clinical trial (RCT) - as the emergence of a scientific paradigm. The full model took a long time to develop, but reached its zenith during the 1960s and 1970s.[9] Most studies, which in fact assess impact as well as quality, use numbers of articles as indicators of the frequency with which trials were performed.[10]

In a well-known study, conducted by Fletcher et al., a random sample was examined of 612 original articles published in 1946, 1956, 1966 and 1976 in three prestigious general medical journals: the Journal of the American Medical Association, the Lancet and the New England Journal of Medicine. The category of all clinical trials as defined by Fletcher et al. includes randomized controlled trials; non-random controlled trials, in which patients are allocated to experimental and control groups by means of some non-random process (e.g., convenience or clinical judgment); and uncontrolled trials, in which there is no control group.

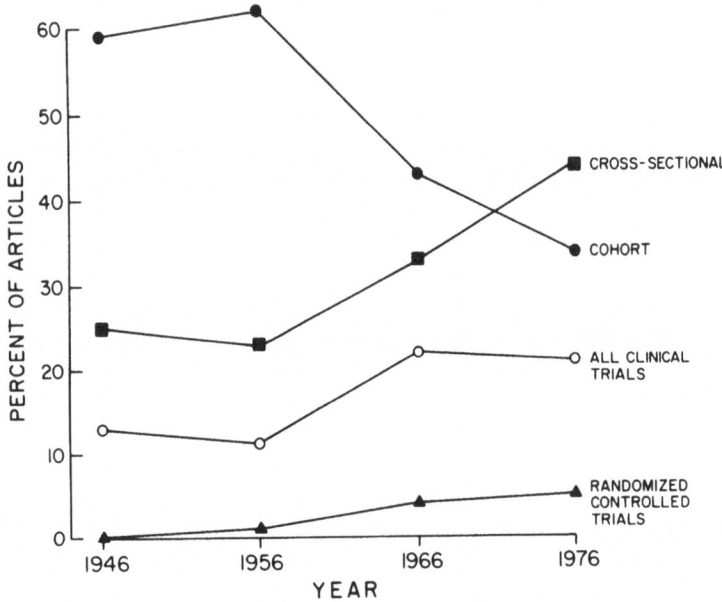

Figure 1.1
Research designs for 612 articles from 1946 to 1976.
Reproduced with permission from Fletcher et al. (1980).

The number of clinical trials increased from 13% to 21%, while the amount of randomized controlled trials rose from 0% to 5% of all investigated articles during this period. Studies by Juhl et al. for the field of gastroenterology and by Mulrow et al. for the field of digitalis treatment show the same pattern.[11]

Though the randomized controlled clinical trial is mainly a post Second World War acquisition, its influence seems to be marginal. Fletcher et al. conclude to their own surprise, *"that with the exception of the small growth in the number of randomized controlled trials, there was no evidence that the predominant research designs used in 1976 were more accurate ways of conducting clinical research than had been used in earlier years".*[12]

Their conclusion reflects a general disappointment in the medical community. Despite many attempts to improve the assessment of therapeutics the gap between theory and practice seems to be as wide as it used to be. However, the gap may be less than suggested.

1. The demarcation between controlled clinical trial and other clinical studies depends on the criteria used; or the type of empirical material collected. Lionel and Herxheimer, for example, studied 141 therapeutic reports, published during 1966-1969 in four British journals. They evaluated these reports by using a comprehensive set of strict criteria such as the use of appropriate controls, random allocation, objective measures (double-blind) and the statistical analysis used. In this way they concluded that 51% of all reports were "acceptable", 33% "unacceptable" and 16% "probably acceptable" (apparently satisfactory but lacking descriptive information to assess their definite validity). These findings differ from those presented above.

2. The impact of the clinical trial differs in distinct medical areas.[13]

Many authors have pointed out that specific areas were very prominent in the application of controlled clinical trials, e.g the fields of bacteriology (antibiotics) and immunology (vaccines), cardiology and oncology.[14] Furthermore, the evolution of the controlled clinical trial interfered with the expansion of pharmaceutical development and drug regulation. In this area many clinical trials are not published. In Finland, for example, the proportion of controlled clinical trials about psychotropic drugs that were not published, increased from 15% in 1965, via 17% in 1970 to 41% in 1974 and 1975. The quality of these unpublished trials seems to be as good, or as bad if preferred, as that of the published ones.[15]

3. Contextual differences are pertinent to the development of the CCT. Cochrane, a strong advocate of the controlled clinical trial, wrote: *"If some such index as the number of RCT's per 1.000 doctors per year for all countries were worked out and a map of the world shaded according to the level of the index (black being the highest), one would see the UK in black, and scattered black patches in Scandinavia, the USA and a few other countries: The rest would be nearly white".*[16] Though this map represents differences in actual research power and other factors, the geographic distribution of CCTs probably reflects differences in the standard of clinical science. A further indication is the finding of Juhl et al. that 40% of the CCTs were published in 10 medical journals, six of which were British. British editorial boards pay substantial attention to this type of clinical research.[17]

4. The studies discussed use frames of reference in a retrospective way. Though these frames conform reasonably well to the accepted definitions of clinical research designs, they originate from prevailing views at a certain time; subsequently they are used to study clinical

research in the foregoing period. Major problems with this approach will rise if shifts in emphasis on criteria took place.

Ross, for example, concluded in 1951 on the basis of his analysis of 100 articles in 5 major American medical journals that 75% assessed treatment incorrectly due to the absence of adequate controls.[18] According to Ross 25% of the reports fulfilled the scientific criteria, a higher amount than the 13% (in 1946) as suggested by Fletcher et al. The crucial point, however, is that Ross emphasized the use of control groups more than randomization.

During the 1940s and 1950s placebo and double-blind controlled trials received most attention in the medical world. In contrast, randomization as a strict criterium was restricted to the specialised circles of biostatisticians and clinical epidemiologists. During the 1940s and 1950s a flood of studies appeared about the placebo-effect.[19] These studies covered a wide range of topics: characteristics of the "placebo reactor", the degree of efficacy of placebo in different therapeutic areas, mechanism of action and toxicological profile of placebo etc.

In the field of anti-anginal treatment, Greiner et al. (1950) and Beecher (1955) estimated that in 35% - 38% of cases in a series of patients - exceeding a thousand - beneficial effects were achieved with placebo therapy. Subsequently, this estimation was taken as a sort of baseline in anti-anginal treatment.

The following quotation is illustrative: *"...if the effectiveness of a substance exceeds 40%, this fact becomes highly significant because it is impossible to exceed this figure with a placebo. In effect, the total subjective effectiveness of a drug is equal to its true effectiveness augmented by that of its placebo which, it is reasoned, represents the beneficial effect which the a priori favorable anticipation associated with the trial of a new treatment can have and actually does have".* [20] This practice was eliminated when control groups were accepted as the norm for therapeutic assessment. This standard implied that in each test separately the effects of the new drug had to be checked with reference to a placebo (or another medication).

How should we evaluate these four critical points? The emphasis of these studies lies in the evaluation of the merits of the clinical trial, not in its historical development. We are far from a clear picture of the historical development of the clinical trial. However, three aspects have to be stressed. Firstly, the clinical trial did not develop uniformly in distinct medical areas and settings. Secondly, the relationship between theory and practice of the clinical trial is much more complex but also closer than generally suggested. Thirdly, shifts in definitions did take place over time.

All three aspects point in the same direction. The advent of the controlled clinical trial was meant to reform medical practice. To understand its impact on medicine a monolithic conception of medical practice is insufficient. Different medical practices reveal a variety of relationships between different methods of gathering and testing medical knowledge.

Science or art?

The introduction of the controlled clinical trial has been perceived to upset the balance between clinical science and clinical experience. On the one hand it was strived for to develop a science of experimental medicine with the patient as its subject.[21] On the other it was claimed that the clinician was *"the field naturalist who cannot treat problems in a ward as the physiologist does rabbits in the laboratory".* [22] Medicine was beyond science, being more like an art. This professional concern originated from a conflict about what counts as the proper subject and method of medical knowledge.[23] A majority view is that the epistemological basis of clinical medicine lies within the limits of the clinical encounter between doctor and patient. Clinical medicine equals knowledge of (individual) patients; its basis is clinical experience that is acquired, taught and applied at the bedside. The controlled clinical trial directly conflicts with this medical self-image.[24] As Ambrose declared in 1950: *"Clinical impression against cold science".* [25]

However, self-images involve more than just medical practice. These images were reactions to the profound changes that took place in medicine after the Second World War. One such profound change was the move from the patient to the laboratory.

Feinstein and his colleagues found that there was a decline in the proportion of "clinical" research projects - that is, those that contain human material, are disease oriented, or are "people centered" - whereas there was an increase in the proportion of research containing non-human material or measuring laboratory values.[26] Furthermore, while the authors concluded that the proportion of therapeutic projects devoted specifically to therapy dropped from 8% to 2%, they simultaneously pointed out that *"many pharmacologic studies of new drugs and of other therapeutics were not classified as therapeutic because the only variables reported and correlated in the response to therapy were such laboratory measurements as blood counts, urinalysis, chemical tests, and X-ray changes".* [27]

Thus, in contrast to what Feinstein and co-workers described, the number of "therapeutic" projects actually rose though this was not overtly apparent. Indeed, the controlled clinical trial moved therapeutic assessment from the bedside to the laboratory. This move from the patient to the laboratory was a general trend in medicine. Ruesch pointed to *"a declining clinical tradition"* that disrupted clinical and medical practice.[28] Pellegrino referred to *"the identity crisis of an ideal".* [29]

This professional concern should not surprise us. The controlled clinical trial was brought to medicine to reform medical practice and therapeutic assessment. The aim was the expulsion of casual experience. Many believed that through the controlled clinical trial not only disease but finally also therapy was in hands of Nature. *"Through strict adherence to a methodologically rigorous research design"*, as Mulrow et al. declared, " *'the whim, the inaccuracies and the blunder' can be eliminated...".* [30]

The rapid development of the pharmaceutical industry during the *"Golden Age of Drug Discovery"* and of drug regulation shortly thereafter interacted with the salient rise of medical and scientific specialization to fit clinical research to the needs of therapeutic innovation. This forms the subject of the next section.

1.3 The implementation of the controlled clinical trial in drug research

A remarkable feature in the history of drug regulation is its slow development, yet it speeded up in response to disasters.[31] An example was the use of the "Elixir of Sulfonamide" which caused a major disaster in 1927 in the United States. This elixir contained, as a solvent, diethylene glycol, that caused death to more than one hundred people. Consequently, a new law was enacted which demanded that industry demonstrate the safety of a new medicinal product before marketing. The basic shortcoming of this law was that it did not require the proof of a drug's effectiveness.[32] The debate about this shortcoming continued for decades, until it was settled as a result of the thalidomide disaster around 1960. This new drug, used as a hypnotic drug in pregnant women, caused gross fetal deformities. This dramatic event aroused great community concern and led to the enactment of the Kefauver-Harris Amendments to the existing Food, Drug and Cosmetic Act in 1962. These Amendments provided the Food and Drug Administration substantial power to control the investigational use of drugs, to demand pre-marketing testing with respect to both efficacy and safety, and to remove unsafe, ineffective or improperly labeled drugs from the market.[33] In other western countries the thalidomide disaster also initiated new drug legislation.[34]

However, regulatory patterns differ widely because of varying regional situations. Firstly, these regional differences are pertinent to the scope , or what Klaes et al. called the "intensity" or "density" of drug regulation.[35] Potential subjects of regulation concern manufacturing conditions, quality control procedures, packaging and marketing issues. Other subjects relevant to this analysis, concern development and investigation: animal studies (scientific and ethical aspects); comparative safety and efficacy in man; clinical trials (protocols, licensing of investigators); efficacy/safety ratio; and adverse reaction monitoring.[36]

In the United States of America the scope of regulation was most extensive; in West-Germany, on the contrary, much less. In Norway, however, legislation that stretched back as far as 1928, incorporated the medical need for licensing of medicines.[37] In principle, this "need clause" formed an extension of the set of well-known criteria such as efficacy, safety and quality.

Secondly, regional differences influenced the extent to which these regulatory matters have been implemented in practice. The role of the FDA has often been contrasted with the British system of drug regulation with its voluntary basis in the 1960s. The FDA prepares and issues guidelines for conducting clinical studies; whereas the federal acts and regulations are mandatory, the guidelines are mostly voluntary, but they enter decision making through the repeated contacts between the FDA and industry.[38]

Thirdly, there were differences in the extent the medical profession agreed with the regulatory process. Though the subject of professional freedom formed a source of counter-pressure, the British and American medical communities were in favour of controlled clinical studies to evaluate drugs. In contrast, German physicians were not eager to have this type of clinical research interfering with medical practice.[39]

Despite these regional differences other factors brought unification to drug regulation with emphasis on the American situation. Firstly, the United States is the biggest market for pharmaceuticals and in preparing clinical studies and marketing plans most pharmaceutical industries primarily take the American situation into consideration. Secondly, internationalization of medicine became prominent in the post-War period, and Anglo-American medicine became the centre of international medicine. Thirdly, international organizations such as the World Health Organization and the World Medical Association committed themselves directly or indirectly to the need for clinical trials.[40]

Hence, through regulation, directly or indirectly, the controlled clinical trial became intricately connected with drug research. Since the United States is widely considered as the model for the implementation of the controlled clinical trial in drug research, this will be discussed in more detail in the following section.

The American way of regulating drugs

Any new drug to be tested in man has to have approval from the Food and Drug Administration. Sufficient preclinical evidence of safety and efficacy is required; extensive toxicity testing on potential teratogenic, mutagenic and carcinogenic hazards has to be performed. When permission has been given by the FDA, the drug is then called an Investigational New Drug (IND). If the required clinical studies are completed, and approval for licensing is applied for, the drug is called a New Drug Application (NDA). Once approved, the drug is coined with the term "NDA-approved". Through the regulations the FDA has promulgated, this phase of clinical testing is divided into four stages which, still following American practice, have become known as Phases I-IV.

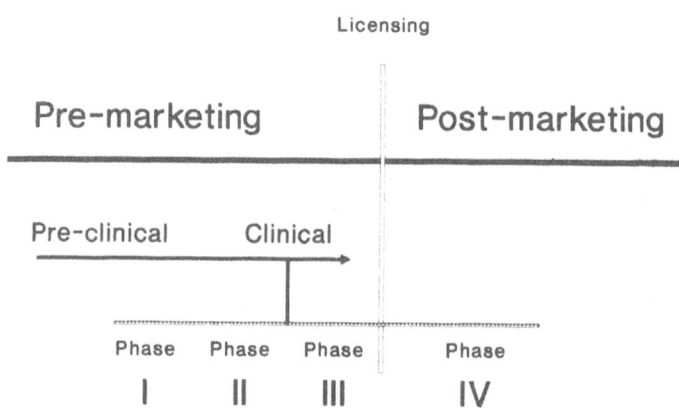

Figure 1.2
Stages of drug development.

During phase I the new drug will be tested in healthy volunteers for efficacy, dose-res-ponse relationship, duration of action, kinetic behaviour and potential hazards. The second phase encompasses studies with small group of patients, selected by strict criteria. Kinetic aspects of the drug, such as resorption, distribution, metabolism and biological availability, are studied in more detail. Also the pharmaceutical aspects are examined. Indications, absolute and relative contra-indications, side-effects, route of administration and precautionary measures are determined.

Subsequently, during phase III, double-blind, randomized controlled clinical studies have to be conducted. According to the guidelines of the FDA, the firm that conducts the IND-program, is required to study the safety and efficacy of each clinical indication in a minimum of two hundred subjects registered in studies supervised by at least two different clinical investigators. Other guidelines are to ensure that all clinical studies are reviewed and approved by an Institutional Review Board, to review and to evaluate all data received from investigators, to make progress reports regarding safety and effectiveness at least annually, and to report hazards immediately. Moreover, the FDA has developed requirements concerning informed consent documents, informed consent procedures, clinical protocols and expertise of clinical investigators , labeling of the IND, and many other aspects relevant to the IND-program.[41]

When sufficient data are collected to support reasonable claims of safety and effectiveness, and the drug is approved, phase IV, e.g. the "Post-Marketing-Surveillance"-phase, starts. In many countries the new drug is marketed without follow-up. Only, if unknown and dramatic hazards are reported, will the drug be evaluated again. The FDA, however, has the power to require from firms, on approval of a new drug application, reports to the FDA quarterly for the first year, semiannually during the second year, and annually thereafter, for as long as the product is marketed.[42]

Two sides of the same coin

That the Kefauver-Harris Amendments gave the FDA power to require evidence about the efficacy of drugs has been considered as somewhat illogical. The thalidomide disaster speeded up the enactment while the major problem with this drug was its toxicity, not its efficacy. Still, the Amendments were in accordance with prevailing views. During a four day meeting on the regulation of drugs in 1963 under the auspices of the Johns Hopkins University, attended by a select audience of pharmaceutical, medical, academic and governmental people in exploring the major problems in making safe and effective drugs, the conferees *were universally committed to the view that the basic features of safety and effectiveness are inseparable and constitute two aspects of the same fundamental properties of a drug".* [43] Safety and efficacy formed two sides of one and the same coin. Drug manu-facturers were also committed to this view. The summary of the comments during this meeting stipulated *"that in the course of the Senate hearings preceding passage of the Drug Amendments of 1962, the majority of the directors of the Pharmaceutical Manufacturers Association favored the inclusion of the effectiveness clause and that the PMA officially testified in favour of this provision".* [44]

However, during the Blatnik and the Kefauver committee hearings pharmaceutical manufac-turers were vigorously battling another issue closely related to it. It was proposed that if a drug available on the market was therapeutically adequate, then no new drugs should be certified for use for the same indication. Pharmaceutical manufacturers contested this proposal because experience in the hands of general practitioners could bring out aspects not fully revealed during initial clinical tests. Thus, physicians-at-large should be given the privilege of working with new drugs, in certain cases at least, even though officials believed that satisfactory drugs were available for the same condition. This view was challenged by other participants who cast serious doubts on the capability of the average physician to contribute significantly to the generation of knowledge about the drug. Manufacturers and the medical profession joined in arguing that the proposal encroached on the professional freedom of the physician. Furthermore, ethical arguments were put forward to state that minor groups of patients would possibly be deprived of drugs which, though in general not more effective than already marketed drugs, would be beneficial for them. These arguments achieved the purpose of keeping the entry to the market as large as possible. Political, ideological and economic factors came to the forefront while the epistemological dimension, i.e. conflicting conceptions about the role of medicine in drug innovation, shifted to the background.

Increasingly, the debate about the factors influencing drug innovation became dominated by two opposing views. The first view was subscribed to by the FDA, notably by the Commissioners Schmidt and Kennedy, and was more or less accepted by a broader, though heterogeneous audience of academic, medical and regulatory people. This view stated that the drop in drug innovation as a worldwide phenomenon was caused by the thought *"we are on a plateau of discovery"* or *"the well has run dry -wait for the millennium"*. [45] The following quotation, retrieved from an address by FDA Commissioner Schmidt in 1974 is typical in this respect: *"That reason begins with the fact that in many areas of biomedical knowledge, we are on a plateau. We have temporarily exhausted the exploitation of known concepts and tools. Truly dramatic new progress in medicine now awaits some basic innovation in molecular science, some breakthrough in our understanding of disease mechanisms, some new therapeutic concept or some new tool"*. [46]

This view, known as the "Knowledge gap hypothesis" or "Research depletion hypothesis", considers the "Golden Age of Drug Discovery" in the 1940s and 1950s to be the result of the dramatic and steady progress in bacteriology and chemistry in the latter part of the 19th and the first half of the 20th century.[47] Subsequently other types of disease, e.g. chronic, degenerative diseases such as cardiovascular distress, cancer and rheumatic arthritis, appeared on the scene. Since these diseases have complex and multifactorial etiology, medical science had to adjust its course to find new directions. There still is a lack of fundamental knowledge in biochemical and physiological processes underlying these diseases. The other view is that drug innovation is slowing down because of regulatory activities. Time, money and creative energy is spent on routine pharmacological and toxicological studies to meet regulatory demands. Together with other governmental measures which negatively influenced price standard, patent protection, and restriction of physician prescription has diminished the return of profits. Hence, this view is called the "Declining profitability hypothesis". [48]

Despite the differences both views have a common concept of drug innovation. While defending the 'declining profitability hypothesis' Clymer described drug discovery as follows: *"By a myriad of pre-clinical research pathways originating years before, often with basic fundamental biological findings that evolved into applied research, synthesis, and animal testing, a new chemical agent reaches the critical decision-making stage. This is the point at which a compound has been identified with a unique pharmacological spectrum, sufficiently active and non-toxic to meet the criteria for potential new therapy. A decision is then made to take it into clinical trial. At this point it becomes a specific, identifiable product candidate, and the discovery phase has been completed"*. [49]

This view of Clymer on drug discovery is basically the same as expressed by Schmidt. Both differ, however, in their explanation of the decline of drug innovation during the 1960s and

1970s. The former attributes this to the suffocation of the discovery process by regulation; the latter to the temporary slackening of the process due to the exhaustion of basic knowledge. One consideration remains: the "declining profitability hypothesis" which conceives of drug innovation as a black box using input and output parameters to establish that the rate of drug innovation has declined. This implies that this hypothesis can be juxtaposed to different views of the discovery process. In practice, however, the black box presupposed by the declining profitability hypothesis, is filled with a view about drug innovation which is essentially the same as that expressed by the knowledge gap hypothesis.

Basic criticism

The role of the FDA has been much discussed during the 1960s and 1970s. The basic criticism of the drug regulatory system was that it was too restrictive, that it was too bureaucratic and too costly, not that it was fundamentally wrong. In the course of the 1970s, however, the controlled clinical trial, the centre-piece of drug regulation, became the target of basic criticism.

During the 1970s the occurrence of new, unexpected and severe adverse drug reactions (ADR's) led to widespread publicity: practolol, SMON, stilbestrol- induced vaginal cancer in the second generation, clozapine associated agranulocytosis and lactic acidosis caused by phenformin. Shortly thereafter therapeutic newcomers such as triazolam, benoxaprofen, zomepirac, osmosin and zimelidine *"once again alarmed the public, physicians, drug regulatory agencies and manufacturers"*, as Idänpään-Heikillä, Chief Medical Officer for Drug Evaluation in Finland commented. He posed the obvious question: *"Why do so many surprises occur in the post-marketing phase despite modern methods of drug development, sophisticated medicine and high technology? Are they avoidable?".* [50] Awareness grew that controlled clinical trials could not pick up these side-effects in the pre-marketing phase.
Simultaneously, another basic criticism appeared: the artificiality of the clinical trial. The majority of all medicines are prescribed by general practitioners in pathological conditions which are hardly ever seen or distinctly differ from those conditions seen in clinics. Moreover the population actually studied in controlled clinical trials concerns a specific and selected group even compared to the clinical population: highly selected patients with clear-cut syndromes while elderly subjects, pregnant women, severely ill patients, children, and other kinds of subgroups of patients are excluded from controlled clinical studies. The conditions under which drugs are marketed and prescribed routinely to patients differ from the clinical trial situation. Awareness grew that *"a drug's actual performance is what we care about, not what it ideally might do".* [51]
The evaluation of a drug in the post-marketing phase was acknowledged as a neglected subject. This led to a renewal of interest in other methods of establishing cause-effect relationships: case-control studies, retrospective analysis, and spontaneous reporting systems - based on the method of casuistic reports. This re-appraisal of methods of gathering medical knowledge was stimulated by the progress in computer sciences, decision theory, clinical epidemiology and pharmaco-epidemiology. The major objective formed the detection of

adverse drug reactions. Gradually, other objectives were added: economic and social assessment of therapeutic outcomes, improvement of drug use, and analysis of prescribing patterns. Recently these post-marketing-surveillance (PMS) systems have been acknowledged as sources of new knowledge about therapeutics.[52]

1.4. Criticism of the classical view of the controlled clinical trial

The horizontal dimension - a linear view on drug development

Oates, professor of medicine and pharmacology at the School of Medicine at the Vanderbilt University, has provided an interesting criticism of the classic view of the controlled clinical trial. In a presidential address to the Association of American Physicians, he dismissed the idea of FDA commissioner Kennedy that the Food and Drug Administration is merely "a regulator of technology transfer" and that therefore attrition of therapeutic innovation cannot be due to the regulatory climate for clinical investigation:

"In these statements Dr. Kennedy unveiled his perception that clinical investigation is not a contributor to new knowledge. So defined, clinical investigation can be regulated without consequence to the discovery process which he conceived as taking place entirely outside of the arena of the Food and Drug Administration's influence. In disclaiming that regulation of clinical research could influence innovation, he proposed that "There has been a decline in basic research", thus emphasizing the construction that clinical investigation is not basic research. When a distinguished biologist does not recognize that clinical investigation also is a discovery discipline, this perception must be rampant among policy makers from nonscientific backgrounds. Accordingly, I have no critique for Donald Kennedy but thank him for his clear articulation of a concept that has become pervasive in Washington". [53]

Thus, Oates wrote cynically, *"each molecule should arrive at the bedside for the first clinical investigation with the package insert already written".* [54]

According to Oates the source of this limited vision is the attitude, widely held in policy circles, that research is a one-way street in which acquisition of fundamental knowledge leads to testing and evaluation of that knowledge, and then to application; basic research is followed by technology transfer. Oates supports his assessment by showing how this limited view which governed American research planning during the 1950s and 1960s influenced biomedical policy. In doing so he refers to his experiences as a medical expert participating in the research program strategy of the National Heart, Lung and Blood Institute (NHLBI) Planning Report of 1973 under the auspices of the National Institute of Health (NIH). The NIH policy was strongly influenced by the Department of Defense strategy towards research policy in the post-War-period. Consequently, a misinterpretation took place during the application into the biomedical sciences (figure 1.3).

The misinterpretation consists of equating the acquisition of fundamental knowledge to research by non-clinical investigators, and of clinical investigation as the evaluation of know-

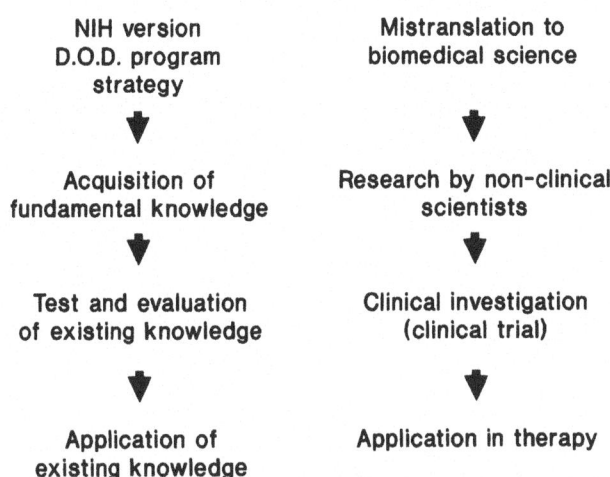

Figure 1.3
Left panel, the "order sequence" describing program strategy in 1973 program planning document of the National Heart, Lung and Blood Institute, a sequence quite similar to that put forward previously by the Department of Defense (D.O.D.). Right panel, Oates' perception of how a restricted view of clinical investigation may have been inferred from such a limited model of program strategy.
Reproduced with permission from Oates (1982).

ledge generated solely from non-clinical research.[55] Oates points out that this misconception matched the classical way antibiotic (and cancer) research proceeded (figure 1.4).

Oates states: *"In this mode of discovery, research in laboratory systems and experimental models leads to a disease-specific potential drug. If it is not too toxic, you then evaluate it in man and, if again it is not full of ill effects, it will become a therapeutic agent. However, I believe this model from the antibiotic is too broadly generalized in terms of drug discovery".* [56]

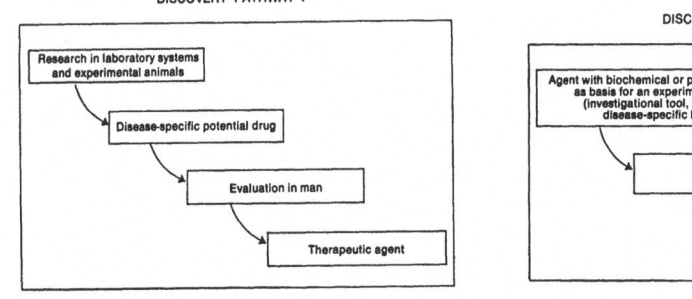
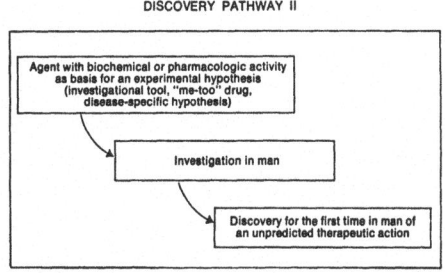

Figure 1.4
Pathways of drug discovery according to Oates.
Reproduced with permission from Helms (1975).

Consequently he stresses another route in drug discovery in which clinical investigation is a prime source of new drugs. This author agrees with Oates in his critique of the classic view and with his attempt to unravel other pathways of drug discovery. In this thesis some examples of these pathways will be provided, including some in detail.

The classic view of the controlled clinical trial, i.e. a linear view on therapeutic innovation can now be summarized: first basic science, then applied science, clinical research and finally medical practice. This will be called the horizontal dimension of the classic view of the controlled clinical trial (figure 1.5).

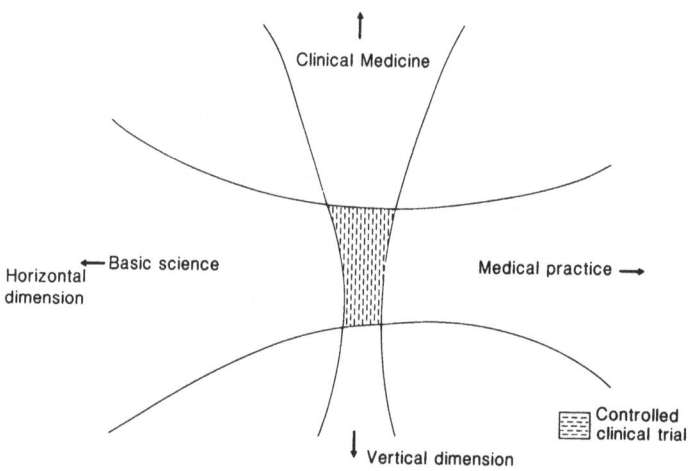

Figure 1.5
Horizontal and vertical dimension of the classic view about the role of clinical medicine in drug discovery.

The vertical dimension - the clinical trial as a particular type of clinical activity

But there is a second characteristic, i.e. the vertical dimension (figure 1.5), which means that clinical medicine is restricted to one particular method. The fact that doctors resort to other sources of knowledge, e.g. observation and retrospective analysis of clinical records, is regarded as an undesirable, although in practice, unavoidable situation. The reason for this is the standard view that the CCT provides the best information for medical therapy. Thus, different forms of medical knowledge are ranked in order of merit or quality with respect to therapeutic knowledge. In practice many interpretations of this normative judgment from weak to strong can be defined but this will be dealt with in chapter 8.

It is remarkable that the discussion over the value of the CCT is directed at the evaluation of therapy but takes place in the context of the development of therapy. In this respect the CCT is a critical test for a hypothesis which is generated from other areas of medical knowledge. It is a means of producing reliable data - not of producing new data, in spite of the fact that during a clinical trial often new aspects of a drug or new areas of application may be discovered. These discoveries are not the result of the CCT itself but rather the unexpected findings during retrospective analysis of the data gathered during the trial. This implies that other forms of medical knowledge are more potent sources of new information than the CCT (figure 1.6).[57]

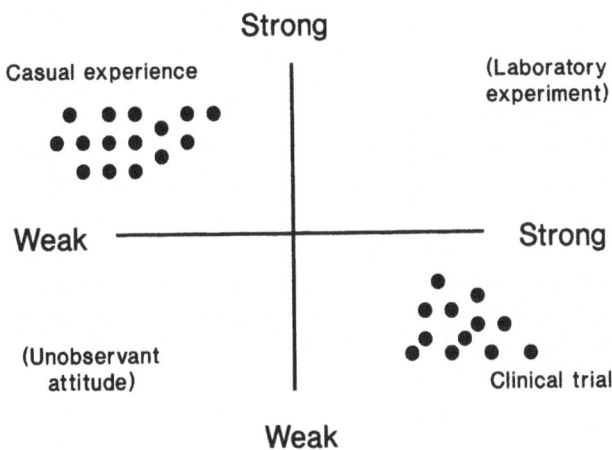

Figure 1.6
Sources of generating and validating medical knowledge project along two axes, i.e. "validation of knowledge" along the X-axis and "generation of knowledge" along the Y-axis.

While the CCT is a strong source for the validation of therapy it is a weak source for discovering new knowledge about the therapy. For unexpected or unplanned findings originating from casual experience the reverse is true. Of course, one could claim that casual experience should be placed in the lower left quarter of the diagram. However, this is incorrect because this source of medical knowledge cannot be interchanged with the unobservant and uncritical attitude which one often finds in practice. The process whereby casual experience leads to new therapies will be discussed in chapter 8.

The generation and validation of therapeutic knowledge

The preceding section shows that the standard view of the CCT is based on a sharp differentiation between the development and the validation of a therapy. The stronger the normative judgment on the controlled trial the more visible is the contrast between generation and validation of knowledge. A good example of this is found in the following passage taken from the book **Clinical Epidemiology. A Basic Science for Clinical**

Medicine written by Sackett, Haynes and Tugwell[58] (emphasis by the authors themselves):

*"Having decided that the patient's sickness **does** warrant treatment and having selected the goal of this treatment, you must now select the specific drug, operation, splint, exercise, or conversation that will best achieve this goal. How (on earth) do you decide which one to prescribe? It seems to us that there are three ways to pick a therapy:*
*1. On the basis of retrospective analysis of your own uncontrolled clinical experience, that of others, or the extension of current concepts of mechanisms of disease you can logically arrive at the therapy that **seems to work** or **ought to work**; we shall call this the method of **induction**.*
*2. On the basis of prospective analysis of formal randomized clinical trials designed to expose worthless or dangerous treatments, you can select the therapies that **successfully withstand formal attempts to demonstrate their worthlessness**; we shall call this the method of **deduction**.*
*3. On the basis of recommendations from your teachers, consultants, colleagues, advertisements, or pharmaceutical representatives you can simply accept a treatment **on faith**; we shall call this the method of **abdication** (or, to fit the rhyme and cadence of the other two, the method of **seduction**).*
*It will, by this point in the book, come as no surprise to learn that we prefer the **deductive** (or, more correctly, the **hypothetico-deductive**) method for selecting specific treatments. The best information on whether a given treatment does more good than harm to patients with a given disorder is the result of a randomized clinical trial (..)".* [59]

The claims put forward by the authors are strong indeed. Do not believe your colleagues or others unless they back up their claims with proper evidence from randomized clinical trials; and do not believe retrospective material which is necessarily unreliable knowledge! The key to the above division lies in the strong separation between development and validation of therapeutic knowledge. This can be best illustrated in the distinction between induction and deduction. The authors say: *"Why are we so hard on the method of induction? After all, this method constitutes the major strategy for nominating the treatment ideas that get tested in randomized clinical trials, and many of these treatment ideas prove to be powerfully efficacious. The fatal flaw in the method of induction is that it is often incapable of exposing erroneous conclusions about efficacy, even when the observations on which it operates are totally accurate".* [60]

At the moment when the development of therapeutic knowledge is raised, the authors call on the power of sources of knowledge other than the CCT. Development and validation form the extremes of a continuum or rather, two aspects of an iterative process in which scientists generate and test hypotheses until finally a critical clinical test is made possible. Phase I and II research, preceding this critical test in phase III should be viewed in this light. During these phases clinical scientists spy out the land of the new therapy. In part they rest on their own experience, in part they feel their way along untrodden paths creating new boundaries. Therefore a laborious process of determining dosage regimens, period of treatment, in- and exclusion of patients, and diagnostic and therapeutic parameters precedes the clinical trial. This occurs against the background knowledge of the therapeutic problem concerned. This is disguised by the rigid dichotomy in generation and validation as two separate spheres of activity, but which relate to the classical view of the controlled clinical trial.

Schaffner who has done much work to develop a logic of discovery in the biomedical sciences, has developed a framework in order to explicate the stages of both the generation and the early evaluation of scientific hypotheses, and not just at their justification subsequent to their having been fully elaborated.[61] In addition he stresses that scientific inquiry always begins in medias res. While employing a spatial metaphor Schaffner argues that surrounding the set of experimental results and the theory or hypothesis that ought to account for these results, which he calls a subdiscipline, lie *"clusters of often entrenched theories which provide relevant background for the subdiscipline. Around the subdiscipline of antibody diversity theorizing, and interacting strongly with it for example, are located theories of genetics, a theory (or theories) of protein synthesis, and evolutionary theory, which serve both as sources of potentially fruitful ideas in the subdiscipline and as constraints: a new theory in the subdiscipline is required to be consistent with these background theories (or at least with the entrenched background theories)".* [62]

Analogous to Schaffner's viewpoint "disease" and "therapy" being the subject of the controlled clinical trial, form nodal points in a maze of background knowledge. However, this maze entails not only theories. This is not to deny that theories about disease (mechanisms) as well as theories about (mechanisms of action of) therapeutics exist. However, the maze entails various types of experimental results not yet accounted for by theories, experiences with particular compounds or patient populations as well as with therapeutic outcomes in different situations.

If we focus on the body of knowledge pertinent to medical therapy clinical medicine addresses itself to a wide range of topics (table 1.1).

Table 1.1
Classification of clinical topics.

Normality	Biology of nondiseased humans
Manifestations	Clinical presentations of disease
Diagnosis	Properties of diagnostic tests
Frequency	Incidence and prevalence of disease frequency
Cause	Factors increasing the risk of disease; pathogenesis (mechanism) of disease
Prognosis	Natural history of disease
Therapy	Value of treatment, risks of treatment, mechanism of action

Reproduced with permission from Fletcher et al. (1980).

Answers to these different questions may lead to new knowledge which directly or indirectly affects therapeutic development. More specifically this knowledge affects the decisions to be taken in order to achieve a critical test of the new drug.

If we focus on the available clinical methods - various types of classifications exist - the controlled clinical trial is merely one method.[63] These methods contribute in their respective ways to the knowledge of disease and treatment. This finds expression in the way the object of study is treated. The clinician emphasizing the study of the "natural history" of angina pectoris, sees patients other than encountered by the clinician evaluating anti-anginal drugs on the basis of the clinical trial.

Russek and co-workers, for example, developed during the 1950s a method - combining the two-step-exercise-test with ECG-registration developed by Master - on the basis of a group of almost two hundred patients being observed for more than ten years. Fewer than forty papers were published in leading medical journals during the 1950s and 1960s.[64] The experience of this group showed that merely one out of fifty patients were suited for this type of investigation. Thus, a specific "angina-patient" forms the subject of their research.

Next to Russek's approach are other types of investigation: clinical lesson, casuistic report, open- and single-patient-studies, and the varieties of clinical-epidemiological research. Each type defines the angina patient differently, and collects in its own way knowledge about the disease.[65] This knowledge is stored with the background knowledge which is not a static entity nor an amorphous mass of data. It is - note the anthropomorphism - a **body** of knowledge with a specific structure but continuously re-shaped in many ways and by various sources.

1.5. Conclusions

The evolution of the controlled clinical trial exhibits a complex history. It is generally appraised as a decisive step forward on a long and laborious pathway towards a rational medical therapy. The apparent clarity and ingenuity of the clinical trial, however, merely proves to be the tip of a complicated iceberg. On the one hand it represents a particular way of organizing medical knowledge and encompasses heterogeneous elements - knowledge, funding, logistics, ethics and social features.[66] On the other hand it reveals the intricate relationships between clinical medicine and drug development. From the epistemological point of view the classic view about the controlled clinical trial consists of five elements:
1. the scientific reform of medical practice aimed at the expulsion of casual experience;
2. the central role attributed to the clinical trial to sift effective from non-effective drugs;
3. the basis of decision making in drug regulation;
4. the strong emphasis on the pre-marketing period in drug innovation and development;
5. the exclusive role ascribed to the clinical trial to establish a rational preference in therapy choice.

During the 1950s and 1960s the classic view of the controlled clinical trial dominated clinical medicine and the pharmaceutical sector. Thereafter this view tends to disintegrate as a result of varying degrees of acceptance and criticism of each element. Emphasis is nowadays more on post-marketing surveillance (elements 3 and 4). Moreover, the exclusive status attributed to the controlled clinical trial in establishing effectiveness and rational preference in therapy choice (elements 2 and 5) is balanced within the spectrum of scientific methods in clinical medicine and epidemiology. Yet, the balance is unstable and the impact of the classic view about the controlled clinical trial is still considerable. This applies in particular to the negative attitude towards casual experience (element 1).

This classic view became amalgamated with a linear view about drug discovery. As a result conceptions of the role of clinical medicine and medical practice in drug discovery have been narrowed down. First, clinical medicine was assigned a specific place in the sequence of events leading to new drugs (horizontal dimension). Secondly, the contribution of clinical medicine to the growth of therapeutic knowledge was curtailed in two particular ways (vertical dimension): 1. the range of topics that clinical medicine addressed itself to, hereby yielding relevant knowledge about diseases and drugs, and thus, directly or indirectly, affecting therapeutic development, was restricted to therapeutic assessment in a narrow sense; 2. the range of clinical methods was restricted to the one that could claim to provide reliable knowledge about medical therapy: the controlled clinical trial.

This by no means implies that the clinical trial cannot figure in an epistemologically adequate conception of the discovery process.[67]

Most striking is that the merits of the clinical trial have been discussed with respect to the evaluation of medical therapy while the trial has also structured, both in theory and practice, the developmental process. Underneath lies the sharp distinction between generation and validation of therapeutic knowledge. This distinction disguises the fact that clinical research workers and physicians are involved in a lengthy and iterative process in which they go back and forth, add new elements to background knowledge, eliminate or transform others, and test certain hypotheses in the light of this background knowledge.

Viewed in that light the apparent simplicity with which protagonists advocated the clinical trial, is an understatement because this simplicity conceals the complex relationship between medical theory and practice. Most striking therefore is that the controlled clinical trial has been discussed in general terms which is not surprising since it has been advocated for medicine as a whole. This monolithic conception of medicine immediately appears to be unrealistic. Not only because medicine consists of a conglomerate of medical practices, but also when we realize that various groups of patients are excluded from clinical trials: elderly people, seriously ill patients, pregnant women, and young children. In all cases the assessment of effectiveness and of toxic effects and the creation of the criteria for proper treatment are dependent upon other methods. Even when the controlled clinical trial is applied to these heterogeneous groups of patients in a satisfactory way, the fundamental problem remains. Every time a trial is set up, we know it is a selected and re-interpreted part of medical practice, but it is never the practice itself. The controlled clinical trial therefore is not an exclusive form of medical thinking and acting; it never has been and it never will be. This historical analysis of the evolution of the controlled clinical trial, specifically in the context of drug development, reveals four closely related topics that form the subject of subsequent chapters:

a. The differential relationships between academic and industrial research, clinical medicine and medical practice;
b. The different pathways of drug discovery;
c. The role of casual experience and other sources of medical knowledge in drug discovery;
d. The structure and change of the body of knowledge of drugs and diseases.

Chapter 2. The architecture of drug discovery

2.1. Introduction

In this chapter an architectural framework of the drug discovery process is developed.
Part 1 discusses basic features of drug discovery by analyzing two sets of philosophical terms,
i.e. basic-applied and rational-empirical, including art and serendipity, used in the pharmaceutical sector (2.2.), and by presenting (2.3.) the view of cognitive science on scientific
creativity. Subsequently, some basic features of the drug discovery process will be analysed
again (2.4.).
In part 2 the concepts of drug (2.5.2.) and disease (2.5.3.) profile will be examined. Part 3
develops a set-theoretical definition of the concept of profile (2.6.) and a set-theoretical
model of the drug discovery process (2.7.).

Part 1. The discovery process

2.2. Current views of drug discovery

2.2.1. Basic concepts in drug discovery

Drug discovery is commonly divided into two stages: the discovery and development phase.
Almost synonymously the terms "lead generation phase" and "lead development phase" are
used. Creativity guides the first phase, and once a new concept is born and a novel compound
found, the second phase starts to bring the drug to the market. The first phase is the more
glamorous of the two, but the second is in fact no less important. Both phases are highly
complex processes in which thousands of different activities are put together. The term
"development" is misleading since it is in fact **research** as Smith nicely puts it, *"using as the
definition of this word 'the seeking for and interpretation of new knowledge'"*.[1] Indeed, each new
drug starts a voyage of discovery through an unmapped terrain which is shrouded in mist
and beset by pitfalls. Moreover, these phases and their basic components, although usually
mapped out sequentially, often occur coincidentally and have constant feedback. However,
since many explorers are involved and many aspects of the drug have to be defined, much
time is involved and critical to the developmental phase is the ability to coordinate
effectively. *"As opposed to drug discovery, where a certain degree and type of disorder is encouraged"*,
Spilker comments, *"drug development has order, organization, and discipline as goals"*.[2]
The creative phase of drug discovery involves finding lead compounds. Every day thousands
of chemical compounds are synthesized in industrial laboratories, but only when a compound with an interesting biological activity is found, is it called a lead compound (or a
chemical lead). The term "lead" suggests on the one hand what the chemical compound

should be or in what direction to search for such a compound, and on the other hand about what the substance should do. If a concept about the biological activity is lacking, one is left with a chemical compound. If there is an interesting concept but no chemical compound, one has a lead. It is very important to any pharmaceutical industry to find such a compound while it can be patented and thus ensure repayment of its development costs.

The term "lead compound" is used to designate the first interesting compound that fits the basic concept of the project. This compound triggers the synthesis of many new compounds until a substance is found which it is hoped will become a drug, e.g. a candidate compound. Usually this marks the end of the discovery phase.[3]

The terms lead and lead compound encompass a time dimension as well. Sometimes, after a phase of dramatic and feverish search, one finally finds a compound with demonstrated biological activity. Alternatively, chemical curiosity may yield a chemical compound which shows interesting activity when tested, and the substance becomes a lead compound.

Many approaches and methods have been proposed for finding leads or lead compounds.[4] In general four ways of searching new lead compounds may be distinguished:
1. screening
2. molecular modification
3. rational approach
4. serendipitous findings, chance observations

Ad 1. Screening

The screening approach consists of making large numbers of new chemical compounds; subsequently testing them in a battery of test-systems to identify their potential action and picking out the candidates with possible usefulness in man. This approach has been variously termed "blind screening", "random screening" and "molecular roulette" and became very popular in pharmaceutical science after the War. Numerous compounds, sometimes exceeding hundreds of thousands, were synthesized and tested but many were rejected. But increasingly more "targeted" (non-random) screening is performed, in which case the frequency of successful discovery is much higher. Hahn estimated the odds in finding leads among synthetic compounds in the chemotherapeutic area is one in several thousand, varying between 1 in 3.000 and 1 in 10.000.[5]

Ad 2. Molecular modification

This approach starts from a given substance with biological activity with the aim of increasing or altering the spectrum of activity, reducing side effects and toxicity, prolonging the duration of action or improving absorption. Very often modification of known drugs is employed. Side-effects for one use of a drug may serve as a new indication for the same drug. More often such problems trigger chemical work to search for related compounds with a more potent action of the desired type.

Many attempts have been made to put this approach on a more rational footing in developing pattern analysis methods to correlate biological activity and structural or physico-chemical parameters more specifically. These methods are also used in the process of lead definition, that is, while having a lead but no compound, defining the desired structural properties to reduce the vast number of chemical possibilities.

This approach has been questioned for its potential of achieving innovative drugs because one departs from known structures and tries to change the basic structure to improve specificity, potency or toxicity.[6] Thus, molecular modification purportedly leads to "me-too" products, not to breakthroughs. However, this view is criticized because drug discovery not only encompasses revolutionary stages but also an incremental process of step-by-step-improvement.

Ad 3. Rational approach

This approach aims at finding a new drug as a rational, or totally planned design. It can sometimes be best explained by contrasting it with what it is not: it is not empirical, serendipitous or random. More often, it covers all the approaches based on knowledge of the physiology and biochemistry of the disease and the chemical nature and mode of action of key substances within the chain of communicative events in the body. The past decade has witnessed an upsurge of interest in this rational approach. The rapid developments in biological sciences and the expanding knowledge of bio-active agents at the molecular level are increasingly perceived as the cornerstone of drug innovation.[7]

There are, however, various routes through which biological knowledge filters through to the drug discovery process. New knowledge may be used to set up new animal models of disease, to hypothesize biological and biochemical key reactions in a particular disease or to disentangle the mechanism of action of drugs.

Ad 4. Serendipitous findings, chance observations

It is difficult to summarize this approach in a few words.[8] Sometimes it designates what is called the "scientific hunch" which is even harder to define. This "flash of insight" or whatever term is suitable to denote this moment of "Eureka" could apply to any scientist, e.g. in the pharmaceutical sector, the chemist, biologist, pharmacologist, etc.

Most often, however, serendipitous findings or chance observations refer to accidental discovery. Then it is the unexpected, unprecedented discovery of a novel chemical that has biological activity, or it is the finding of a biological activity of an unanticipated type during any stage of drug discovery and in any laboratory. The elucidation of a new clinical activity during human studies or in clinical practice belongs to this category as well.

Difficulties in categorizing drug discovery methods

The categories in this review of basic approaches in drug discovery, are unsatisfactory for various, interrelated reasons. It is unclear to what the terms apply: the process or basic components of it; the results of this process or the prime mover? Furthermore, it is unclear at which level of the pharmaceutical sector - laboratory, company or industry - these terms operate while their purpose is also unspecified. Moreover, the categories are not exclusive, and hereby loose their significance.

However, these categories attempt to grasp the essential features of the drug discovery process and underneath lies the question of what kind of knowledge is pivotal to the discovery process. For this reason two epistemologies in the pharmaceutical area will be discussed in more detail in the next section.

2.2.2. Basic epistemologies in drug discovery

Members of directory boards, managerial drug decision makers, directors of scientific, medical and sales departments address themselves at business and professional meetings to the basic principles of the drug discovery process. These addresses are often cast in philosophical terms. True, these addresses form the rhetoric of the pharmaceutical enterprise, but they also reflect a genuine view on the role of scientific knowledge. Two sets of philosophical terms are relevant to the therapeutic enterprise. The first relates to the distinction between 'basic' and 'applied' science; the second to the 'rational-empirical' distinction.

Basic and applied research

In its strongest sense, the term "basic" designates the type of research which is fundamental or exploratory without any clearly identifiable usefulness. In contrast, applied research is targeted and makes use of the knowledge acquired in the basic sciences.

These terms originated from the positivist philosophy of science which regards the formulation of theories the ultimate objective of science, and which takes physics as the classic example of real science. The general principles that comprise the body of physical knowledge may be "applied" to particular events in nature. From this epistemological tradition stems the logical sequence of hypothesizing, gathering data, testing, establishing universal laws and again deriving new hypotheses for gathering data and testing.

The issue as to what extent basic or applied research contributed to drug discovery and how much of each type of research should be conducted within the company became a much debated issue during the 1950s and 1960s. Many examples were given of innovations which originated either from academic or industrial laboratories and either side could make a good case for whether it was academia or industry that could monopolize the role of true innovator.[9]

During this period the conventional view about drug innovation emerged which Maxwell has aptly described as the "prime mover" model (figure 2.1).

Pharmacological research → Exploitable knowledge → Screening → New drugs
(nonindustrial, basic)   (industrial, applied)

Figure 2.1
The "prime mover" model of drug discovery.
Reproduced with permission from Maxwell (1984).

Non-industrial research yields the body of basic knowledge which will be applied to chemical screening and pharmacological testing systems. According to this view basic, academic research is the prime mover of drug discovery. This view confuses epistemology with sociology. The type of research (basic-applied) is conceived of as synonymous with the institutional setting (academic - industrial) in which it is conducted. According to Maxwell this prime-mover model is insufficient. It is too much based on textbook and educational science. To cite Maxwell:

"These perceptions (of the prime mover, RV) are often advertently passed on to succeeding genera-tions via the professor-student relationship. Inadvertently, they are passed on in the medical school or graduate student classroom by the didactic convenience of teaching a coherent, logical story. For example, the physiology of the sympathetic nervous system is logically taught: preganglionic neuron acetylcholine postganglionic neuron norepinephrine effector cell; the details of the biochemistry of norepinephrine at nerve terminals are then presented. Once this scheme is in mind, in the same order we learn; preganglionic neuron inhibitors (nicotine, hexamethonium) postganglionic neuron, inhibitor (guanethidine) effector cell, inhibitors (phentolamine, propranolol); the drugs that influence the biochemistry of norepinephrine in and at the nerve endings are then presented (cocaine, reserpine, desmethylimipramine, MAO inhibitors). Unfortunately, this mnemonically appealing picture tacitly teaches that this body of pharmacologic knowledge was developed in the same orderly fashion. The reality, however, is much different from the linear model".[10]

Here, Maxwell touches upon the difference between the process of discovery and the intellectual products of it. The results of this discovery process will be validated and stored as accepted knowledge. This body of knowledge forms the background of new discoveries and serves the purpose of educating students and young scientists and of passing it to allied fields and disciplines. Hence, this knowledge has become detached from the context of scientific change, and it is insufficient to characterize the discovery process itself. Thus, the conventional view overlooks the fact that drugs are frequently developed first and thus precede basic knowledge being ex post facto explanations. Furthermore, it forgets that drugs are sensitive research tools and lead to an accumulation of biochemical and pharmacological knowledge.

Therefore, Maxwell has good reason to question this view and to propose another model that probably comes closer to reality (figure 2.2)

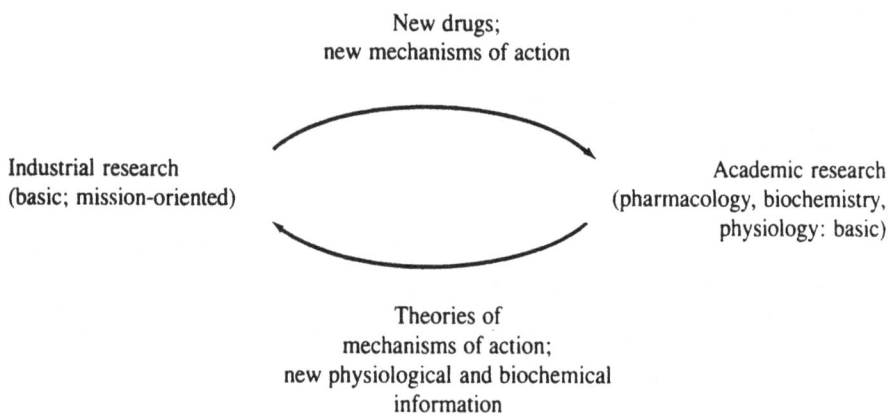

New drugs;
new mechanisms of action

Industrial research   Academic research
(basic; mission-oriented)   (pharmacology, biochemistry,
                                                                                                          physiology: basic)

Theories of
mechanisms of action;
new physiological and biochemical
information

Figure 2.2
The "interaction" model of drug discovery.
Reproduced with permission from Maxwell (1984).

Figure 2.2 expresses a symbiotic relationship between industrial drug discovery and academic research with each segment nurturing the other to mutual benefit. In Maxwell's model, the confusion of the epistemological with the sociological is resolved. Further, the terms basic and applied are relaxed to some extent. Hence, industrial research apparently encompasses both types of research but this seems not to apply to academic research.[11] Moreover, the model is asymmetric in what is transferred from one context to the other. There is good reason to presuppose that industrial research generates theories of mechanisms of action, and new physiological and biochemical information as well.

One important assumption still applies to Maxwell's model: clinical medicine and medical practice are excluded from the domain of discovery. In this sense Maxwell's revised model does not repair the damage caused by the misuse of the notions basic and applied in the biomedical field.

Obviously, there is much more to say about the categories of basic and applied research than discussed here.[12] Nowadays, these categories are rendered obsolete, and more refined classifications now cover the range of research activities conducted in both contexts.[13] To the extent that these classifications have rendered the distinction between science and technology itself obsolete, the distinction is dispersed into a much broader taxonomy of scientific and technological discovery.[14] However, many classifications still relate to this distinction between basic and applied, and reflect the dominance of theory-oriented epistemology.[15]

Rational and empirical drug discovery

The distinction "rational" versus "empirical" functions on the conceptual and methodological level. The methodological level concerns the methods for actually finding and creating a new lead. The preceding section described several of such methods ranging from empirical screening methods to rational procedures. In this respect a pragmatic attitude guides pharmaceutical science. All methods are used while differences in emphasis depend on laboratory culture, managerial style and the area of research. Whenever the methodological discussion permeates the debate about traditional and modern approaches in drug innovation we immediately reach the conceptual level which will be discussed in more detail.

The topic rational drug design is the centre point of interest in the pharmaceutical sector. Rational drug design aims at correlating conformational or other basic features of molecular structures with changes in biological activity on a highly predictive level. The ultimate interest is to achieve such a degree of prediction and sophistication that rational design may depart from first principles. The term design brings no semantic difficulty because it denotes shaping of the kind of substances suggested by the rationale. For quite some time this view has fluctuated between hope and reality and nowadays hopes are high that rational design is no longer a dream.[16] Rapid developments in computer sciences, molecular biology and biotechnology greatly influence these high expectations.

Rational drug design is very often juxtaposed to the rational approach in drug discovery, though they are not similar. The former concerns the rationale underlying the shaping of the desired molecules. The latter, in contrast, designates a rationale of the desired biological activity. The rational approach is also called the "biological" approach. Detailed knowledge of intracellular processes is needed to identify the key mechanisms in disease. However, terminology is fuzzy, and sometimes one expression overlaps another.

Both are concealed in the idea of specificity which actually has a long tradition in medicine and therapeutics.[17] One approach of this concept is the attempt to localize disease, that is, to identify the target for therapy. The other is therapeutic specificity or in modern terms: selectivity. There may be many possibilities for intervention, but each intervention it is hoped will reach its target selectively and replace mediators, switch off transducer and messenger systems by disturbing the normal physiological mechanisms as little as possible. The old dream of the "Magic Bullet" has its modern equivalent in this idea of selectivity. It is the rational drug designer's task to make the bullet, i.e. to shape this selectively acting molecule. It is the rational biologist's task to mark the selective path the bullet should take to hit the mark.

This rational way of thinking is balanced by its opposite: empiricism. To these opposite concepts Biel and Martin address themselves as follows: *"Our young graduates (medicinal chemists, RV) have become increasingly reluctant toward the 'instinctive' empirical approach of molecular modification. They are much more inclined toward the rational, mathematical, and computer oriented type of research. This is fine as long as it is based on sound biochemical and pharmacological principles and is not oblivious to the fact that there still is a living organism to be treated that is sufficiently complex to defy mathematical typing. Over-reliance on pure rationale is as dangerous as blind adherence to indiscriminate and unsophisticated molecular modification. Properly balanced, the two styles of research are eminently compatible".[18]*

But this balance is an unstable equilibrium. It is acknowledged that the history of therapeutic discoveries is in large measure a tribute to empirical observations and random discovery but this reflects a lack of intellectual power. Drug research finds itself in a situation of underdevelopment. *"There is no mystery about this situation"*, as Lasagna argues, for *"it is simply that the state of the science does not permit us the luxury of thoroughly rational drug development and will not for a long time to come. This is not to say that we should spurn progress achieved by any route, that we need to be anti-rational, or that it is wrong to be as rational as we can be".[19]* Lasagna expresses a majority point of view in pharmaceutical industry. The empirical approach is a reflection of the present state of incapacity in science and medicine. The most appreciation empiricism seems to get is to make a virtue of this necessity. This implicit feeling of inferiority and subordination easily leads to disdain about empiricism in drug research as terms like "molecular roulette", "molecular manipulation", "blind screening" and "random or chance discovery" might suggest.

Empiricism, however, enjoys a re-evaluation when connected with the terms "art" and "serendipity". Drug research resembles art because the discovery process needs the experience and expertise of chemists and biologists. Hence it will be governed by rules and preferences similar to those of an artistic vision at a given period of time, style, and innovative experimentation.[20] Thus, the nature of the chemist's or biologist's work resembles the artist's or craftsman's practical grasp. This practical grasp is necessary because the basic difficulty in drug research is that biological systems not only interact with drug molecules, but also form the living context in which these interactions do take place.[21]

From the chemist's perspective this difficulty implies the creation of relatively small molecules that must react with target molecules that are enormous and convoluted structures. Drug design therefore resembles shadow boxing; the target is there but can be barely discerned.[22] It is largely a process of making good guesses, relying on intuition and exploiting one's skills to trace the mark. Just as for the artist, the essence of the chemist's job lies between shaping what is imaginable and imagining what is shapeable. And probably many in pharmaceutical science would agree that drug discovery is an art rather than a science.[23]

The term serendipity strikes a somewhat different tone. Most often it refers to accidental discovery. A pure chance event attracts the attention of a scientist and points to a new direction in science. It is the ingenious and bold scientist who is prepared to take up the new possibility and carry it over the border of scepticism and unbelief.

Thus, the terms of art and serendipity express a basic route in drug discovery because it is an epistemology per se. It restores the imbalance between rational and empirical.

Evaluation of the sets of philosophical terms

Two sets of philosophical terms have been discussed both affecting current views on the drug discovery process in two ways.

Firstly, both sets act in a normative way because of ranking different types of knowledge in order of merit. At this point it is not argued that there are no good arguments to do so, but it is merely accepted as a fact.[24] The first set of terms, i.e. basic and applied, emphasizes the relationships between academia and pharmaceutical industry. In this respect it excludes clinical medicine and medical practice from the centre of scientific progress and drug discovery. Evidently, this exclusion is incomplete because it does not apply to those areas of medicine which are research oriented, use scientific methodology and explore the mechanisms of disease. But casuistics, the study of the natural history of disease and continuous adjustment of therapy to the needs of individual patients are not incorporated. At best they are considered useful in applying scientific knowledge and therapeutics in a rational way. In the same normative way, the other set of terms, i.e. rational and empirical, operates. However, a balanced picture is evolved when passing from the terms of rationalism and empiricism to that of serendipity and art.

The other mechanism acts on the descriptive level. Terms derived from these epistemologies are used by participants to describe the crucial episodes. As far as their limitations go, terms like "theory", "empirical generalizations", "laws", "experiments" and "observations", selectively focus on certain aspects of the discovery process. The same applies to the categories of art and serendipity with interrelated terms such as accidental discovery, chance observation, and serendipity.[25]

Most striking is that these expressions other than those related to art and serendipity stem from philosophy of science whereas many philosophers believe that discovery lies outside philosophical inquiry. What distinguishes science from art or any other creative activity is the insistence on testing, on subjecting knowledge to the most intense scrutiny, and to objectify knowledge with the help of empirical evidence. Emphasis is on verification, not on generation of knowledge. The following section will therefore deal with that scientific discipline in which scientific discovery has been identified as a proper subject of analysis, i.e. cognitive science.

2.3. Scientific discovery from the viewpoint of cognitive science

The scientific study of the discovery process has become the subject of cognitive psychology, artificial intelligence and cognitive science. The objective of this section is not to give a comprehensive review of the developments in these scientific fields but to touch on some topics relevant to any study of the discovery process and to place this thesis in a broader perspective of the study of scientific discovery. To do so frequent reference will be made to the book **Scientific Discovery: Computational Explorations of the Creative Processes** by Langley, Simon, Bradshaw and Zytkow.[26]

The following passage expresses the purpose of the book: *"However romantic and heroic we find the moment of discovery, we cannot believe either that the events leading up to that moment are entirely random and chaotic or that they require genius that can be understood only by congenial minds. We believe that finding order in the world must itself be a process impregnated with purpose and reason. We believe that the process of discovery can be described and modeled, and that there are better and worse routes to discovery - more or less efficient paths".[27]*

In this way the central challenge is posed. The authors think that discovery is amenable to rational explanation. In this respect they distinguish between a descriptive and a normative theory of discovery.[28] The former relates to a theory of the mechanisms that are implied in the discovery process, the latter undertakes to provide rules for actually making discovery. Specifically, such a theory proposes and evaluates a substantial number of heuristics that facilitate and speed up the discovery process - the "How To Make Discoveries Book".[29] Though emphasis lies on the elaboration of the descriptive theory by developing computer programs that simulate the discovery process, the foundations for a normative theory are explicitly strived for and discussed.

Langley and his colleagues take the view that discovery is a special case of human problem solving. In a sense problem solving involves a process of pattern seeking. Consider the alphabetical string as follows:

A B M C D M F E M ....

The pattern concealed in the string forms the problem to be solved. Thus, a possible solution is that the characters are ranked in alphabetical order, being interrupted by an **M** at the third, and every subsequent third position. This pattern can be represented by a formula such as $A(nMn)^*$, where n represents "next character of the alphabet", A and M denote themselves, and the asterisk denotes infinite repetition. By seeking for relationships such as "similarity", "sequence", "difference" or "inverse order" human beings quickly find such problems. Problem solving does not occur at random but is guided by rules that limit the range of possibilities. To the above-mentioned problem in which the seeking period is limited to a few seconds, the sequence of searching, testing, storing the result, again searching, etcetera until a satisfactory solution is found, also applies.

The **problem space** which is searched for, involves all conceivable patterns of characters; this space is also called the **space of instances**. When searching through this infinite space human beings use **rules** to produce candidate-patterns. The formula described above - whether it is correct, however, is another question - is an example of such-like rules which are stored in the **space of rules**. The process of problem solving can now be represented as a searching process within the space of rules to find the rule that generates the correct pattern. Subsequently, a check is made as to whether the generated pattern compares with the one given.

The essence of this searching process is that the seeking for rules is guided by rules as well. In the case of inductive, data-driven discovery these rules are inductively taken from the problem space.[30] If, for example, it is recognized that B follows A then by induction, the hypothesis arises that a rule implying alphabetical order should be searched for; this information is transferred to the space of rules. In other words, during inductive discovery the data not merely form the test-case for (interim) results of the searching process but also act as a direction-finder.

In short, the basic components of the model of scientific discovery developed by Langley and colleagues are:

1. There is a space of possible locations which they call the problem space. This space is composed of a set of states that can be occupied at any given time;

2. Within this set there exists a special state from which one begins the search process; this is the initial state;

3. There is a goal state that one wants to achieve;

4. There are operators (rules) that allow one to generate new states from the current state. Such states may be generated in an exhaustive fashion, and this is where heuristics come into play. Heuristics provide suggestions for 'cutting of' routes and to determine to what extent realized states meet the goal state.

This framework has been used to develop computer programs capable of making scientific discoveries by performing several search strategies on bodies of data. A number of computer programs have been constructed to discover scientific laws and concepts. Well-known laws such as those of Kepler, Ohm, Coulomb and Snell were re-discovered making use of the original body of raw data on which these scientists performed their creative activities. Some new laws were developed as well.

A simple example provided by the authors themselves, is instructive. The example concerns Kepler's third law of planetary motion: The cube of a planet's distance from the Sun is proportional to the square of its period. This law can be restated as $D^3/P^2 = c$, where D is the distance, P is the period, and c is a constant.

The authors provide the following three simple heuristics:

1. If the values of a term are constant, then infer that the term always has that value;

2. If the values of two numerical terms increase together, then consider their ratio;

3. If the values of one term increase as those of another decrease, then consider their product.

Table 2.1
Computational discovery of a scientific law.

Data obeying Kepler's third law of planetary motion.

Planet	Distance (D)	Period (P)	Term-1 (D/P)	Term-2 (D^2/P)	Term-3 (D^3/P^2)
A	1.0	1.0	1.0	1.0	1.0
B	4.0	8.0	0.5	2.0	1.0
C	9.0	27.0	0.333	3.0	1.0

The three planets considered in table 2.1 represent Kepler's third law in which the constant is 1. Since the names of the planets are the independent variables we have to consider the values of the dependent terms, i.e. of D and P. When considering the second and third column, we see that D increases with P. Therefore, in applying the second heuristic principle, the ratio of D and P (D/P) has to be calculated, the result of which is represented in the fourth column - called Term-1.

While D increases as Term-1 decreases, the third heuristic may be applied which yields Term-2, i.e. D^2/P. Consequently, while applying the same rule with respect to Term-1 and Term-2, Term-3 is obtained.

In this way, by using a small set of idealized data and applying three simple heuristic rules, Kepler's third law of planetary motion has been rediscovered.

This example illustrates the model. There is a problem space in which to seek for a pattern. The initial state is formed by a series of data to which heuristic rules and operators - the formulas to calculate the products and ratios - are applied to generate the next state. Following a pair of intermediate states the goal state is achieved: the desired pattern, in this case a law, has been found.[31]

To represent the various states cognitive science has developed symbolic structures such as **list structures** and **list processes** which form the basis of the majority of current expert systems. Noteworthy is that here the term representation denotes storage (list structures) as well as the use (list processes) of information.

A particular knowledge area is represented by objects, properties of objects, relations between objects and changes in these relational structures. Objects form elements of lists of objects, properties are part of lists of values attributed to objects, and relations are components of lists of relationships. Alternatively, (sets of) rules to manipulate objects, properties of and relations between objects are components of list processes.

These symbolic structures are important in representing various routes of discovery. A good example is the finding of Fleming that a mold lysed some bacteria. This observation, as Langley et al. argue, can be represented by L(m,b), where **m** is a mold, **b** a culture of bacteria, and **L** the relation that **m** lysed **b**:

*"From this representation, a series of research problems can be defined: to find the range of molds that can produce these effects, to find the range of bacteria or other organisms that are affected, and to study how the intensity of the effect depends on the pair (m,b). This is, in fact, a part of the research program that Fleming carried out after his accidental discovery of the phenomenon. Of course, to apply this problem-generation strategy one must be able to designate candidates for the sets to which **m** and **b** belong. Generally, prior knowledge in the form of classifications (the relation is **a**) will provide candidates. For example, the fact that **Penicillium**, the organism originally observed, **is a** mold suggests extending the experiment to other molds. The fact that the target organism **is a** species of bacteria suggests generalization to other bacteria. Every developed field of knowledge has its taxonomies and criteria of similarity that can be used as a basis for generalization and for consequent generation of candidates".*[32]

Thus, the objects **m** and **b** are elements of lists of similar objects. The properties of these objects, and their relations are part of list structures too while list processes contain the rules and formulas to manipulate objects. The concept of list must be understood literally as in the case of a telephone-book; in passing down the column with our finger ("pointer") we stop when the element of this list has been found. In the same way lists of scientific objects, of their properties and relations, can be turned over until the object, property or relation is found. Moreover, rules can be imagined to change these lists by adding, changing or removing elements; or to seek better and more quickly.

The assumption of Langley and colleagues is that list structures and processes simulate the structure and function of the human mind. In this context the question arises of other forms of representation of (scientific) knowledge. Two important forms are discussed by the authors: "sentential" and "pictorial" representations. According to the idea of sentential (or propositional) representation it is claimed that scientists think in "sentences". Knowledge is stored and used in the form of sentences from a natural or artificial language. In contrast, the view of pictorial representation claims that scientists think in "images". These forms of representation including list-structure are considered to be the fundamental forms of the human capacity of representing.

2.4. The drug discovery process revisited

Two sets of philosophical terms, i.e that of basic-applied and rational-empirical, have been discussed in order to clarify the basic features of the drug discovery process. They address the issue of the source of discovery and emphasize theory-driven discovery. However, the terms rational and empirical express a more balanced view between theory-driven and data-driven discovery when the epistemology of art and serendipity appears on the scene.[33] This epistemology involves, as described, inter-related terms such as accidental discovery, chance observation, and serendipity. It might be useful to clarify some of these terms and it is convenient to start with the term of accidental discovery.

In this context Langley et al. note: *"Accidental discovery requires both prepared minds to notice the phenomena and 'prepared' laboratories to originate them. It is not accidental that such discoveries often happen in laboratories equipped with instruments or concerned with newly discovered substances. There is nothing exceptional or unexplainable in accidental discovery. In the presence of new substances and instruments and new experimental arrangements, the simple goal of exploring a new domain systematically can generate reasonable research problems"*.[34]

Where experiments are performed, where nature is manipulated, there such phenomena will occur. Bacon, the philosopher of experiment, emphasized that experimenting is to *"shake out the folds of nature"* or *"to twist the lion's tail"*.[35] According to Hacking positivist philosophy has lost sight of this, literally, creative, aspect of experimenting. With its emphasis on theory, philosophy has split up scientific activity into theory and observation, and experiments merely serve the purpose of providing the empirical evidence for the theories under scrutiny. Philosophers neglect that experimentation has a life of its own.[36] In fact, as Hacking notes, contrasting theory with experiment tends to neglect that both have variable shapes rather than being an uniform kind of thing.[37] Thus, there is much more in the no man's land between theory and data driven discovery: the production of phenomena, the improvement of measurement, the invention of techniques, the explorations of new scientific domains, to mention some examples.[38] Consequently, differential relationships between theory and experiment have to be identified: *"Theory and experiment have different relationships in different sciences at different stages of development. There is no right answer to the question: Which comes first, experiment, theory, invention, technology,.....?"*.[39]

Closely related to this generative, creative side of experimenting, which Hacking terms "intervening", is the concept of observation.[40] Observations in experimenting are not merely used to test theories. Observations also refer to the sharp-sightedness of the experimenter and to his skills of enhancing what is of interest to him, and in eliminating the distortions of what he sees. Noticing may be a better alternative to observing in this respect. In this context Hacking points to an important kind of observation, less noticed by philosophers but essential to experimentation: *"The good experimenter is often the observant one who sees the instructive quirks or unexpected outcomes of this or that bit of the equipment. (..) Sometimes persistent attention to an oddity that would have been dismissed by a lesser experimenter is precisely what leads to new knowledge"*.[41] In other words, Hacking emphasizes what is coined with the term "prepared mind" by Langley et al. in the passage quoted above, and by pharmaceutical scientists when using the vocabulary of serendipity. At each step in the discovery process scientists have to notice the phenomena which are being studied or which profess to be novel.

At this point the model of scientific discovery elaborated by Langley et al. provides intriguing insights about the role of recognition and representation in science. Discovery is an incremental process which consists of thousands of mostly minor, and sometimes larger steps. At each step the recognition of phenomena plays a crucial role as well as heuristic procedures to decide upon how to proceed further. The recognition of new phenomena occurs against the background of known regularities, generalizations, laws and theories. The sources of new phenomenons are various; new problems are generated; new instruments and methods developed; and new generalizations, laws and theories are suggested. Still, the novel phenomena derive their meaning from current knowledge and their recognition occurs in the field of tension between the known and unknown, or the familiar and unfamiliar.

The issue of representing knowledge raises fundamental questions. In part, these questions are the subject of controversy, for example, the pictorial-versus-propositional controversy.[42] Intriguing is that in these controversies classic philosophical positions are pulled down and new positions taken up. Thus, Hacking rejects theory-oriented philosophy and pleas for a "Back-to-Bacon-Movement" emphasizing the role of experiment in science. Langley and colleagues also reject theory-oriented philosophy suggesting that the distinction between the context of discovery and justification is not as sharp, and much more complex and diverse than widely acknowledged.

The various methods of storing and using knowledge is therefore the subject of the study of the discovery process. To draw a parallel with computers: scientists use all kinds of data bases, and use various sorts of software programs for storing, retrieving and manipulating data. Philosophy has become a philosophy of scientific theory loosing sight of this wealth of methods for storage and retrieval of information. The terms "body of knowledge" and "background knowledge" which are used by philosophers camouflage this deficiency but are in themselves significant.

If there is a body of knowledge, it is plausible to suggest that this body of knowledge is as complex as the human body. As the human body is characterized by all shades of homeostatic mechanisms, stores, transport and communication processes, so is the "body of knowledge" a multi-layered system consisting of hierarchical structures for information storage, retrieval and manipulation and of a variety of feedback mechanisms. The following sections will deal with an important type of representing knowledge in drug research and biomedicine, namely drug and disease profiles.

Part 2. The representation of knowledge about drugs and diseases

2.5. An epistemological analysis of the concept of drug and disease profiles

2.5.1. Introduction

The central activity of any scientist and physician involves both data gathering and looking for a pattern or form in the data. The concept of profile refers to the latter aspect of pattern-seeking as an attempt to classify a drug or a patient.
The term profile forms a central part of daily communication between scientists and physicians. Scientific and medical literature use it liberally, usually in connection with some adjective: "biochemical profile", "pharmacological profile", "chemical-pharmacological profile", "clinical profile", "toxicological profile". This term therefore provides a common base for communication and understanding in contemporary science and medicine.
The aim of this section is to investigate the epistemological characteristics of the concepts of drug profile (2.5.2.) and disease profile (2.5.3.).

2.5.2. The concept of drug profile

2.5.2.1. The classification of drugs

In arriving at a more precise definition of the concept of drug profile we may start by giving an example of how scientists represent their knowledge about drugs. The following table (2.2) is derived from a comprehensive review article in which Zsoter and Church discuss the classification of the calcium antagonists.[43]

Table 2.2
The concept of drug profile - profiles of verapamil, nifedipine and diltiazem.

Action	Verapamil	Nifedipine	Diltiazem
Effect on fast channels	+	0	+
Local anaesthetic effect	+	0	+
Slowing of AV conduction	+	0	+
Prolongation of refractory period in AV node	+	0	+
Vascular O_2 consumption	↓	0	↑
Negative inotropic/negative chronotropic effect	> 1	≫1	< 1
Peripheral vasodilator effect	+	++	+
Activation of baroreceptor reflexes	+	++	+

Reproduced with permission from Zsoter and Church (1983).

The table represents a common way of depicting the characteristics of some compounds within a particular class of drugs.

An important aspect is the use of heterogeneous elements. The action of verapamil, for example, on "fast channels" - i.e. certain holes in membranes for ion fluxes -, is quite distinct from the peripheral vasodilator effect, i.e. a dilation of blood vessels. The former relates to a biochemically defined action, the latter to a hemodynamically determined effect. Some aspects characterize the effects of the drugs on the contractile function of the heart, others on the rhythmic function of the heart or other parts of the cardiovascular system. The sixth characteristic is interesting because it represents the ratio of two characteristics: negative inotropic/negative chronotropic action.

Furthermore, these characteristics are provided with values represented by mathematical symbolism. Each symbol represents a property which can be measured and can be given numerical values. But here the wide ranges of numerical values are reduced to some principal ranges which are designated by symbols. The symbol of the arrow, for example, is typical in this respect. The arrow down, in the case of the effect of verapamil on vascular O_2-consumption, represents that verapamil decreases oxygen consumption. In contrast, diltiazem increases vascular oxygen consumption, hence the arrow pointing upwards. The same applies to the sixth characteristic: the ratio is expressed as a combination of a numeric value and a symbol, i.e. '>1', '>>1' and '<1' for verapamil, nifedipine and diltiazem respectively.

Usage of the symbols '+', '++' and '0' is more difficult to understand. With respect to the first two characteristics the symbols '+' and '0' are used to denote the absence or presence of these characteristics: verapamil and diltiazem have an effect on fast channels and possess a local anaesthetic effect while nifedipine has not. In contrast, the third and fourth characteristic express a value as well but this is camouflaged by the expressions in the first column: slowing of AV conduction, and prolongation of refractory period in AV node. These characteristics may be reasonably translated into:

slowing of AV conduction = AV conduction: slowing
prolongation of refractory period in AV node = refractory period in AV node: prolonged

Alternative values are "acceleration" or "no alteration". It is not a problem to attribute suitable symbols to the values: slowing and prolongation may be represented by arrows pointing downward, acceleration and shortening by arrow upwards, and no alternation by the symbol '='.

With respect to the last two characteristics the symbols '+' and '++' clearly designate the strength of the effects, i.e. represent three types of values: no effect (= 0 or absent), a moderate and strong positive effect. The absence/presence of characteristics is a matter of values as well. Now, the wide ranges of possible values is reduced to a borderline above which a particular effect is conceived of as present, and below which as absent.

When using 0 and 1 to denote the absence/presence of characteristics, + and ++ to denote the degree of the effects of the compounds, and the arrows to designate the direction into which the effects of the compounds point, the following reconstructed profiles result (table 2.3).

Table 2.3
Reconstructed profiles of verapamil, nifedipine and diltiazem.

Action	V	N	D
Effect on fast channels	1	0	1
Local anaesthetic effect	1	0	1
AV conduction	↑	↔	↑
Refractory period AV node	↑	↔	↑
Vascular O_2 consumption	↓	↔	↑
Negative inotropic/chronotropic effect	>1	>>1	<1
Peripheral vasodilator effect	+	++	+
Activation baroreceptor reflexes	+	++	+

V = verapamil; N = nifedipine; D = diltiazem.

Accordingly, three profiles are obtained that express two basic characteristics: the absence/presence of characteristics; and the values of these characteristics.

The profiles of the three compounds serve different purposes. One purpose obviously is the comparison between the compounds. Taking the first four characteristics separately - which assess the effects on the rhythmic function of the heart - then verapamil and diltiazem appear to be similar compounds but nifedipine is clearly different. The same applies to the last two characteristics. If the profiles were constructed on the basis of these six characteristics, two profiles had to be discerned: one representing nifedipine, the other simultaneously representing verapamil and diltiazem. In this respect the fifth and sixth characteristic are decisive in distinguishing between verapamil and diltiazem. In addition, the three compounds have many more properties than listed but merely eight are presented. The presented list is therefore the result of a selection procedure based on ranking properties in order of merit. Thus apart from the presence or absence, and the values of characteristics, profiles have a third important feature: ranking of characteristics.

Another purpose is the representation of prototypes within one particular class of drugs. The calcium antagonists encompass a class of drugs of which, at present, verapamil, nifedipine and diltiazem are conceived of as prototypes. Each represents a subclass within the general class of calcium antagonists. In this way the position of existing or newly developed compounds in the class of calcium antagonists can be identified rather precisely.

The classification of classes of drugs

The concept of profile also enables scientists to classify classes of drugs, not only of single compounds within a class. In table 2.4, taken from the same review article of Zsoter and Church, the calcium antagonists are compared with digitalis and the beta blockers.

All the symbols used designate values and the absence/presence of characteristics does not play a role in this case. The table raises the same issues regarding the values as discussed above. However, some other aspects are noteworthy.

In some cases the symbols are depicted between brackets while in others notes are added to specify the location of the effect, the circumstances in which the effects occur or the compounds concerned. To some extent these specifications result from uncertainties in the body of knowledge; this applies especially to the symbols between the brackets; the most extreme example is the question-mark with regard to the second characteristic of the beta blockers.[44] Also these specifications are the result of over-simplification due to the process of the classification itself: the comparison between classes of drugs. However, this over-simplification is asymmetrical. The table clearly disregards the differences between related

Table 2.4
The classification of classes of drugs.

Action	Digitalis	Calcium antagonist drugs	β-Adrenoceptor blocking drugs (propranolol)
Ca^{++} influx into cells	↑	↓	↓
Na$^+$, K$^+$-ATPase	↓	(↑)^2	?
Cardiac contractility	↑	↓ (↑)^2	↓
Myocardial O$_2$ consumption	↑	↓	↓
Heart rate	↓	↓ (↑)^2	↓
AV conduction	↓	↓	↓
AV refractoriness	↑	↑^{3}	↑
Excitability	↑	↓	↑
Coronary artery	(C)	D	(C)
Peripheral vessels	(C)	D	(C)

1   In vessels by diltiazem.
2   *In vivo.*
3   Verapamil and diltiazem only.
C = constricted.
D = dilated.

Reproduced with permission from Zsoter and Church (1983).

compounds within the class of "digitalis-like" compounds and the beta blockers. Digitalis is used as the prototype of agents that are used to strengthen the force of contraction of the heart, and propranolol is used to represent the class of beta blocking agents. In contrast, the table attempts to capture the similarities and dissimilarities between verapamil, nifedipine and diltiazem.

In comparison with the former table some characteristics are left out in the second, i.e. the local anaesthetic effect and the activation of the baroreceptor reflexes. Some others left out in fact reappear in another form. The characteristic "effect on fast channels" is related to that of "Na$^+$,K$^+$-ATPase", the latter representing the enzyme involved in the sodium and kalium pump pertinent to the fast channels in the heart. The ratio negative inotropic/negative chronotropic activity has disappeared, but is replaced by adding the characteristics "cardiac contractility" and "heart rate" separately into the second profile. While some characteristics have remained the same, other characteristics have been added to the second table, i.e. calcium influx into cells, excitability and coronary artery dilation/constriction.

2.5.2.2. Incursion of drug profiles into disease profiles

As more drugs become used in disease therapy, knowledge about drugs grows, and will be incorporated into drug profiles. An example illustrates this point.

The blockade of sympathetic over-activity by beta blockers during myocardial infarction (MI) on arrhythmias and infarct size led to enthusiasm amongst cardiologists to try beta blockers in the prevention of early mortality in the post-myocardial-infarction-phase. Subsequent experience showed that application of these drugs is justified by the therapeutic desire to reduce pain, arrhythmias and infarct size, but not mortality per se. Additional investigations showed that patients with infarction in particular areas of the heart and with higher rhythmic rates but without overt heart failure were most likely to benefit.

Table 2.5 Incursion of drug profiles into disease profiles. Advantages of early vs. late initiation of beta blockade (metoprolol) in acute myocardial infarction (MI).

Endpoint	Subgroup	
	Therapy ≤ 12 hr after pain onset	Therapy > 12 hr after pain onset
1. Mortality (90d)	35% ↓	35% ↓
2. Enzymatic infarct size	↓10% overall ↓16% if ↑ HR initially ($P < 0.02$)	
3. Ventricular arrhythmias	Reduced (↓)	Reduced (↓)
4. Chest pain	Reduced (↓)	Reduced (↓)
5. Severity of CHF	Reduced (↓) (furosemide ↓40%)	No change (→)
6. Hospital stay	Shorter stay (↓1-2 days)	Longer stay
7. Late MI	↓Late MI (vs. placebo)	↓Late MI (vs. placebo)

Reproduced with permission from Anderson (1986).

Table 2.5 shows the results of treatment with beta blockers within twelve hours after MI and longer than twelve hours after MI.

Both groups reveal no differences regarding mortality but the former group reacted positively with respect to the therapeutic goals 2), 5) and 6). With respect to the other goals there are no differences. If we suppose that these results are accepted by the cardiological community as significant and representative, in what way does this knowledge affect the drug profile of the beta blockers?

Characteristics of the beta blockers involve all six therapeutic goals but in addition an attempt is made to decide whether the moment of drug administration is relevant to therapeutic success. Hence, the time point of administration becomes a characteristic of the drug itself. But it is not as simple as that.

The outstanding feature of this table is that two **subsets** of patients are characterized, one subset associated with a myocardial infarction which did not last for twelve hours, a "fresh" infarction, and one subset of patients with a longer-lasting infarction. In the former case the reduction of all pathological features of MI patients is realized while in the latter case this was the case for therapeutic goals 1), 3), 4), and 7) but not 2), 5) and 6). The point is that previously, based on the knowledge about myocardial infarction, cardiologists set these seven goals as requirements which any post-myocardial infarction therapy had to meet. That is any therapy should at least reduce mortality, enzymatic infarct size, and so forth. To some extent the therapeutic results were satisfactory but then it appeared that by splitting up the whole category of MI patients into two subsets, the treatment with beta blockers gave more success in the one subset than in the other.

This shows that the incursion of drug profiles into disease profiles is a complex issue. Here it suffices to mark some points. Firstly, there is a difference between the route of discovery and the outcome of the discovery process. The outcome, however, remains the same: there are two subsets of MI patients and treatment of one subset is more successful than that of the other. Secondly, the clinically relevant features shown in the scheme clearly differ from the effects on biochemical processes or other technical and experimental aspects of the disease listed in the preceding profiles.

2.5.2.3. The nature of drug characteristics

The preceding section discussed the characteristics of drugs and the formation of drug profiles. To clarify this problem it is convenient to start with a simple definition of a drug.

Definition: **A drug is a remedy to treat disease**

Three concepts are concealed in this definition.

First, the term "remedy" refers to a means which is in this case a compound. This implies that such a means can be characterized by certain properties which are of a physical and chemical nature: molecular structure, geometry, lipophilic or hydrophilic aspects, acidity, etc. Henceforth such properties will be called **structural** characteristics of drugs. The term "structural" is used because such characteristics determine the "make up" of the drugs.[45]

Secondly, the term "disease" is essential. In the following section the concept of disease profile will be discussed but for the moment it suffices to state that a disease is a pathological condition of the patient, and that **disease** characteristics are the essential components of medical knowledge about disease.

Thirdly, the term "treat": in its broadest sense it encompasses every legitimate therapeutic goal: the relief of pain, the ease of symptoms, palliation, prevention and cure. The least this term implies is a change in the organism of the patient. For example, a drug should relieve headache in the case of a patient with headache and must therefore induce a variety of responses in the organism, e.g. constriction of blood vessels in the head and suppression of certain nervous pathways. These changes in the organism which are induced by the drug, are called **therapeutic** characteristics. The term therapeutic denotes that these characteristics are related to some therapeutic goal.

This simple definition of a drug has produced three types of characteristics: structural, therapeutic and disease characteristics. The following example examines these in more detail (table 2.6).

Table 2.6 Characteristics of a drug.

Structural	Therapeutic	Disease
Nitrite	Reduction of O_2 demand	Pain in the chest

The characteristics in the three columns are presented without any connection. Undoubtedly, a connection immediately suggests itself: is the structural characteristic "nitrite" responsible for the reduction of the oxygen demand of the heart which in its turn relieves the pain in the chest experienced by some patient?

Suppose such a connection exists, then still, the distinction between the three characteristics makes sense. A "nitrite" is a particular molecular structure which may be characterized by a variety of physico-chemical parameters which are not necessarily specific for reducing oxygen demand. There may be many compounds with quite different structures that reduce oxygen demand.

Let us accept this for a moment and return to the distinction between therapeutic and disease characteristics. The difference is obvious and no one would deny the difference between "reduction of O_2 demand" and "pain in the chest". However, the clinician might argue that reducing the oxygen demand of the heart is a therapeutic goal as is the relief of pain in the chest, particularly because both goals are causally related. Thus, the difference is not quite so clear as suggested and the following improvement may be made (table 2.7).

Table 2.7
Therapeutic and disease characteristics.

Therapeutic	Disease
Reduction of O_2 demand	Increase of O_2 demand
Relief of pain in the chest	Pain in the chest

This particular disease is characterized by an increased oxygen demand and pain in the chest whence two therapeutic goals are desirable. However, therapeutic and disease characteristics are still different things. Therapeutic characteristics determine what a drug **should do**, disease characteristics determine what a disease **is**.

Now, suppose a drug has in addition to the two characteristics described above, some others as well, for example, the dilation of the gall bladder. Then clearly this is not a structural characteristic. It is an effect in the organism but neither is it a therapeutic characteristic. So, a drug produces a variety of effects in the organism but some are judged as therapeutically useful and others as useless. This judgment is always considered with respect to a particular disease or a range of diseases. Henceforth, the effects of drugs on the organism will be called **operational functional** characteristics. The term "functional" is chosen in contrast to "structural" to denote the difference between the make-up and the function of the drug. The term "operational" refers to a drug actually having certain effects on the organism. Functional characteristics which are considered as therapeutically useful, are desirable features; henceforth these are termed **"wished for"** characteristics.

The distinction between wished for and operational is crucial. It is an empirical matter what the effects of a drug are. However, to treat a disease implies that we wish the treatment to have particular characteristics, that is, we wish a drug to act in a certain way. We may test a certain drug and find that it has the beneficial effects to be expected; and again, we might determine with the help of sophisticated techniques and methodologies that the drug really is efficacious, and all this would be a matter of empirics. But any time we treat the disease we would wish the drug to act in a certain way. If we lived in a world in which a drug could act first this way and then that way, it would be clear that we literally want a drug to act in a particular way. In other domains of real life we experience similar situations often. When our car runs out of petrol or our bike has a punctured tire, we suddenly become aware of the insufferable difference between what we continuously want a car or bike to perform and what they actually do, and we become angry.

If a drug possesses the characteristics wished for, it is a good drug; if this is not the case, then it is a bad drug or not a drug at all. But it would be ridiculous to suggest that such a compound doesn't induce any changes in the human body. The only thing we can say is that these are not wished for, that we don't desire them if we administer the drug to a particular patient. In this sense two patterns of characteristics are pertinent to any drug. One pattern, i.e. the set of wished for (functional) characteristics, expresses what we desire of a particular drug. The other pattern, i.e. the set of operational (functional) characteristics, represents what a drug actually does. The extent to which these patterns fit, determines our judgment of the drug.

Similarly we may apply the distinction between operational and wished for to the structural characteristics.[46] An example illustrates this and provides additional evidence of the usefulness of the distinction.

Suppose, we have a lipophilic drug. In contrast to a hydrophilic drug such a compound is to be expected to pass the blood-brain-barrier rather easily. If the therapeutic use of that drug in some disease is severely restricted by its central nervous effects, clearly a hydrophilic compound is preferable. If we demand that a drug not pass the blood-brain-barrier we set requirements for the structural make-up of the drug, i.e. it should be hydrophilic, not lipophilic.

However, when searching for a compound that preferably exerts its beneficial effect in the central nervous system, for example, in the case of Parkinson' disease, then a lipophilic compound is desired. If that compound exerts central nervous side-effects as well, there is a conflict between what is desired and what is not, or better, between what is desired and what a drug actually does. Scientists will look for other ways to meet the requirements. If they don't succeed, they have to adjust their goals, that is they have to be satisfied with a less perfect match between the two patterns described above. However, in this case, there are two pairs of patterns. One pair concerns what we wish a drug to do and what it actually does: the set of wished for and operational functional characteristics respectively. The other pair concerns what we wish a drug's make up should be and what it actually is: the set of wished for and operational structural characteristics respectively. In other words, what we desire depends upon the intended application which determines what kind of structural and functional characteristics we wish. The extent to which we are satisfied with what is actually found, depends upon many circumstances: available therapy, the severity of the disease to be treated, and goals of medical therapy.

2.5.3. The concept of disease profile

2.5.3.1. Disease profiles as pigeon-holes of medical knowledge

A central activity in medicine is to delineate disease entities by the clustering of symptoms and signs, events in natural history and therapeutic outcome, and by discovering that apparently unrelated phenomena have the same causes. Such identification of disease entities, called "syndromes", is of immediate practical interest to the diagnostic process of the physician in order to provide an appropriate prognosis and treatment of the patient. Hence, taxonomy, or nosology, seems to be as old as medicine itself. Feinstein describes this basic clinical activity as follows: *"As the main language of clinical communication, diagnostic labels transmit a rapid understanding of the contents of the package; diagnostic categories provide names for the intellectual locations in which clinicians store the observations of clinical experience. The taxonomy used for diagnosis will thus inevitably establish the patterns in which clinicians observe, think, remember and act".* [47]

Disease profiles are therefore the pigeon-holes in which physicians store their knowledge and experiences. The features discussed with respect to drug profiles apply to disease profiles as well, and it suffices to discuss one example which is taken from the medical literature.

Developing a classification system of angina pectoris Wartak et al. employed arrays made up of numerals that designate five important parameters (see figure 2.3).

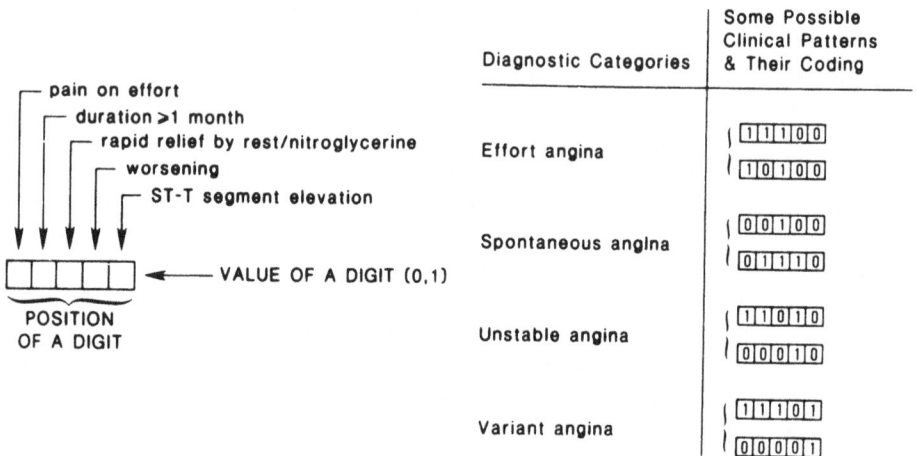

Figure 2.3
Numerical coding of pectoris. Left: the principle of constructing the numerical code. Right: numerical codes for various clinical patterns of angina within diagnostic categories presently distinguished.
Reproduced with permission from Wartak et al. (1984).

These parameters are: (1) pain on effort, (2) duration > 1 month, (3) rapid relief by rest/ nitroglycerine, (4) worsening, and (5) ST-T segment elevation. The presence of a given factor can be coded as "1", while the absence of that factor can be coded by a "0". As the result, one obtains an array of 1's and 0's or a binary vector for a given clinical pattern of angina pectoris. Four main diagnostic categories of angina pectoris are established, each with a pair of clinical patterns to match.

The clinical patterns listed by the authors reveal the features and difficulties which have been discussed with respect to the concept of drug profile, i.e. absence/presence, values and priorities of characteristics.

In this system of numerical coding, knowledge about angina pectoris is reduced to the mere absence or presence of characteristics - indicated by the binary digits. However, if we look at the second parameter, the time period during which the patient suffers from the disease, this parameter is formulated in terms of a value: "duration ≥ 1 month". Once again, this illustrates that by splitting up all the possible ranges of values of this parameter into two classes, a binary interpretation of values is generated: either the characteristic is absent or present.

In figure 2.3 the feature of ranking takes a somewhat different form. An example of this is seen in the two clinical patterns; the upper one which belongs to the disease category spontaneous angina and the one below belonging to the category variant angina. The mere presence of the third parameter is sufficient to distinguish spontaneous angina, the mere presence of the fifth parameter to make the diagnosis variant angina.

Also important to note is that underneath this system of numerical coding lies the supposition that the absence of a characteristic is as important as the presence. This seems to be somewhat awkward but it makes sense. The presence of pain of effort is an important aspect of effort angina; actually this aspect signifies this sub-type of angina. In contrast, the absence of pain of effort is a significant symptom of spontaneous angina; the term "spontaneous" denotes that the pain (in the chest) is experienced at rest like a bolt from the blue. Effort angina is characterized both by the presence of pain on effort and the absence of pain at rest. Similarly, spontaneous angina is characterized both by the presence of pain at rest and the absence of pain on effort. There is no principal difficulty in formulating the absence of certain features as "positive properties".

There are two additional points to note, particularly because they reveal basic problems in the classification of disease:

1. Obviously, a numerical classification might be developed that extends beyond the five parameters just described. Thus, Wartak et al. suggest that a binary vector should be included to represent the results of the angiogram, a technique to assess atherosclerosis of the blood vessels in the heart. The coding of angiographic patterns would be helpful in identifying high-risk sub-sets of patients who benefit from bypass surgery. Such a coding would also help to distinguish between the patients suffering from stable, unstable, or variant angina with normal and damaged coronary arteries. To the extent that a mere enlargement of the number of characteristics is involved, is not a problem. However, in two other respects, it is.

First, what kind of characteristics do clinicians allow to form components of the classifica-tion; secondly, for what reasons do they do so? In both ways the fundamental basis of the classification system is challenged.

2. An array of five binary digits can produce numerous patterns but only some of these are identified as representing subtypes of angina pectoris. Under each diagnostic heading merely two patterns are distinguished. But what about a patient with the pattern "0,1,1,0,0"? Such a patient poses a problem to the clinician when using the system of numerical coding developed by Wartak and colleagues. This addresses a central problem of medicine: the tension between general and particular knowledge.

2.5.3.2. The fundamental basis of taxonomy in medicine

Since taxonomy is as old as medicine, each generation of physicians will "split" and "lump" to suit its own purposes.[48]
Nosologists of the eighteenth century, for example, were complaint-oriented. Under the influence of Thomas Sydenham's (1624-1689) concept of the natural history of diseases clinicians classified diseases according to the complaints of patients as they appeared to the clinician. Late 19th and early 20th century nosologies explicitly aimed for a topographical and morphological classification. Concurrent disease classifications, however, mix together categories derived from pathology, microbiology and physiology.[49] The categories are therefore heterogeneous but they still signal, just as the former nosologies did, normative judgments in two, interrelated respects.

The first normative judgment concerns the purpose of the classification. Nosology serves not only the purpose of coherent data collection but that of therapeutic decision-making as well.
Consider, for example, whether one lists tuberculosis as an infectious disease, a genetic disease, an environmental disease, or one of defective immunity. We signal tuberculosis as an infectious disease in that this appears to indicate the most efficient mode of treating and preventing the condition. There is evidence, however, that there are genetic variations in the susceptibility of populations to tuberculosis, and in any case a eugenics program aimed at increasing resistance to tuberculosis would very likely be more dangerous than would be justified. Similar considerations influence the categorization as an immunological failure or as a disease due to social conditions. With regard to the latter, for instance, there is a great deal of information that general social variables bearing on housing and nutrition affect the morbidity and mortality patterns of tuberculosis. The point here is that nosologies of disease can signal where or how one should think about treatment or prevention.[50] Even so, the purpose of the classification affects what kind of medical knowledge is stored into disease profiles.

This leads to the second normative judgment which concerns the types of categories included in nosology. Much of Feinstein's work, for example, consists of developing a disease classification based on bedside clinical procedures, not on laboratory and other medical-technical techniques. Feinstein opposes the dominance of pathophysiology and technology in contemporary nosology.

The latter points attest to the various sorts of disease characteristics: biochemical, pathological, physiological, technical and patient-oriented. Here two fundamental types of disease characteristics will be distinguished, i.e. experimental and clinical.

Symptoms and signs observed in human subjects are clinical disease characteristics. In contrast, information about disease gathered from investigations in non-human material - cell and tissue cultures, animals and the like - are experimental disease characteristics. The same applies to data gathered from biopsy, autopsy, amputation of limbs, or otherwise extracted human material: organs, blood, sputum, skin, hair and nails.

The categories experimental and clinical are not absolute but a matter of degree. In most cases it will be clear whether experimental or clinical disease characteristics are investigated. In addition, the clinician might wonder whether to focus on symptoms or signs. Actually, when the technological character of contemporary medicine is debated, the current emphasis on signs available through the use of sophisticated medical techniques, is criticized. It is argued that medicine should pay more attention to symptoms but the distinction proposed here, i.e. between experimental and clinical, avoids the basic question. There is no problem in distinguishing between symptoms and signs within the category of clinical characteristics.

2.5.3.3. Convergent and divergent forces in clinical taxonomy

Clinicians have studied hundreds of thousands of patients to seek for regularities and similarities in order to build up medical science. None of these patients were ever completely identical regarding the constellation of symptoms and signs they presented.[51] Thus, in practice, clinicians are confronted again and again with patients whose clinical patterns deviate from the ones established as diagnostic categories. Accordingly, clinicians make use of rules, formally or informally settled, to solve the problems. If, however, many patients were encountered with a particular pattern, clinicians might decide to include this pattern into clinical taxonomy.

This points to the tension between general and particular knowledge in medicine. Essential to the latter type of knowledge is that it particularizes its object. Each individual patient to be encountered by the physician represents a specific arrangement of signs and symptoms that one way or the other will not fit the generalized clinical pattern. Every doctor-patient interaction, each therapeutic decision, and each act of intervention in sick people challenges clinical taxonomy. The individuality of patients and the complexity of real life medical practice forms a rich source of variation and deviation. Disease concepts loose fixed meanings in daily practice of clinical diagnosis and treatment.

This type of medicine therefore may be conceived of as a divergent force in nosology opposite to the convergent force of that type of medicine which seeks general knowledge. This tension between divergent and convergent forces generates the vocabulary, described by Fleck, of pseudo- and para-determinations of disease that is so characteristic for medicine. We may encounter: Typhus-Paratyphus; Psoriasis-Parapsoriasis; Anemia-Pseu-doanemia; Pseudobulbairparalysis; Pseudocroup; Pseudonervitis optica; Pseudosclerosis; and Pseudotabes; and many other look-alikes of varying shades and degrees.[52]

This shows that disease profiles are continuously being shaped and re-shaped. This iterative process is not merely confined to theoretical developments about the etiology and mechanism of disease. It is also generated at a deeper epistemological level and is a tribute to the feedback of clinical practice to medical science - this will be discussed in detail in chapter 8 and 9.

The practical significance of this tension is related to the translation of daily medical language into disease profiles. This practical significance is perhaps illustrated most clearly by the following examples[53]:

    i) "Effort usually precipitates pain"
    ii) "Emotional upset frequently produces pain"

The sentences i) and ii) express characteristics of effort angina. But what do the terms 'usually' and 'frequently' express? Two interpretations are possible.

1. A universal law is involved which has, in this case, the form of a simple universal condition: "For any x, if x is A then x is B". For example, in case of sentence i: "For each patient, if the patient has pain on exertion, then this patient suffers from angina pectoris". The profile of effort angina can be translated into a profile with two characteristics: effort produces pain (in the chest) and so does emotional upset. Nevertheless, patients are found without this characteristic but such patients still have to be classified as effort angina. Accordingly, clinicians should posses additional rules to assess clinical patterns that deviate from this universal pattern. Such a rule might be: "If a patient has pain with emotional upset, but not with effort, then it is still probably a patient with angina pectoris".

2. Both sentences express a frequential probability, though in a quantitatively inexact manner. Suppose it is widely accepted that in 70% of all cases patients suffering from angina pectoris have pain in the chest on effort, what does such a probabilistic statement mean? If it expresses a disease characteristic, the disease profile of effort angina encompasses something like "70% likelihood of chest pain on effort". This makes no sense from the viewpoint of the clinician facing his individual patient. This patient might have any clinical pattern, but either this patient has pain on effort, or not.

It is more reasonable therefore to suggest that there are in fact two clinical patterns, one associated with the presence of the characteristic pain on effort, the other with the absence of it. In addition, a likelihood is expressed with which both patterns may be encountered in reality, one in 70% of the cases, the other in 30% of all patients. Somehow this knowledge about the distribution of profiles is captured in a rule or set of rules.

However, from the viewpoint of the clinician facing his individual patient, the probabilistic structure of medical knowledge poses more fundamental problems. Firstly, the clinician pays attention to this individual patient in an inclusive way: all characteristics which affect the life of his patient will be considered, many of which are not incorporated in the general clinical pattern. Thus, right from the beginning the clinician creates a particular constellation of symptoms, signs and features of the patient that will not fit the general pattern, at least not entirely. Whenever the individual history is critical to diagnosis, then somehow the clinician has to use additional rules to match the pattern identified to the general pattern. Secondly, the clinician starts by building up the profile of the individual patient from scratch. After having identified a small set of symptoms and signs, the clinician must decide whether or not this particular patient matches a general pattern. While the clinical scientist builds up disease profiles, hence identifies disease characteristics given there is a disease - or given there is no disease, the clinical practitioner starts by asking whether, given some symptoms and signs, there is a disease. This problem is a central part of current research into diagnostic reasoning, using Bayes' theorem. This theorem enables the clinician to assess the probability a particular patient has a disease on the basis of the symptoms and signs identified in this particular patient, and the known frequential probabilities about the occurrence of symptoms and signs given the presence or absence of the disease.

Since a great part of medical knowledge is probabilistic in nature, the second interpretation seems to be the best candidate. However, underneath lies the problem of diverse threads of knowledge in medicine. The question is whether the language of disease profiles is neutral with respect to the various types of medical knowledge. The author's hypothesis is that the language can be further specified in order to meet the peculiarities of each type of knowledge. In the scope of this thesis this fundamental issue will be put between brackets, and reserved for further investigation. This implies that a methodological decision has to be taken how to treat terms like "usually", "frequently", "very often", or "mostly" in medical knowledge. This forms the subject of the next section.

2.5.3.4. The translation of everyday medical language into the structure of profiles

The purpose of the preceding section was also to illustrate the problem of translating sentences of everyday medical language into the structure of profiles. A necessary condition for this translation is that medical knowledge expressed by clinicians or scientists, either informally or formally in text-books and articles, has to be reduced to the three basic components of profiles identified above.

Table 2.8 represents five characteristics of two forms of angina distinguished by Prinzmetal and co-workers in 1959, i.e. the classic form of angina (= angina of effort) and the variant form of angina (see for the complete profiles chapter 6).
The expressions illustrate what has been said in the preceding section - note that the examples presented in that section represent the first two characteristics of the classic form of angina pectoris.

Table 2.8
Differences between the variant and classic form of angina pectoris
regarding to five clinical characteristics selected from the profiles
published by Prinzmetal et al. (1960).

Variant Form	Classic form
Exertion usually does not precipitate pain	Exertion usually precipitates pain
Emotional upset does not produce pain	Emotional upset frequently produces pain
Pain is frequently more severe and of longer duration than in classic angina	Pain is usually less severe and of shorter duration than in variant form
Attack often consists of series of pain, occurring in cyclic and remarkably regular pattern	Pain is not cyclic
If pain is not cyclic, period of increasing pain is equal to period of decreasing pain	Period of increasing pain is longer than period of decreasing pain

The expressions underscore the difference between general and particular knowledge, and relate to the probabilistic structure of medical knowledge. However, from the viewpoint of general knowledge there is a clear-cut difference between variant and classic angina. In the former case exertion does not precipitate pain whereas in the latter exertion does. The term "usually" in this example refers to the problem of the clinician facing an individual patient - other patterns may be encountered.

Since the creation of general knowledge forms the subject of this study it was decided to eliminate this probabilistic terminology. This applies also to similar expressions in the table: "often", "frequently", "generally", "(not) as common" and "(not) regularly".

Table 2.9 represents the first five characteristics of both disease profiles as reconstructed in terms of the theory of profiles.

The first characteristic of both disease entities listed by Prinzmetal and co-workers have been translated into two pairs of characteristics. It might be argued that in fact there are just

Table 2.9
Reconstructed profiles of angina of effort and variant form of angina.

Variant form		Classic form	
(v_1)	Exertion does not produce pain	(c_1)	Exertion precipitates pain
(v_2)	Pain at rest	(c_2)	No pain at rest
(v_3)	Emotion does not precipitate pain	(c_3)	Emotion produces pain
(v_4)	Intensity of pain (severe)	(c_4)	Intensity of pain (mild)
(v_5)	Duration of pain (long)	(c_5)	Duration of pain (short)
(v_6)	Series of pain cyclic/regular	(c_6)	Series of pain not cyclic

two characteristics, i.e. pain at rest (v_1) and pain on exertion (c_1), where: $v_1 \in V$, $v_1 \notin C$, $c_1 \in C$ and $c_1 \notin V$. However, the mere absence of the characteristic "pain at rest" in case of exertional angina or "exertion precipitates pain" is understating the case. The presence of one characteristic was almost as typical as the absence of the other. The same argument applies to the relationship between emotion and pain and the (non)cyclic character of anginal attacks. The characteristics with respect to the nature of pain, i.e. intensity and duration, are in both cases the same, yet their values differ (severe-mild, long-short). This table may be easily extended to cover all characteristics of both disease forms.

2.5.4. Conclusions

One special and important way of gathering information and finding a pattern in a set of data has been identified; the use of drug and disease profiles by scientists and clinicians. A profile is a pattern and as such it enables scientists to recognize something and to set it apart from other things. There is a rationale for denoting such patterns, e.g. the arrangement of attributes of any drug or disease, as the profile of that drug or disease. As a profile of a man's face characterizes that particular man amongst a crowd of people, so the profile of some drug or disease brings out that drug or disease from a chaotic spectrum of objects in full relief.

From the epistemological point of view a profile has three basic features: a) the absence-presence of a characteristic; b) the value of a characteristic; and c) the priority of a characteristic.

The proposal that profiles are open for translation into the language of set theory will be examined in the following section. The aim is to provide a model for modeling the drug discovery process, and to elucidate, formally, the concepts of drug and disease profiles as cognitive structures in drug research.

Part 3. A set-theoretical model of drug discovery

2.6. A definition of the concept of profile in terms of set theory

2.6.1. Introduction

The preceding analysis of the concept of profile ended with a proposal to translate the concept of profile into the language of set theory. This section attempts to show how this can be done and the set-theoretical definition of profile should include the three identified components.

2.6.2. The first aspect of a profile: membership

Disease profiles can be considered as (finite) sets of disease characteristics.[54] Let b denote breathlessness, c congestion and h headache. The lower case letters b and c represent well-known characteristics of heart failure, a disease entity represented by P. In contrast, h symbolizes a complaint not characteristic for this disease. If we presume P possesses no characteristics other than b and c, then:

i) $b \in P$
ii) $c \in P$
iii) $h \notin P$
iv) $P = \{b, c\}$

The clinician's comment might be that congestion actually represents a complex of other characteristics, for example: enlargement of the liver (l), peripheral edema (e) and increased jugular pressure (i). Then:

v) $c = \{l, e, i\}$
vi) $P = \{b, \{l, e, i\}\}$

Clause vi) shows that members of sets can also be sets. In principle, disease profiles can be constructed as sets, sets of sets, and so forth thereby constructing towers of sets of great height and complexity.

The clinician's comment is interesting for another reason. The fore-mentioned symptoms are the result of congestion. Congestion of the liver leads to enlargement of the liver while accumulation of fluid in the blood circulation might cause engorged veins in the neck and edema in the legs. Similarly retention of fluid in the lungs leads to breathlessness which occurs as a consequence of the excessive work of the respiratory muscles required to inflate the lungs.[55]

Thus, knowledge of physiological and biochemical processes enhances the understanding of the relationships between symptoms and signs of a disease. In the ideal case, when a theory describes all characteristics of a particular disease entity and their relationships, it is worthwhile representing knowledge in terms of set theory.[56]

However, medical reality is more complex and medical knowledge is incomplete. Still, these unsolved features of the disease are clinically relevant to establish prognosis and treatment, and they can be included in disease profiles.

The domain is the set of all conceivable disease characteristics. In the preceding analysis two categories were distinguished: experimental and clinical. Let C be the set of all (conceivable) disease characteristics, EC the set of all experimental, and CC the set of all clinical disease characteristics while P denotes a disease profile. Then[57]:

i) $EC \subseteq C$
ii) $CC \subseteq C$
iii) $C = EC \cup CC; EC \cap CC = \emptyset$
iv) $P \subseteq C$

Clause i) indicates that the set of all experimental disease characteristics is a subset of C; similarly the second clause states the same with respect to the set of all clinical disease characteristics. Clause iii) expresses that the union of both subsets equals the set of all disease characteristics and that their intersection is empty. Clause iv) states that disease profile P is a subset of C.

In a similar way other classifications of disease characteristics (etiological, precipitating factors, or therapeutic goals) can be dealt with.

In conclusion, the first aspect of the concept of disease profile can be defined as follows: a disease profile is a set of which the elements are (sets of) disease characteristics.

The comparison between profiles

To enable us to compare profiles in different ways we can employ an operation comprising the determination of the **symmetric difference** between two profiles, say P and Q (figure 2.4).

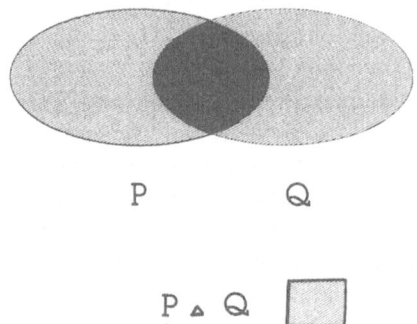

Figure 2.4
The symmetric difference between profiles P and Q.

The symmetric difference between P and Q is represented by the shaded area in this figure, and contains that part of Q that has no overlap with P, as well as that part of P that has no overlap with Q. The notation (P ∆ Q) will be used to denote the symmetric difference between sets P and Q which is a set as well. To denote the absolute number of elements of the set (P∆ Q), we write |P ∆ Q|.

Let us take the comparison of profiles one step further, i.e. the comparison of two profiles with respect to a third (figure 2.5.). Let P be a disease profile composed of five disease characteristics: P = {a, b, c, d, e}. Let further Q and R be disease profiles, for example, of two patients, where: Q = {a, b, c, f}; and: R = {a, b, f, g}.

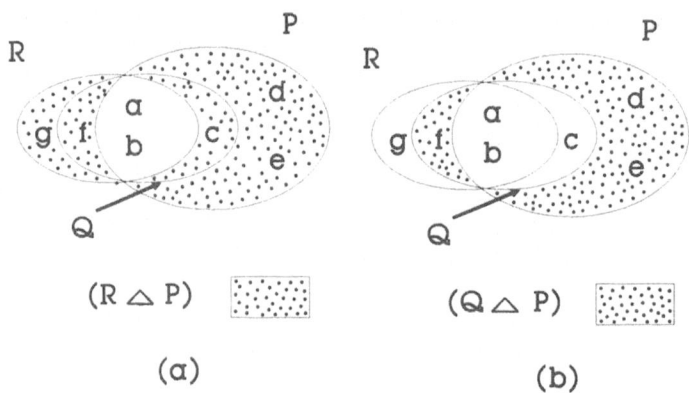

Figure 2.5
Comparison of profiles on the basis of the symmetric difference.

Then:

i) $(Q \vartriangle P) = \{d, e, f\}$
ii) $(R \vartriangle P) = \{c, d, e, f, g\}$
iii) $(Q \vartriangle P) \subset (R \vartriangle P)$

Given the definition of the symmetric difference, i) and ii) are self-explanatory; iii) follows from i) and ii) on the basis of the definition of **inclusion**.[58]

Definition 2.1:

X looks **qualitatively** more like Z than Y:= $(X \vartriangle Z) \subset (Y \vartriangle Z)$

Given definition 2.1 and iii) it is true that Q looks qualitatively more like P than R. We write

iv) $(Q \vartriangle P) \subset (R \vartriangle P)$

In contrast to the example presented, this definition proves to be too strong in practice. Therefore it is convenient to have recourse to a **quantitative** definition.

Definition 2.2:

X looks **quantitatively** more like Z than Y:= $|X \vartriangle Z| < |Y \vartriangle Z|$.

Given definition 2.2 and clause iii) it is true that Q looks quantitatively more like P than R, because iii) implies:

v) $|Q \vartriangle P| < |R \vartriangle P|$

On closer inspection of figure 2.5. the first term of the equation in clause iv) contains three elements, the second term five elements: $|Q \vartriangle P| = 3$; and $|R \vartriangle P| = 5$.
From the definitions given it follows that the quantitative definition is weaker than the qualitative one. However, the former is useful: Q scores more often with respect to P than R. The quantitative definition could compel us to draw conclusions we don't like: one fault is not the same as the other while the quantitative definition treats all faults alike.[59]

2.6.3. The second aspect of the concept of profile: values of the disease characteristics

The second aspect, namely values of disease characteristics, has been treated implicitly in 2.6.2. The definition presented assumes that each characteristic has two values: 1 (yes) or 0 (no). In reality disease characteristics possess more values.[60]

An example helps to illustrate the translation of this aspect in the language of set theory. Suppose that P still is a disease profile composed of five characteristics: $p_1, ..., p_5$; P again represents the disease entity heart failure. Let us further suppose that the values of the characteristics concerned are numerical, where v_i denotes the value of each characteristic p_i of P - in this case i is 1 up to and including 5. Figure 2.6. represents one possible situation q with respect to the values of the elements of P.

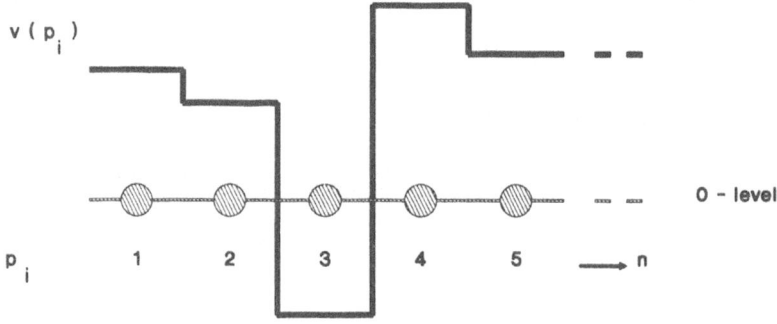

Figure 2.6
Representation of a specific profile of P, i.e. a specific combination of values of characteristics

The horizontal line represents the 0-level of the numerical values that disease characteristics might possess. Above this level values are positive, below negative. The circles denote a disease characteristic of P.

The line in bold type represents, literally, one particular version of profile P:

$$q = <v_1, v_2, v_3, v_4, v_5>.$$

In this case q represents one possible combination of values regarding P, that is, an ordered five-tuple: one specific value for each disease characteristic. Such a specific combination of values will be called a **specific profile**. The notation < > indicates an ordered n-tuple of elements.[61]
In practice disease characteristics will possess more than one particular value. Let V_i be the space of possible values of p_i. Then the resulting product

$$V = V_1 \times V_2 \times V_3 \times V_4 \times V_5$$

represents all possible combinations of values of P, hence the set of all possible specific profiles.[62] Strictly speaking a disease profile P is composed of a set of specific profiles; such a set will be called a **global profile**. Each patient who suffers from heart failure, is characterized by a specific profile that is an element of V.

Suppose now three "value levels" of P; that is, specific profiles, r, s, t $\in$ V, associated with increasing values all along the line; and suppose that these three levels lie above the 0-level (figure 2.7.).

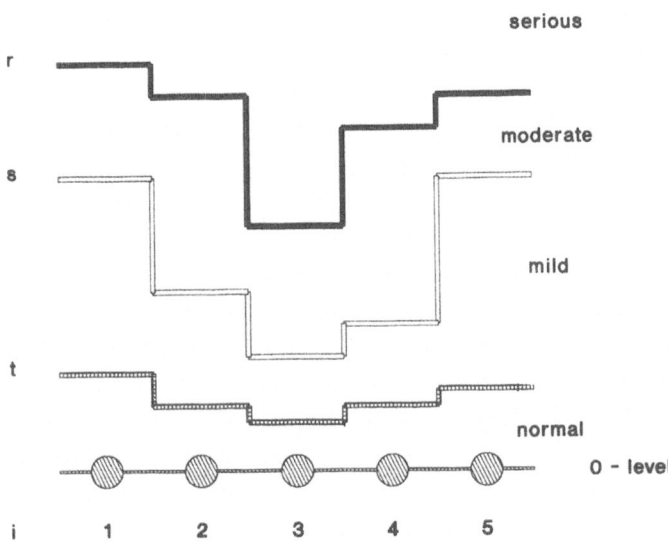

Figure 2.7
Representation of subsets of heart failure on the basis of "value levels" of disease characteristics.

Suppose clinicians distinguish three categories of heart failure: a serious (X), moderate (Y) and mild (Z) form; and further the normal condition (N). Let us assume further that the serious form of heart failure is represented by the area above r, the moderate form by the area between r and s, and the mild form by the area between s and t; the area below the t-level concerns the normal condition. These "value-areas" lead with regard to p_i to a space of values V^*_i which is "coarse" in comparison with V_i:

$V^*i = \{a_i, b_i, c_i, d_i\}$, on the basis of the next

Definition 2.3:

$$a_i = (r_i, +\infty) \quad =: \{x \,|\, \text{for all } i: r_i < x < +\infty\}$$
$$b_i = (s_i, r_i] \quad =: \{x \,|\, \text{for all } i: s_i < x \leq r_i\}$$
$$c_i = (t_i, s_i] \quad =: \{x \,|\, \text{for all } i: t_i < x \leq s_i\}$$
$$d_i = (-\infty, t_i] \quad =: \{x \,|\, \text{for all } i: -\infty < x \leq t_i\}$$

The original space of values V_i is divided into four global values as it were. As a result a new product V' follows associated with new, "coarsened" specific profiles amongst which four specific profiles, the **"category-profiles"**, e.g. as follows:

Definition 2.4:

$$V'i =: V'_1 \times V'_2 \times V'_3 \times V'_4 \times V'_5$$

X	=: < a_1, a_2, a_3, a_4, a_5 >	(serious heart failure)
Y	=: < b_1, b_2, b_3, b_4, b_5 >	(moderate heart failure)
Z	=: < c_1, c_2, c_3, c_4, c_5 >	(mild heart failure)
N	=: < d_1, d_2, d_3, d_4, d_5 >	(normal condition).[63]

In this way a large set of values has been reduced to a small number.[64] Physicians continuously apply such reductions to keep their complex world of data about diseases and drugs conveniently arranged. In our case, i.e. the diagnosis of heart failure, the clinician merely needs to make allowance for 1024 **specific** profiles - V' contains 4^5 possibilities - which can be compared with the four **category**-profiles X, Y, Z, and N.[65] Alternatively, this illustrates that a rather simple disease profile composed of five elements each having four values at the most, i.e. a, b, c, and d, yields a reasonable number of combinations. Here are six examples:

(1) < a_1, a_2, a_3, a_4, a_5 >
(2) < a_1, a_2, b_3, a_4, a_5 >
(3) < a_1, b_2, b_3, b_4, a_5 >
(4) < a_1, a_2, b_3, b_4, d_5 >
(5) < a_1, b_2, b_3, d_4, d_5 >
(6) < a_1, d_2, d_3, d_4, d_5 >

Patient (with profile) (1) represents the serious form of heart failure, and will be treated accordingly. Patients (2) and (3) pose a classification problem. Patient (2) has four characteristics in common with the serious form of heart failure; the third element of the set, however, belongs to the moderate form. With regard to patient (3) the problem is more complex; the first and last element belong to the serious form, the other three elements to the moderate form of heart failure (figure 2.8).

How should the clinician classify this patient?
A common solution is to make the diagnosis "moderate to serious heart failure". Sometimes however, this is not sufficient. If, for example, treatment of the moderate form strongly differs from that of serious heart failure, a choice has to be made. Naturally, other aspects of the patient's situation can be taken into account such as the social state, psychical constitution or clinical condition - which can be included as characteristics into a disease profile. However, if the clinician has to decide on the basis of the situation described above, he needs to introduce additional rules, for example: "If a set A has **at least** three elements in common with X, Y or Z, then A might be equalized with X, Y or Z respectively". Following this rule patient (2) should be classified as serious, patient (3) as moderate heart

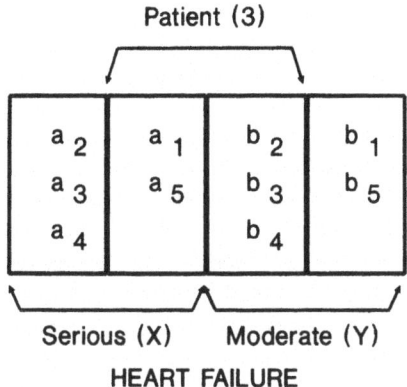

Figure 2.8
Classification problem and the "logic of profiles".

failure. In contrast, patients (4), (5) and (6) will be considered as not suffering from heart failure. From a clinical point of view this may be unsatisfactory, hence the rule has to be modified. What if a similar rule is chosen but now with the restriction that A and X, Y or Z should have at least **two** elements in common to be equalized? Patients (5) and (6) pose no problem, patient (4) obviously does.

With patient (4) the last rule leads to a stalemate. The clinician avoids it by introducing additional rules, for example, the rule: "Choose in case of indecision between two (sub)types of diseases for the most serious affection". The clinician keeps on the safe side, and makes the diagnosis serious heart failure. On the basis of another rule, e.g. "Choose in case of indecision between two (sub)types of diseases for the one which first choice of treatment causes the smallest harm", patient (4) will be classified as a patient with moderate heart failure.

From this follows that rules for solving classification problems are complex, that is, are composed of two or more rules. In particular, this applies to the rules formulated in the preceding paragraph. Moreover, these rules are of a general nature, and therefore applicable to any disease profile. In contrast, the rules formulated in the last paragraph but one are specific with regard to disease profiles X, Y and Z. In both cases rules are not purely logically motivated; therefore the term **heuristic principle** will be used. The actual construction of such principles falls outside the scope of the "logic of profiles", and are the subject of heuristics and statistics. This implies that the heuristic principles can be described only partially in the language of set theory.

To continue with the diagnostic problem posed by patient (4), what happens if he possesses two characteristics lying "high in the value-area of serious heart failure", and two characteristics lying "high in the b-zone"? Clinicians will be more inclined to classify such a patient as suffering from serious heart failure than a patient with two characteristics "low in the a-zone" and two "low in the b-zone". More often clinicians decide on a pragmatic basis by introducing additional rules as illustrated above.

However, if clinicians increasingly encounter patients with some characteristics "high in the b-zone" and other features "low in the a-zone", they may want to reconsider the original classification. Other sources of medical knowledge like new theories, or complementary information collected by new techniques, might stimulate this process of reconsideration. In fact clinicians descend to a lower level to judge previous decisions according to their merits, and possibly altering them.
Summarizing sections 2.6.2. and 2.6.3. together, this reciprocal relationship between representation of knowledge (into profiles) and decision rules to use the knowledge, is found at different levels. At the lowest level the characteristics of heart failure with the large set of values occur; elements (first aspect, 2.6.2.) and values of elements (second aspect, 2.6.3.) can be represented in disease profiles. At this level the rule is formulated to distinguish three subtypes of heart failure, that is, the value-areas of disease characteristics are divided into four "parts". As a result, three disease profiles and a profile representing the normal condition, appeared; and additional rules to solve the classification problems are proposed. Consequently, this may influence, at another level, the way disease profiles are reconstructed and rules are formulated.

2.6.4. The third aspect of the concept of profile: ranking order of characteristics

Patient (4) presented in the preceding section, might represent another problem, i.e. the ranking (or priority) of disease characteristics. Some features are considered more characteristic than others. When the clinician classifies patient (4) as serious heart failure because of the elements a_1 and a_2, this indicates that the two elements have a higher priority than the other elements. The most extreme example of this is the "pathognomonic" sign, a complaint or aberration so peculiar for a particular disease that any patient with this sign is immediately labeled as suffering from that disease. If element a_1 represents a pathognomonic sign of serious heart failure, patient (6) from the example in the preceding section has to be considered as having serious heart failure.
The decision problem posed by patient (4) is of a twofold nature: either it is a value-problem or a problem of priority. The aspect of ranking is a central part of daily medical practice. Though disease profiles contain tens or hundreds of characteristics, a small number of features is sufficient to make the diagnosis. In scientific research this aspect of priority also plays an important role while from the historian's point of view, shifts in scientific and clinical views are crucial.
Two comments on this aspect of priority can be made. The **first** is that important aspects of a disease entity form central nodes in the maze of medical knowledge. Since many aspects are part and parcel of these central nodes, a characteristic ranked high represents a variety of variables and parameters. This is disguised by the examples used in this analysis. In reality disease profiles contain, as described, tens, even hundreds or thousands of elements, and no

great effort is needed to imagine the large numbers of possible permutations. The problem of order dissolves as it were in the first aspect of the concept of profile, that is, in terms of membership. For not all possible variables and parameters are assigned the status of membership when ranked in order. However, if these variables and parameters were taken up as elements into profiles, the quantitative operation of symmetric difference would be applicable.

The **second** is that order seems to be more like a means to use knowledge than a feature of the representation of knowledge. It serves to reduce a finite but large number of elements to a small(er) set of important elements which is easy in operation. Just as with the rules in the preceding section, some rules may be given a formally tenable interpretation, whereas this is not the case for other rules.

Both comments are inadequate to sufficiently extenuate or eliminate the aspect of priority. If this aspect is left from the analysis, the formal elaboration of the concept of profile becomes artificial and removed from daily practice.[66] The question emerges as to whether logical methods are available to compare profiles including the aspect of ranking. The positive answer to this question is complex, and falls outside the scope of this study; a proposal for such an elaboration is sketched in appendix I.

2.6.5. Conclusions

A set theory definition of the concept of profile has been given. Without difficulty the first and second aspect of the concept of profile can be defined; but the third aspect is not so simple. The definition proposed therefore partially meets the condition of encompassing the three aspects.

This partial success can be viewed optimistically, however. Firstly, the aim was to make the proposal plausible; in this respect we have been reasonably successful. Secondly, the definition of the first two aspects of the concept of profile enables the description of developments in medical views. Thirdly, some problems with respect to the concept profile have been clarified. Thus, the distinction but also close relationship between representation and use of knowledge has been touched upon. In this respect the difference between formally tenable and heuristic principles to compare profiles and to solve classification problems, has been highlighted.

The formal analysis is performed with respect to the concept of disease profile. Since the drug and disease profiles are basically similar, the results achieved also apply to the concept of drug profile.

2.7. The drug discovery process - a set-theoretical model

2.7.1. Introduction

It is convenient to start with a fundamental concept from the drug innovation literature: the concept of **a lead (compound)**. As described (2.2.1.), this concept indicates the basis of the discovery process: a mere compound is insufficient, rather it should possess an interesting biological activity. On the one hand this concerns the material or some global idea about it, on the other the application or a class of applications, however vaguely formulated. This corresponds to the distinction between the operational (the actual properties of the material) and wished for (the intended application of a material) characteristics.

On this basis a naive definition can be given of the concepts of a lead and a lead compound in the language of set theory; the term "naive" denotes that this definition will be adjusted.[67]

2.7.2. A naive definition

Let K be the (finite) domain of all relevant drug characteristics, w the set of all wished for properties (wished for profile), and $o(x)$ the profile of compound x (figure 2.9); the symbol "o" denotes operational, that is: the profile of x as it really is.

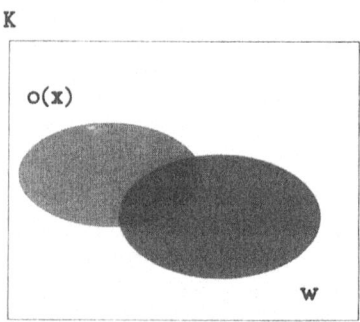

Figure 2.9
The domain K of all relevant characteristics of drugs: operational and wished for drug profiles.

The most plausible interpretation seems to be that $o(x)$ concerns a chemical compound, and w the lead. What now is the lead compound? At first sight the lead compound seems to be represented by the intersection of $o(x)$ and w, but this interpretation is not very satisfactory. Since a lead compound is the starting-point for further research, positive features have to be improved and negative features eliminated or minimized. Therefore the symmetric difference between $o(x)$ and w represents a reasonable interpretation of the concept of lead compound. This concept comprises three aspects:
1) the set of operational characteristics ($= o(x)$);
2) the set of wished for characteristics ($= w$);
3) the symmetric difference between $o(x)$ and w ($= (o(x) \Delta w)$).

In an elementary form the discovery and development of drugs can be described as a process of **rapprochement** between drugs and diseases.

The searching process in fact does not occur without having an idea about the applicability of the compound searched for. This implies that one has in mind one or more reference compounds ($o(x)$) in order to determine whether the new compound improves upon standard therapy.

Definition 2.5: x_2 is a **qualitative** improvement of x_1 with respect to w:=

$$(o(x_2) \vartriangle w) \subset (o(x_1) \vartriangle w)$$

Definition 2.6: x_2 is a **quantitative** improvement of x_1 with respect to w:=

$$|o(x_2) \vartriangle w| < |o(x_1) \vartriangle w|$$

Notice that 5 implies 6, and that the terms "qualitative" and "quantitative" possess a formal meaning. A drug x_2 which is quantitatively better than x_1 but not qualitatively in a formal sense, may be from an informally therapeutic viewpoint a qualitative improvement; or even a stronger thing to say, such a drug might be a therapeutic breakthrough.

The definitions given are based on the assumption that the wished for profile remains identical throughout the developmental process, but this need not be the case. Thus, it is quite possible that new insights result in certain properties initially being wished for, being placed in an unfavourable light. And the reverse is also possible. In both cases the wished for profile w changes which may lead to important changes in the comparison with $o(x)$.

Definition 2.7: w_2 is a **qualitative** concession to x with respect to w_1:=

$$(o(x) \vartriangle w_2) \subset (o(x) \vartriangle w_1)$$

Definition 2.8: w_2 is a **quantitative** concession to x with respect to w_1:=

$$|o(x) \vartriangle w_2| < |o(x) \vartriangle w_1|$$

2.7.3. First adjustment of the naive definition: structural and functional characteristics of drugs

Two fundamental types of properties of drugs have been distinguished: structural and functional. When incorporating this distinction in the definition of the searching process for new drugs (2.7.2.) a first refinement of the naive definition will be achieved. In terms of set theory two sets of drug characteristics are at stake:
1) A set of **structural** characteristics;
2) A set of **functional** characteristics.
Both are considered as "fixed sets", namely as two separate domains so that:

i)   K = domain of all relevant drug characteristics
ii)   S = domain of structural characteristics
iii)   F = domain of functional characteristics
iv)   S and F do not intersect, and their union is K, i.e. $S \cap F = \emptyset$, $S \cup F = K$.

The consequences of the naive definition can be summarized by the following clauses (figure 2.10):

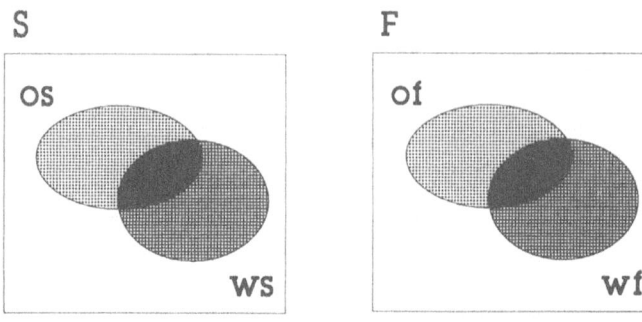

Figure 2.10
Domains of structural and functional characteristics of drugs.

v) $o(x) \subseteq K$
vi) $os(x) \subseteq S$
vii) $of(x) \subseteq F$
viii) $os(x) \cup of(x) = o(x)$
ix) $w \subseteq K$
x) $ws \subseteq S$
xi) $wf \subseteq F$
xii) $ws \cup wf = w$

Henceforth os(x) will be called the **operational structural profile**, and of(x) the **operational functional profile**. Furthermore, ws will be called the **wished for structural profile**, and wf the **wished for functional profile**.

A fictitious example: the development of Eurrhythmic

Now it is time to give flesh and blood to the defined concepts by connecting these with the reality of drug research. For this purpose a fictitious example will be used that presumably is realistic and recognizable.

The story starts from the molecular modification of an ubiquitously appreciated drug "Eurrhythmic" that is applied successfully in the treatment of cardiac arrhythmias. Research within the company selling this drug, found that the therapeutic action of Eurrhythmic is associated with the presence of a certain chemical group R_2 in the molecular structure. This finding is the result of structure-activity-relationship (SAR) research. It was surprising because it departed from the general doctrine in the field that a chemical substituent R_1 at another site in the molecule is responsible for the therapeutic effects of the drug. Fevered attempts were made to confirm this finding. The scientists manipulated the chemical groups R_1 and R_2 in many ways, synthesized various series of substances, and tested these but all the evidence pointed in one direction: compounds with the substituent R_2 have an improved therapeutic activity (potency, specificity, or whatever). Finally, the project appears to be successful, and some years later a novel drug is introduced.

This story can be used to clarify the basic concepts formulated above.
Why did the results in the industrial laboratory provoke curiosity? Presumably because the structural profile of Eurrhythmic differed considerably from that of the new compound but their functional profiles were remarkably similar. The scientists were therefore perplexed because their finding conflicted with the general view at the time (figure 2.11).

S: structural   F: functional

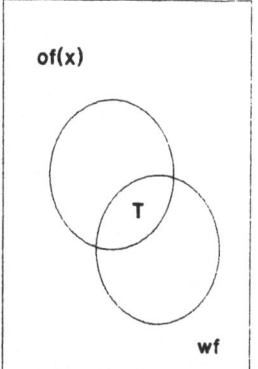

os(x)   of(x)

Y 2

Y 1   T

ws   wf

Figure 2.11
Conflict about the compound Eurrhythmic:

General opinion in the field:
$y_1 = R_1$ and $y_2 = R_2$;
New observation in the company:
$y_2 = R_1$ and $y_1 = R_2$.

The character "T" denotes the therapeutic action, and the symbols R_1 and R_2 are the chemical groups. Notice that these elements in their turn might represent a variety of characteristics. The prevailing view is that the structural characteristic R_1 belongs to os(x) but also to ws, while R_2 is a member of os(x) but not of ws. Further, t is an element of of(x) but also of wf.
This view might have been **generated** from different sources. Perhaps, it is the result of a theory about the conformational structure of the receptor to which the compound attaches. This theory explains why a chemical group R_1 given a certain molecular structure perfectly "fits" the receptor concerned. In addition this theory may have been a prime force in developing Eurrhythmic but it might also have been an ex-post-facto explanation. It is quite possible that the same theory explains why a substituent like R_2 is never able to fit the receptor. Consequently, the observation of the research team means not only a novel drug but also the end of a widely accepted theory.
At this point the obvious question rises. Why did the industrial scientists find what others in the field had not, or had rejected? The answer lies in what the chemical groups R_1 and R_2 in fact represent. Without doubt other scientists have manipulated the molecular structure

of Eurrhythmic. They have replaced R_1 by various groups largely deviating from the one in the chemical structure of the drug Eurrhythmic; in each case the result was the effectiveness of Eurrhythmic, the ineffectiveness of the other compounds. Undoubtedly attempts were made to introduce small changes into the chemical group R_1, considered crucial to the activity of Eurrhythmic. Each time it was found that the biological activity increased or decreased slightly but never disappeared, thus enforcing the view that the group R_1 was the decisive site of action.

In short, whenever the structural profiles of the manipulated compounds mimicked that of Eurrhythmic, an operational functional profile was found very similar to that of the widely used drug. Manipulation of R_2 showed that, though structural profiles of the compounds obtained were very different from that of Eurrhythmic, the functional profiles remained similar to that of the drug. There was no immediate cause to attribute an important role to the chemical group R_2.

Then the scientists in the industrial laboratory made their big discovery. Perhaps someone replaced R_1 in the molecule of this compound Eurrhythmic by some substituent in which an interesting biological activity had been noticed. Maybe the substituted chemical group was so absurd that only by mere accident due to a failure during the synthesis, this compound was discovered. Additional investigation revealed, for example, that this compound was very much similar to a chemical structure that combined the groups R_1 and R_2.

However, it might have fared quite differently. Perhaps the chemist applied a new, controversial theory to his problem, hence capable of looking at the conformational structure in a completely different way; or maybe he studied aspects hitherto neglected. The investigation yielded a structural profile strongly differing from that of Eurrhythmic while the functional profiles of both types of compounds were remarkably similar.

In general two possibilities exist. Either the scientist finds the new compound first, i.e. the structural profile, concludes - to his surprise - that it meets the activity wished for, and corrects the wished for structural profile. Or the scientist follows the reverse procedure. He might have been involved in a research project on the role of particular chemical substances in disturbing the rhythm of the heart, mapped out a wished for structural profile, and consequently gained insight into the possibility of chemical structures different from that of Eurrhythmic.

However, another possibility is that a new theory about the therapeutic action of Eurrhythmic may suggest a particular functional characteristic, for example, the blockade of a certain receptor, being of little importance to the beneficial effect produced by the drug. As a result, the wished for functional profile is adjusted and new avenues are opened up to search for other patterns of activity, hence for other chemical structures. However, it might have so happened that a clinician applied another drug than Eurrhythmic to a patient suffering from (a particular form of) cardiac dysrhythm, and unexpectedly found a beneficial effect. The operational functional profile of this compound was basically different from that of Eurrhythmic.

This fictitious story about Eurrhythmic illustrates the introduced concepts but also that new observations merely manifest themselves against the background of accepted conceptions, either about operational and wished for functional profiles or about operational and wished for structural profiles of drugs. Further, it shows that different relationships between profiles, both within and between the domains of drug characteristics, exist.

The relations within domains, i.e. between operational profiles mutually and with respect to the wished for profile, have already been discussed. The relations between domains, as illustrated by the Eurrhythmic-story, are much more complex, and can not be expressed in formally tenable principles. Therefore, as said earlier, **heuristic principles** (HP), of importance to the searching process will be discussed. Our analysis is restricted to the qualitative formulated heuristic principles but quantitative versions can be similarly derived.

HP1:=

Structural similarity implies functional similarity, that is, if x_2 looks structurally more like ws than x_1, then x_2 looks functionally more like wf than x_1:

$$os(x_2) \triangle ws \subset os(x_1) \triangle ws \quad \rightarrow \quad of(x_2) \triangle wf \subset of(x_1) \triangle wf.$$

HP2:=

Functional similarity implies structural similarity, that is, if x_2 looks functionally more like wf than x_1, x_2 looks structurally more like ws than x_1:

$$of(x_2) \triangle wf \subset of(x_1) \triangle wf \quad \rightarrow \quad os(x_2) \triangle ws \subset os(x_1) \triangle ws.$$

Both heuristic principles played their role in the development of an alternative drug for Eurrhythmic; they also form the basis of SAR-research.

2.7.4. Second adjustment of the naive definition: disease characteristics

When taking the concept of disease profile into account, a third domain, i.e. that of disease characteristics, has to be included into the analysis (figure 2.12).

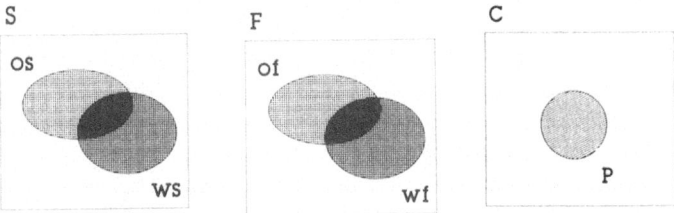

Figure 2.12
The three domains of structural (S) and functional (F) drug characteristics, and disease characteristics (C).

The processes within the domain of disease characteristics have been discussed extensively in the analysis of the concept of disease profile. The relation between the domain of structural respectively and functional characteristics on the one hand and the domain of disease characteristics on the other hand needs some illumination. The wished for profile w will normally be formulated with respect to the disease profile P. This formulation originates from theory, experience, or practical know-how and the precise mechanism through which w, hence ws and wf, is derived from P is not implied by the model.

In the preceding history of Eurrhythmic the possible changes in the functional profile leading to the discovery of new drugs were touched on. Functional profiles might also change due to the fact that disease profiles are changing. Two additional heuristic principles can be formulated:

HP3:=

Similarity of disease profiles implies functional similarity, e.g. of the treatments of the disease entities concerned, that is: if $P(y_2)$ looks more like $P(y_3)$ than $P(y_1)$, then $wf(y_2)$ looks more like $wf(y_3)$ than $wf(y_1)$, where y_1, y_2 and y_3 denote three disease entities $(y_1 \neq y_2 \neq y_3)$:

$$P(y_2) \vartriangle P(y_3) \subset P(y_1) \vartriangle P(y_3) \quad \rightarrow \quad wf(y_2) \vartriangle wf(y_3) \subset wf(y_1) \vartriangle wf(y_3)$$

The reverse is also plausible:

HP4:=

Similarity of functional profiles implies similarity of disease profiles, that is: if $wf(y_2)$ looks more like $wf(y_3)$ than $wf(y_1)$, then $P(y_2)$ looks more like $P(y_3)$ than $P(y_1)$:

$$wf(y_2) \vartriangle wf(y_3) \subset wf(y_1) \vartriangle wf(y_3) \quad \rightarrow \quad P(y_2) \vartriangle P(y_3) \subset P(y_1) \vartriangle P(y_3)$$

Both heuristic principles are important and realistic.[68] Suppose that on the basis of new insights rheumatoid arthritis (y_2) and hyperactive action of the thyroid (y_3), originally being conceived of as two separate disease entities, are considered as the manifestation of the same derailment of the immunological system. Then both disease entities may be distinguished from a disease associated with another type of immunological disorder (y_1).

On the basis of the heuristic principle 3), the drugs producing beneficial effects in the treatment of rheumatoid arthritis can be hypothesized as being more effective in the treatment of the hyperactive thyroid, then of the other disease involved. Reversely, on the basis of the heuristic principle 4): similarity of the treatment results in different disease entities yields insights about the similarity of the diseases concerned.

2.7.5. The improvement of toxic effects of drugs: positive and negative aspects and their judgment

Therapeutic properties of drugs pose no problem to the theory because they are considered as "wished for" properties, hence can be conceived of as elements of the wished for drug profile. When a novel drug produces more beneficial effects than standard therapy, then it clearly improves medical therapy. What now if side-effects of the drug are manifested? Side-effects involve undesirable effects, hence are not included into the wished for drug profile! How then can a new drug producing fewer side-effects than current therapy be evaluated? This section discusses a solution to this problem without greatly changing the model.[69]

When administrating a beta blocker to a patient with angina pectoris (A) a side-effect such as heart failure (P) might occur. Let A and P be two disease profiles composed of merely one element:

angina pectoris: $A = \{e\}$, e = exercise tolerance;
heart failure : $P = \{c\}$, c = cardiac output.

Further suppose that each characteristic might show three values: low (= l), medium (= m), or high (= h); the value is written as a subscript to the character that represents the disease characteristic concerned; thus a high value of c is written as c_h.[70] Then the following specific profiles are possible:

$A_l = \{e_l\}$
$A_m = \{e_m\}$
$A_h = \{e_h\}$

$P_l = \{c_l\}$
$P_m = \{c_m\}$
$P_h = \{c_h\}$

Given the above-mentioned profiles, A_l represents the patient with angina pectoris because of having a decreased exercise tolerance; A_m indicates the healthy subject, and A_h, for example, the athlete.[71]
Further, P_l represents heart failure because of the decreased cardiac output, while P_m and P_h represent the healthy and trained human being respectively.
The wished for drug profiles in a functional sense have to be mapped out with respect to A_l and P_l respectively. Ideally spoken, a therapy suitable for the treatment of angina pectoris should increase exercise tolerance; a perfect therapy for heart failure, however, should increase cardiac output:

$wf(A_l) = \{e_h\}$
$wf(P_l) = \{c_h\}$

However, these are wished for profiles for each disease separately. Suppose that it is a question of a combination of angina pectoris and heart failure: $AP = <e_l, c_l>$.[72] The disease profile AP is composed of two elements, one characterizing the decreased exercise tolerance, the other the decreased cardiac output. Accordingly, the wished for functional drug profile with respect to AP would be:

$$wf(AP) = <e_h, c_h>.[73]$$

Still, this inadequately describes the issue we are interested in. In case of a side-effect there is no question of a patient with angina pectoris associated with heart failure. On the contrary, the angina patient might have a cardiac output which is normal ("m") or even increased ("h"), but which is decreased by the drug **itself**. The perfect drug in the treatment of angina pectoris is a drug which increases exercise tolerance but does not cause heart failure! The wished for functional drug profile with respect to angina pectoris, is therefore:

$$wf(A'_l) = <e_h, c_{m \vee h}> , \text{ where } c_{m \vee h} \text{ denotes } c_m \text{ or } c_h.$$

This states that the drug, in addition to the desired therapeutic effect regarding exercise tolerance, may affect cardiac output variably **except decreasing it**. These variable effects except the undesirable one(s) can be considered as desired properties; the decrease as an undesirable property.

Let x_1 and x_2 be available anti-anginal drugs: $of(x_1) = <e_h, c_l>$; $of(x_2) = <e_h, c_{m \vee h}>$, then it is clear that $of(x_2)$ is preferable to $of(x_1)$ on the basis of the symmetric difference criterion. Drug x_2 scores two times "good", whereas drug x_1 scores one time "good", but also one time "fault". If drug x_2 has been developed to improve on the toxic effects of the standard therapy x_1, then x_2 is indeed an improvement.

2.7.6. Conclusions

The process of rapprochement of drugs and diseases has been reduced to the interaction between profiles within and between three domains which can be described in the language of set theory. The processes within the domains can be characterized with the help of formally tenable principles and heuristic principles. The processes between the domains are governed by heuristic principles.

The distinction between formally tenable and heuristic principles is crucial. With respect to the processes which can be characterized by formally tenable principles the model developed can generate normative claims. However, heuristic principles and rules can only partly be described by the language of set theory and cannot support normative claims.[74]

CHAPTER 3. Experimental and therapeutic profiling in drug innovation: the early history of the beta blockers

3.1. Introduction

Current views share the assumption that drug innovation involves the flow of ideas from research laboratories (academic or industrial) into the various medical professional settings, with therapeutic practice determining the success of these ideas. The consequences of this way of analyzing drug innovation are underestimating the possibility of therapeutic practice acting as an important stimulus to innovative drug research and the extent to which it contributes to our knowledge of drugs and of the pathophysiological conditions to be treated. By using the story of the early history of the beta blockers the view will be developed that both clinical research and the therapeutic context are integrally involved in drug innovation. The other purpose of this analysis is to set the stage for the historical developments that form the subject of subsequent chapters.

3.2. Historical overview of the development of the beta blockers

The catecholamines, noradrenaline and adrenaline, are key regulators of many physiological processes in man. As we now know, noradrenaline acts primarily as a neurotransmitter released from sympathetic nerve terminals and adrenaline functions as a circulating hormone released from the adrenaline medulla. These catecholamines then interact with receptors in the tissues and the end result of the transmitter-receptor interaction is the biological response of the tissue. Electrical stimulation of sympathetic nerves as well as injected catecholamines, e.g. (nor)adrenaline-like-compounds, produce their effects in the same way. The concept that catecholamines bind to specific receptors in various tissues, that this binding initiates the physiological response and that there are two types of tissue receptors, excitatory and inhibitory, was first suggested by Langley in 1905.[1]

However, most historical reviews of beta blockers start with Sir Henry Dale's experimental work. Dale (1906) observed that, while the excitatory actions of adrenaline, e.g. vasoconstriction and contraction of smooth muscle in other tissues, were blocked by ergot alkaloids, the inhibitory effects like vasodilatation and relaxation of bronchial muscle in the lungs were not.[2] Thus he provided evidence for Langley's hypothesis.

It remained for Ahlquist (1948) to propose a new receptor classification.[3] He differentiated between two adrenoceptor populations by their responses in a variety of tissues. Ahlquist found only two orders of potency and therefore proposed the existence of two types of adrenergic receptors which he named alpha and beta. In general, stimulation of alpha receptors resulted in such excitatory responses as vasoconstriction and contraction of smooth muscle in various tissues while beta receptor stimulation resulted in the inhibitory responses such as vasodilation, bronchial muscle relaxation and relaxation of the womb.

A crucial exception to this general rule was in the heart. Cardiac excitatory responses, the increase in rate and force of contraction, were attributed by Ahlquist to the beta receptors. In this way Ahlquist classified cardiac excitatory responses along with the inhibitory responses of other tissues. Since at that time drug receptor interactions at the cell level were poorly understood, the significance of Ahlquist's contribution is that he proposed an operational classification in which the cardiac adrenergic receptors were considered functionally homologous to the adrenergic inhibitory receptors of other tissues.

Ahlquist's theory became the model for the pharmacological and physiological study of the sympathetic nervous system, and his terminology has been extended to the realm of adrenergic drugs. They can now be designated according to the receptor for which they have the greatest affinity and according to the type of response which they induce. Hence, alpha-stimulating, alpha-blocking, beta-stimulating and beta-blocking drugs could be developed. Little attention was paid to Ahlquist's theory for over 10 years. However in 1958 the situation changed dramatically with the discovery of dichloroisoproterenol (DCI) by Powell and Slater at Eli Lilly (USA).[4] They were searching for a long-acting and specific bronchodilator to compete with isoprenaline, which at that time was a leading drug for the treatment of asthma. They hoped that chemical manipulation of isoprenaline would yield a new and better drug. DCI however exhibited some unexpected effects. The substance could block adrenergic inhibitory actions on smooth muscle, and thus DCI was launched in academic circles as an interesting pharmacological tool to study adrenergic mechanisms. Most authors regard the action of DCI as an accidental discovery, a chance observation which unfortunately did not alert the Lilly research team.[5] Powell and Slater had missed the blocking action of DCI on the heart, i.e. the blockade of excitatory responses which were supposed to be mediated by "excitatory receptors" according to Dale's classification. It remained for Moran and Perkins in 1958 to demonstrate that the effects of DCI supported Ahlquist's theory.[6]

Initially DCI and its analogous were considered to be laboratory curiosities or drugs looking for a disease.[7] No one seemed able to envision its therapeutic value. It was Black, working at Imperial Chemical Industries (ICI), who first saw the real clinical potential of DCI and ultimately succeeded in bringing pronethalol, the first beta blocker, to the market in 1962.[8] Pronethalol, which proved to be carcinogenic in mice, was followed by propranolol, marketed by ICI in 1964. ICI was closely followed by AB Hassle (Astra Sweden) with alprenolol and Ciba-Geigy with oxprenolol, both around 1966. Propranolol remains the most widely used beta blocker and the prototype of the so-called first generation. Metoprolol (AB Hassle, Ciba-Geigy) and atenolol (ICI) are the major representatives of the cardioselective, second generation beta blockers, which are presumed to block the cardiac receptors more selectively than those of the bronchi. The use of beta blockers became a major advance in cardiovascular treatment, initially for angina pectoris and cardiac arrhythmias and later on for hypertension.[9]

3.3. From Dale to Ahlquist: a new methodology in pharmacology

At the turn of this century, physiologists were familiar with the fact that many bodily functions were regulated autonomically. The various responses of the automatic nervous system, divided into an (ortho)sympathetic (adrenergic) and a parasympathetic (cholinergic) part with often opposed effects on the various organs, were mapped out by means of electrical or similar stimuli.

These classification schemes became the conceptual framework in which pharmacologically active compounds were studied. Compounds were called "sympathomimetic" when they stimulated physiological responses whether "excitatory" or "inhibitory". Compounds were called "'sympatholytic" when they blocked physiological responses, whether "excitatory" or "inhibitory". For example, a compound that stimulated the relaxation of smooth muscle in the bronchi - an "inhibitory" response while constriction would be an "excitatory" response - was therefore called a "sympathomimetic agent". A compound which prevented, i.e. blocked relaxation of smooth muscle in the bronchi, was called a "sympatholytic agent". This resulted in two major lines of research in pharmacology.

Within the first line of research physiological effects of a number of synthetic amines, closely related to adrenaline, were studied. In their article in 1910 - a first example of what is known now as structure-activity-relation (SAR) research - Barger and Dale coined the term "sympathomimetic" because these amines mimicked the responses to the classical physiological stimulus, i.e. electrical stimulation of nerves.[10] Although these sympathomimetic amines did not show all types of responses in the same degree, it was widely accepted that sympathomimetic amines caused qualitatively, but not quantitatively, similar effects. Despite some doubts expressed by pharmacologists adrenaline remained the reference compound. It was considered to represent the physiological stimulus.

The second line of research focussed on sympatholytic agents. This was initiated by Dale's work on ergot that dominated pharmacological research during the following decades. So strong was Dale's influence that as recently as 1949 Nickerson stated: *"Over forty years ago, Dale clearly defined the action of ergot in blocking and 'reversing' many responses to circulating adrenaline and sympathetic nerve stimulation, but subsequent progress in the field has been slow"*.[11] Dale showed how ergot-alkaloids inhibited many, but not all physiological responses of adrenaline and sympathetic nerve stimulation: the "adrenergic blockade". To explain these differences he differentiated between two types of "receptors" for adrenaline: one type as a site for adrenaline resulting in excitatory responses blocked ("paralysed") by ergot, the other one as a site for adrenaline, resulting in inhibitory responses not blocked by ergot.[12] Dale's research provided a standard methodology for pharmacological research. The ergot-alkaloids were used as pharmacological tools to classify the several effects of adrenaline and sympathetic nerve stimulation. Subsequently other groups of agents which inhibited the excitatory responses of the sympathetic nervous system, became available: yohimbine and analogous (1925), phenoxyethylamines (1929), benzodioxanes (1933), imidazolines (1939) and beta-haloalkylamines (1945).[13] Since both Dale and Ahlquist used the receptor concept, it is tempting to assume a continuum with no revolutionary change from the early part of the 20th century to 1948. However receptors did not mean the same thing in 1906, in 1948 or indeed 1958. In the 1940s and 1950s the concepts of sympathomimetic and sympatholytic agents were replaced by agonists and antagonists. This change of terminology was accompanied by an important shift in meaning.

3.4. Change in the concepts of agonist and antagonist

The antagonist concept was developed in the 1940s following the spectacular discovery of the mode of action of Prontosil, a compound which heralded the era of sulpha drugs. Prontosil appeared to be reduced by the host' organism to sulfanilamide that interfered selectively with the metabolism of the micro-organism because of its structural similarity with one of the bacterial metabolites. As with any dramatic change, it took a while for researchers to realize the magnitude of this finding. However it yielded the idea that effective drugs could be looked for among compounds that interfered with normal biochemical and enzymatic mechanisms of micro-organisms. And why would not the same mechanism apply to human regulatory systems as well? This notion was proposed by Fildes, in a paper entitled 'A rational Approach to Chemotherapy', into a general theory of drugs as metabolic antagonists.[14] Enzyme chemists took up the new concept and developed it into a fundamental structure: the theory of competition with and displacement of essential metabolites in an organism by substances with similar structure and composition.[15]

This theory of biological antagonism, had more far-reaching effects than ushering in the modern era of chemotherapy. It extended to other possible therapeutic domains. Consequently experimental drug research ramified into the field of medicinal and organic chemistry, biochemistry and pharmacology. The resulting new science cuts across the lines of biochemistry, pharmacology, physiology chemotherapy, immunology, and others. It is a science based upon fundamental concepts not upon lines drawn in the cloudy sphere of didactic definition.[16]

Pharmacologists in their own way elaborated the concept of antagonism based on Clark's quantitative expressions of the relation between drug concentration and biological effect.[17] Gaddum and Schild in the 1940s pursued the idea that two drugs compete in a reversible way for one single receptor site: the idea of competitive antagonism.[18] This was the era of occupation theories: the observed biological response was a function of the number of receptors occupied by the particular drug. Thus the concept of antagonism had acquired a two-fold meaning. Firstly, antagonists could be considered as potential therapeutic agents extending the domain of potential drugs. Secondly, antagonism had also become a sharply defined and substantial part of a research methodology. Both meanings acquired a central role by pharmacologists in industry testing compounds in animal systems and studying the pharmacodynamic principles of these compounds and their derivatives.

The occupancy theory seemed satisfactory for describing the action of most "inhibitors", but was found lacking with respect to agonists. To cite Albert: *"As a statement of the action of most inhibitors, as important for work in chemotherapy and agriculture, this simple occupation theory can hardly be bettered. However it has been found inadequate to explain the kinetics of agents which elicit a positive response (our emphasis)".*[19]

This notion was pursued in the studies of Ariens, Stephenson, Furchgott and Nickerson. In the 1950s they independently showed that drug action should be understood in terms of two functions rather than one, either affinity of occupancy. In the case of Clark's theory affinity meant the ability of a compound to attach to a certain receptor thereby blocking the action of the agonist; intrinsic activity meant that attachment to a receptor elicits a positive response. Thus compounds could possess in varying degrees both agonistic and antagonistic properties. Subsequently, a new experimental practice emerged to dissect the agonistic and antagonistic properties of compounds. In this way a new understanding of the drug-receptor-interaction allowed pharmacologists to conceive agonists and antagonists as experimental tools as well as potential drugs.

Ahlquist's theory

Ahlquist studied adrenaline- and ephedrine-like compounds. He observed that different amines stimulating heart frequency and constriction of blood vessels - "a typical sympathomimetic effect" - sometimes gave rise to an unexpected blood pressure fall (depressor response), due to vasodilation. This was a surprising observation because at the time the terms sympathomimetic and "vasoconstrictor" were regarded as synonymous.[20] These results led him to the question whether the adrenergic receptors could be classified simply as excitatory and inhibitory.

He accordingly carried out a comparative study of a series of six sympathomimetic amines in several test systems which he considered an adequate measure for the function of the adrenergic receptor itself. The results yielded two orders of relative potency. He therefore concluded that those effector-response differences must be the consequence of differences between two types of receptors. He called the first type the alpha receptor and the second type the beta receptor. The adrenergic receptor became a functional concept, i.e. the receptor was described only in terms of effector response to drug application.[21]

Neither Ahlquist's experimental work nor his new concept was promptly accepted by the research community. His 1948 article was rejected by the Journal of Pharmacology and Experimental Therapeutics. His friend and colleague W.F. Hamilton, editor of the Journal of Physiology, had to intervene in order for the article to be published in this journal. Contrary to Carrier and Shlafer who suggest that "heresy and audacity, not science, were the crux of the controversy", Ahlquist's work was rejected, at least partially, because of the experimental approach which he employed.[22] Two points were made by the critics.

Firstly, on the basis of his experimental findings, Ahlquist concluded that adrenaline must be the mediator. This conclusion was contrary to Von Euler's (1946) who proposed noradrenaline to be the one and only transmitter of the sympathetic nervous system. The point here is that Ahlquist's work had not met the standards for experimental work which had been raised by the introduction of biochemical techniques and new specific antagonists exemplified by the experimental work of Von Euler.

Secondly, Ahlquist made no use of experimental systems which used pressor responses to evaluate the activity of catecholamines on adrenergic receptors, because he appreciated that the arterial pressure represents the resultant of a number of factors.[23] Although it was well recognized that pressor-depressor test systems were not suited to establish the physiological role of the underlying mechanism, they were nonetheless a standard methodological tool to classify sympathomimetic and sympatholytic agents.

However the key issue was that Ahlquist's work implied a conceptual change, because he interpreted the physiological test systems pharmacologically, stating that "in order to study each type of receptor (our emphasis) it was necessary to work with more or less isolated parts of the cardiovascular system.[24] He conceived these isolated parts of the cardiovascular system as input-output-systems which could serve as a model of the function of the receptor. The receptor itself thus became the object of scientific interest.

In the same period, through their work on agonists and antagonists, pharmacologists became painfully aware of the fact that they did not have the faintest notion of how catecholamines operated at the cellular level, Furchgott asked *"Where are these adrenergic receptors located in the effector cells?"*, *"What is their chemical and physical nature?"* and *"How lead the reactions between them and the catecholamines to the responses which we observe and measure?".*[25] This discussion lasted until the early sixties, when a cluster of four methodological principles was generally accepted: (1) an agonist should interact directly with the receptor; (2) a suitable antagonist must be available to antagonize agonists selectively; (3) active (re)uptake of the agonist must be precluded; (4) controls should be performed to exclude the possibility of classifying physiological reflex responses as drug effects.
Ahlquist followed only the first of these rules by using a series of sympathomimetic agents to identify the adrenergic receptors. He assumed that these compounds acted directly, but employed no experiments to support the assumption. Systematic use of antagonists to selectively block agonists was not done. Available biochemical techniques to satisfy the third requirement were not used; nor did he exclude the possibility that physiological reflexes played a role in the responses he observed. The penetrating aspect of his work was the result of his classifying adrenergic receptors by means of studying the effects of agonists.
The striking feature of this early history was a complex process of disciplinary transformation. Ahlquist's theory became only a paradigm for the experimental study of adrenergic receptors after the cognitive matrix of this research area - the concepts of agonist and antagonist and a set of methodological principles - emerged. Although the discovery of DCI might be said to be accidental, its recognition as a compound with a deviant pattern of action was not an observation by chance as is often said in historical accounts of the beta blockers. Only within this new cognitive matrix of experimental work were scientists able to recognize DCI as the exemplar of a new class of bio-active compounds.

3.5. Experimental and therapeutic profiling in drug innovation

3.5.1. Cardiac arrhythmias

When Moran and Perkins in 1958 interpreted the action of DCI as a confirmation of Ahlquist's theory, it was obvious that it would have great impact on the conceptual frameworks of pharmacology and physiology. The concept of alpha and beta receptors was then rapidly accepted. However its influence on experimental drug research was not immediately evident. With the benefit of hindsight, it is clear that Ahlquist's theory could have changed these research practices at one specific point: the cardiac adrenergic receptor, because this theory gave the cardiac adrenergic receptor a new pharmacological meaning. This change did take place at the moment pharmacologists recognized DCI as an interesting compound because of its deviant pattern of action. It was tested systematically in various experimental systems, and attempts were made to fit the properties of DCI into a pharmacological profile. New questions arose:1.the specificity of beta blockade and its distinction from other types of pharmacological actions; 2. the contribution of beta blockade to normal and pathological mechanisms; 3. the intrinsic sympathomimetic activity; 4. its membrane stabilizing activity. These questions led to research on scattered fronts, because each could only be posed within a specific therapeutic context. The membrane stabilizing activity of DCI, for example, could only be recognized because DCI was tested in experimental systems relevant to various types of cardiac arrhythmias.[26]

DCI was conceived of as a compound with anti-arrhythmic properties despite prevailing views about the pathological role of cardiac excitatory responses. Research on cardiac arrhythmias was structured in such a way that the cardiac adrenergic receptors whether classified as "excitatory" of "beta" were assumed to play no major role. Thus in 1962 Moran and his colleagues pointed out that according to Ahlquist's theory there were two types of adrenergic receptor relevant to the cardiovascular system. Beta receptors mediated the inotropic and chronotropic responses of the heart, and alpha receptors mediated the ectopic excitation by sympathetic stimuli responsible for cardiac arrhythmias. Nickerson in 1959 had divided these responses into "physiological" and "pathological" responses.[27] Thus, pharmacologists held to the view that the "excitatory" cardiac responses played no major role in the pathogenesis of cardiac arrhythmias. Accordingly it was not Ahlquist's theory that changed this concept, but the way pharmacologists developed a profile of DCI.

So, an essential feature of drug development is to establish the contribution of the pharmacological properties of a compound to its biological effects, whether presupposed, ascertained or desired for. This process is called pharmacological profiling. Through this process concepts and tools are pushed into therapeutic contexts which give a therapeutic relevant meaning to these basic findings.

3.5.2. Angina pectoris

For Black and his team at ICI around 1960 there were no "theoretical problems", only "practical ones". They were to reduce intrinsic sympathetic activity to zero, consider the property of membrane stabilizing activity as a threat to the desired drug profile, choose the right test systems out of the field with a high turnover for chemical and pharmacological screening and bring pronethalol to the clinic as quickly as possible. He put the ICI-team to work on these practical problems by moving another clinical problem area into the field of the adrenergic receptors. He was not socialized in the physiology and pharmacology of the adrenergic receptors. Nor was he versed in that train of physiological thought that determined the pathophysiological significance of cardiac adrenergic receptors in connection with cardiac arrhythmias. He had received his scientific training in experimental cardiovascular physiology and was particularly interested in research on anginal attacks, cardiac necrosis and exercise tolerance.

For a long time this field had been dominated by the conception that coronary vasodilation was the choice method for the treatment of angina pectoris. This concept was the basis for therapeutic practice with nitrites and their established effectiveness in the treatment of angina pectoris. The success of the nitrites led to the search for other vasodilator compounds, initially with some success; but with time disappointment grew.[28] The time was ripe for a therapeutic re-orientation as stated by Winbury: *"There must be a re-evaluation of the concepts and theories regarding the mechanisms involved in angina pectoris and the approaches to the development of drugs for treatment of the disease".*[29]

Black and others recognized that DCI had therapeutic potential as a chemical knife to damp the sympathetic drive of the heart. The cardiac adrenergic receptors were thus connected with a straightforward therapeutic goal. The burden of proof was now reversed. The question was no longer which pharmacological properties did DCI possess and what were their therapeutic significance. Instead Black focussed on what was desired from DCI in a therapeutic setting and how this activity could be enhanced. He thus encouraged the ICI-team to use a chemical structure-activity approach, to see which modifications would improve DCI as the chemical knife desired.

Black thus moved the pharmacology of adrenergic blocking agents to the therapeutic context of angina. By developing pronethalol in 1962 and propranolol two years later, he established leadership in the field. He integrated the therapeutic contexts of angina and of cardiac arrhythmias. He asked questions like: *"Will conditions such as atrial fibrillation and atrial and ventricular tachycardia be helped by reducing the cardiac sympathomimetic responses to anxiety, emotion and exercise?"; "Will myocardial adrenergic blockade reduce the myocardial demand for oxygen?"* and, *if so: "Will this be helpful to patients with angina?".*[30] It is as if he would say: "I think these questions have to be answered with yes. But if you want to address these questions you need pronethalol while it is a tool and a therapeutic modality".

The use of pronethalol and later propranolol in specific therapeutic settings yielded information about their clinically relevant properties and about the conditions essential for enhancing the well-being of patients. This second type of process is called therapeutic profiling. The emanating profiles enable clinicians to mark the therapeutic objectives at stake and to translate basic findings into meaningful medical effects.

3.6. Conclusions

The early history of the development of beta-adrenergic blocking drugs is not only interesting in its own right. It demonstrates the interaction of physiologists, biochemists, pharmacologists and clinical scientists in the development of effective therapeutic agents. As is often (but not always) true, the early contributions of fundamental scientists were paramount. However, these contributions are not isolated events; they are embedded in experimental practice. Furthermore, at a critical point, the transition from the experimental to the clinical context required the creativity of the clinical scientist who visualized the potential solution to an important problem.

Emphasis has been given to the process in which experimental and clinical characteristics of drugs are revealed. The importance of creatively filling the profiles has been demonstrated in this early history of the evolution of the beta blocking pharmaceuticals. This illustrates that through assessing the appropriateness of therapeutic practices therapeutic needs and objectives for future drug development are modelled. These needs and objectives can be conceived of as demands made upon the "new drug" which have to be met in the lead generation and development process by industrial researchers.

Chapter 4. Industrial research and beta blockade

4.1. Introduction

The previous chapter described how the concept of beta blockade became transformed into a therapeutically meaningful concept. Evidence was provided for the hypothesis that this transformation was not possible without clinical practice that studied cardiac arrhythmias, anginal attacks, exercise tolerance, cardiac failure, bradycardia and bronchial spasm in asthma and bronchitis. The aim of this chapter is to substantiate this hypothesis more firmly by showing that clinical issues have structured industrial research and yielded specific targets for industrial scientists to profile their compounds experimentally.

For this purpose some industrial research projects will be described. Around 1960 several industrial laboratories were involved in the study of adrenergic mechanisms. Some programs were successful; others were not. Other companies may have searched for beta blocking compounds too, but not succeeding they have disappeared in the realm of the therapeutic past. Undoubtedly, many industrial scientists tested dichloroisoprenaline and related compounds as is common in industry, but they did not publish their results neither did they enter the field. Therefore the description of industrial research into beta blocking compounds must be necessarily selective. In this chapter five projects are described, i.e. the projects of Imperial Chemical Industries (4.2.), Eli Lilly & Co. (4.3.), Mead Johnson (4.4.), AB Hässle (4.5.) and Ciba (4.6.).

The development of the beta blocker projects of Imperial Chemical Industries and AB Hässle will be described at length to gain insight into the ways clinical perceptions affect industrial research. Academic research will be described with reference to particular developments in industrial research.

4.2. Beta blocker research at Imperial Chemical Industries (ICI)

4.2.1. The early phase

In 1957 Black made a request to the Pharmaceutical Division of ICI for money and support to elaborate a new approach in the treatment of coronary heart disease. Davey, who was in charge of the Biological Research Department, asked him to come to work at the department in Alderley Edge, near Manchester to where the Pharmaceutical Division of ICI had just moved. Time was apparently favorable for novel and risky ideas and Black was certainly the type of person who could persuade people to see his point of view. However, the research project started in an atmosphere of great scepticism and Black's unconventional ideas were in need of Davey's support, the more so since at several times the project seemed to have reached a dead-lock. No lead compound was found up till 1960 and laborious technical work had to be performed, e.g. the building of test-systems and electronic apparatus.

These activities coincided with the attempts of ICI to alter course in the cardiovascular area since the cardiovascular research team at ICI was completing their ganglion-blocker project.[1]

At this point it was already obvious that there would not be much future for this type of compound as other types of anti-hypertensive agents with less grave side-effects became available. The team moved from the peripherally acting ganglion blocking agents to the centrally-active anti-hypertensive drugs but this change of course was beset with pitfalls. In fact, a compound was found but it failed the toxicology tests.

After qualifying in medicine and having worked at the Department of Physiology, first at St. Andrew's, then in Malaya, Black joined the Department of Physiology at the Veterinary School in Glasgow in 1950. The department had contacts with various laboratories, and also with the Departments of Cardiovascular Surgery at Edinburgh and Aberdeen. George Smith, professor of surgery in Aberdeen, was an important person in Black's professional career.[2] Smith, holding a Rockefeller Scholarship, had become familiar with American cardiovascular physiology and surgery and through him Black became familiar with concepts and methods from both areas.

The laboratory at Glasgow studied an important technique to improve coronary artery disease. Exposing animals to hyperbaric oxygen they attempted to prevent or reverse ventricular fibrillation, a serious complication in case of a heart in oxygen distress. Gregg, a key figure in cardiovascular physiology, had established that only a very small increase in blood flow was needed to avoid damage to the heart. So, the idea arose whether a small decrease in oxygen demand would produce a similar beneficial effect.[3] Since it was known that the sympathetic nervous system mediated stress, and hence regulated the demand of the heart, Black became interested in the role of the sympathetic nervous system in coronary artery disease.

As early as in 1940 Raab had put forward his theory, that the triggering factors in angina pectoris such as effort, emotion, cold, and stress, caused a condition of hypersymphathicotony, i.e. a hyperactive state of the sympathetic system associated with excessive release of catecholamines from the supra-renal glands and the sympathetic nerve endings in the heart.[4] The catecholamines were supposed to produce an excessive and superfluous myocardial oxygen consumption: their so-called 'oxygen-wasting effects'. Throughout his life Raab defended his theory and gradually many scientists and clinicians began to follow Raab's ideas.[5] Based on this theory "anti-adrenergic" measures became advocated as a rational treatment in coronary heart disease. Indeed, the anti-adrenergic' measure was the key-notion that underlies Black's hypothesis.

During the 1950s Black studied a commercial extract of bovine heart muscle, for which a variety of therapeutic claims with respect to coronary heart disease had been made. Several studies had shown that the extract exhibited an anti-adrenergic activity in the heart and Black observed that it protected the rabbit heart against the damaging effects of oxygen shortage.[6] This observation initiated Black's decision to develop anti-adrenergic compounds.[7]

In part, his desire to find an anti-adrenergic drug fitted common medical knowledge. Patients told their doctors under which stressful conditions their complaints were evoked and how they could control their distress through re-organising daily life. In the same way physicians told their patients how to adapt their daily stress and emotions to the signals of their hearts. Hence, anginal pain was not only a sign of the disease's progress, but also the starting-point of therapeutic measures.[8] But this practice was far removed from attributing a pathological role to the sympathetic nervous system.

Black refers, in the following, to the long tradition in physiology and medicine that perceived the sympathetic nervous system as a beautiful mechanism of adaptive behaviour: *"Then the influence of W.B. Cannon (Cannon, 1932) with the sheer success of his work in the twenties in formulating his doctrine of homeostasis and the emergency theory of the function of the sympathetic nervous system - the mediation of the fight, fright and flight reaction - apparently imprinted the minds of generations of biologists with images of a system beautifully adapted to survival with its activity ebbing and flowing in a unitary pattern, harmoniously reciprocating with the parasympathetic system. There was not much room in these theories for the idea that the activity of the sympathetic nervous system would not necessarily or always (in cardiac disease, for example) have survival value".*[9]

However much this classic view may have dominated physiology and pharmacology, it was ambivalent in its practical meaning. It did not hinder the introduction of the therapeutic principle of controlling cardiac disease by interfering with the sympathetic nervous system. One example is the introduction of the ganglion blocking drugs which essentially try to control hypertensive disease by cutting the sympathetic nerves. In this respect strikingly different medical practices are seen. In the United Kingdom, for example, ganglion blocking agents became very popular whereas they were rarely prescribed in other countries.[10] The extent to which this therapeutic principle was applied in medical practice, varied accordingly. Another example is surgical sympathectomy in hypertension but this treatment was superseded by the use of ganglion blocking drugs.[11]

Several therapeutic measures therefore showed that if cardiovascular disease could not be conceptualized as a dysfunction of the sympathetic system, then in any case it could be controlled by interference with adrenergic control.

It is striking to see how Black extracted such heterogeneous elements from different backgrounds into this straightforward objective: "Find an anti-adrenergic substance". From the pharmacological perspective, however, this was a controversial idea. The pharmacological literature was filled with attempts to find anti-adrenergic drugs, but there was much confusion and little success.

Black recalls how he screened textbooks of pharmacology and then found the Ahlquist's paper on alpha and beta receptors in Drill's textbook **Pharmacology in Medicine** .[12] In this paper he found what he was looking for: that action of adrenaline in the heart was refractory to blockade, and apparently there was a different receptor in the heart. It was a straightforward way of thinking. Black was determined to find a compound that annulled the effects of adrenaline on the heart, not to solve the intriguing puzzle of the heart as an anomaly to medical theory. Unhindered by classic beliefs and the frustrating experiences in the field, he drew a connection between the therapeutic goal and the adrenergic receptor in the heart.

Though developed within the particular context of ventricular fibrillation, this goal was broadly formulated: complete blockade of the cardiac adrenergic receptor because sympathetic (over)activity is detrimental to the patient's condition in the case of heart disease. This attests to Black's personal view on the drug discovery process: *"I am more interested in offering a compound with a new type of pharmacological action than in finding a treatment for an experimentally induced disease in animals".*[13] The therapeutic target, however, would become angina pectoris. Shanks commented: *"Looking back in the reports that had been written internally at ICI, he (Black, RV) talked initially about 'coronary heart disease' and then the clinical trials worked out by Dornhorst and Robinson were in angina pectoris. So somewhere the change occurred and I am not sure where it did".*[14]

4.2.2. The birth of pronethalol

Black started the project without any formal basis. Black was the pharmacologist and John Stephenson the chemist, working in a section managed by Crowther. One of the major screening tests used was the Langendorff isolated guinea-pig heart preparation. In searching for adrenaline antagonists Black and Stephenson decided to follow up the ideas of Fourneau who had done much research into this area at the Pasteur Institute (Paris) during the 1930s. This strategy was interrupted by the discovery of DCI. In january 1959 the **Project Team Report** summarized: *"There are two clearly differentiated sympathetic receptors - α receptors associated with excitatory effects on blood vessels and smooth muscle and ß-receptors associated with inhibitory effects on smooth muscle and possibly cardiac muscle. All the known adrenolytic agents are α receptor inhibitors. Presumably the unknown factor in heart muscle is a ß receptor inhibitor and recently, the dichloro analogue of isoprenaline has been shown to be a powerful ß receptor inhibitor. The question of whether this latter compound will effectively block the cardiac sympathetic responses remains to be satisfactory answered".*[15]

The finding of DCI evoked confusion and discussion. The ICI team received the crucial papers early in 1959.[16] Black immediately recognized the significance of DCI, yet remained hesitant.[17] Though Moran and Perkins interpreted the effects of DCI in terms of Ahlquist's theory, Black was doubtful because of the strain-gauge-arch-technique used by the authors. Two years earlier Moran and colleagues had published an article claiming that phenoxybenzamine blocked the actions of adrenaline on the heart.[18] According to Black phenoxybenzamine did not exhibit this action, and the technique might be the decisive factor. When subsequently testing DCI in his own Langendorff preparation Black *"found it to be about as active as isoprenaline as a cardiac stimulant and rejected it as a suitable compound for antagonizing the cardiac actions of catecholamines".*[19]

Consequently, dichloroisoprenaline was rejected as a lead-compound. The search for other types of compounds continued but progress was slow. The development of the test-systems turned out to be a laborious undertaking.[20] Late in 1959 the technical problems were solved and Black calibrated the new set-up with the compounds that had been used in the old test system. In this new test system more than a hundred compounds were screened, and some were active but none as much as DCI.[21]

It was decided to take DCI as the lead-compound and in february 1960 Stephenson went straight to pronethalol. In march 1960 a phase of intensive testing started. The ICI scientists took an optimistic view, and the compound became an all-absorbing topic of investigation.[22] High priority was given to the project and antihypertensives-research was dropped.

4.2.3. The demise of pronethalol

The patent on pronetholol was applied for in May 1960. Stephenson left ICI about the same time, and chemical work was supervised by Crowther while Howe and Smith performed the patent completion work and structure-activity studies. When pronethalol was marketed in November 1963, about 800 compounds had been synthesized. A number of substances were potential candidates for further development and the chemists were aware that it would be very hard to keep competitors out of the field.

This period was crucial in two respects. At the chemical-pharmacological level the search for active compounds was performed at fever-speed to keep out competitors in the field. At the clinical-pharmacological level studies in animals and man were performed. The relationship between both levels of activity was bi-directional. The chemists turned up with a whole array of compounds providing the tools for further screening and delivering keys to biological and clinical studies. On the other hand, biological and clinical investigations revealed fundamental problems that formed targets for chemical research.

A critical stage of the research process was reached when clinical trials started in late 1961. In the middle of 1962 the first results were published in The Lancet. The articles reported studies with pronethalol relating to the cardiovascular effects on normal subjects and anginal patients, at rest and during exercise, as well as the effects on glucose and fatty-acid release in man. In 1963 more studies were published in the British Medical Journal. These were small clinical trials establishing the effectiveness of pronethalol in the relief of anginal pain, and also in some types of cardiac arrhythmias. The atmosphere of the project was positive. Clinicians became actively involved in the investigation and many clinicians were receptive to this new approach in cardiovascular disease. However, some problems emerged that threatened the project.

In an early phase, probably as early as in 1961, experiences with pronethalol in cats and dogs showed effects on the central nervous system. Black wrote in the **Project Team Report** (January 1962) *"that analogues of ICI 38174 (pronethalol) were being tested to find a compound which (...) showed less penetration of the central nervous system"*.[23]

Clinical studies performed by Dornhorst, Rosenheim and others revealed these central effects in man too. The side-effects of central nervous origin consisted of paraesthesia, 'walking on air', visual disturbances, dreams, fatigue, nausea, vomiting and dizziness.[24] It was suggested that these side-effects were not due to the beta blocking activity itself but to the high lipid solubility of pronethalol allowing easy passage across the blood-brain barrier.[25]

The clinical reports necessitated that the team find another compound: *"The downside was that this very first drug (pronethalol, RV) caused vomiting at just about the therapeutic dose. So, a lot of people were nauseated by it, I can tell you that and it became quickly apparent that that one wasn't going to do"*.[26] High lipid solubility became an undesirable property of beta blocking compounds and attempts were made to synthesize compounds without this characteristic.

To scientists outside the firm it was a surprise that ICI came up with another compound so quickly[27] but in fact it took a year before a decisive breakthrough came. Shanks who had worked at Belfast and who joined ICI because of his expertise in cardiovascular hemodynamics became deeply involved in this successful event. In November 1962 he performed one of his first experiments administering ICI 45520 (propranolol) to a cat. The compound proved to be about 10 times more potent than pronethalol. In contrast, the dose required to produce toxic effects, particularly the neurological symptoms, was about the same as the toxic dose of pronethalol. Hence the therapeutic ratio (therapeutic dose/toxic dose) was markedly increased.[28] Shanks describes how Crowther and Smith were *"varying the distance of the CHOH group from the aromatic ring by the insertion of different groups; one of the groups selected was -OCH$_2$. This normally would have been done by a reaction involving ß-naphthol but as α-naphthol was available Smith used this instead, and obtained ICI 45520; the compound made from ß-naphthol is less active".*[29]

However, the chemists were aware that activity could be found in both α- and ß-naphthyl derivatives from their work in the pronethalol area.[30] Thus, the compound ICI 45520 was a happy discovery but not accidental. Furthermore, the neurological problems stimulated the team to search for potent compounds.[31] Insights from structure-activity-relationship (SAR) research, though far from being a theoretical guide to the chemist, none the less outlined routes of chemical manipulation. Biological systems were specific enough to pick up the desired compounds of whatever chemical type. Even if the synthesis of ICI 45520 would have been a fortunate event, the recognition of its interesting biological activity was certainly not a happy chance.

This compound (propranolol) was not the solution to the whole problem in that its high lipid solubility still allowed it to penetrate nervous tissue. In 1963 this property became a major problem leading to theoretical and methodological discussions in the field. In the mean time work on pronethalol had continued. Gill and Vaughan Williams reported that pronethalol acted in the same way as quinidine, an anti-arrhythmic agent, and as procaine, a local anaesthetic: *"Experiments (...)indicated that pronethalol was an anti-arrhythmic agent approximately twice as potent as quinidine and **with a similar mode of action**. Since many anti-arrhythmic agents are **also local anaesthetics**, it was of interest to discover whether pronethalol also could produce local anaesthesia. (...) It was found that pronethalol is 1.8 times as active as procaine (...). Pronethalol is **very closely related to** a series of compounds studied as local anaesthetics by MacIntosh and Work".*[32]

The emphasis in this quotation has been added to stress that in this way knowledge about profiles of anti-arrhythmic agents was transferred to the field of beta blocking drugs.[33] A fundamental discussion about the basic action of pronethalol began. Was it the beta blocking action or that other type of activity similar to that of quinidine the essential feature of the anti-fibrillatory action? This basic question also involved the anti-anginal area. Was it the beta blocking action or the "local anaesthetic" action similar to that of procaine the key activity that relieved anginal **pain?** This report therefore disturbed the ICI team because the beneficial effects of pronethalol could possibly be attributed to a property other than beta-blocking activity.[34]

Different terms have been used interchangeably to denote this aspect of the drug: "quinidine-like action", "local anaesthetic activity" and "membrane stabilizing activity" (MSA).[35] In due course the latter term became the preferred one to denote this ancillary property of beta blocking compounds. The high lipid solubility was purportedly reflected in this local anaesthetic or quinidine-like activity. Lipophilic beta blockers were supposed to be compounds with membrane stabilizing activity whereas hydrophilic beta blockers were agents without this undesirable property. The crucial point is that this property was not merely related to toxicological actions but to the therapeutic effects, i.e. the anti-arrhythmic and anti-anginal action, as well.

In this context clinicians posed another problem that to some extent also affected the discussion about the local anaesthetic activity of pronethalol. Stock, a cardiologist in Stoke-on-Trent, reported other than beneficial effects in cardiac arrhythmias: *"The aggravation or precipitation of heart failure by pronethalol is disturbing. We certainly feel that the drug should be given with great caution in the presence of established or incipient heart failure"*.[36]

Two explanations were provided. First, patients near the borderline of heart failure appeared to be in urgent need of the compensating activity of the sympathetic drive that strengthened the force of contraction of the heart. Since beta blockers eliminated the sympathetic drive, they precipitate or even initiate cardiac failure. Second, beta blockers exhibited a direct cardio-depressive action. In fact, local anaesthetics were known to be cardio-depressive agents and beta blockers possessed a local anaesthetic activity. The first explanation dominated the field but throughout the 1960s the "direct cardio-depressive" action of pronethalol, propranolol and other compounds also entered the discussion.

These toxicological problems, however, were surpassed by another finding that dramatically affected the course of the project.[37] During testing for long-term toxicity in mice carcinogenic activity was found. The tumours found in these mice were most commonly in the thymus but other tumours also appeared. Pronethalol was marketed but its use was restricted to *"conditions which themselves threaten life immediately, or cause such morbidity that only short survival may be expected"*.[38] Subsequently many further long term tests were performed in mice, rats, guinea pigs, dogs and monkeys but no carcinogenic effect was observed in any species other than that "Alderley Park strain of mouse" as ICI-scientists cynically expressed. This formulation reflects the psychology of the industrial scientist. For indeed, it is terrible to lose a compound in which so much time and energy has been invested. But it also reflects the strong beliefs and high hopes attributed to that drug.

So, while pronethalol embodied the expectations of a winning team, two dramatic events - the discovery of the carcinogenic effect and the quinidine-like activity - rapidly culminated in an anti-climax: *"It came as a shock to us; it was a disaster"*, as Barrett described the state of mind of the ICI team.[39] Both events wrenched the ICI team out of its routine activity. The demise of pronethalol started and it was replaced by propranolol. Admittedly, it was easy to drop pronethalol *"as propranolol had already been discovered and no tumours had developed in a chronic toxicity study in mice (..)"*.[40]

This dramatic period coincided with the departure of Black who started a new project at Smith, Kline & French that would lead to the famous gastrointestinal drug cimetidine (Tagamet). However, the crucial problems related to pronethalol demanded the utmost exertion of ICI's scientists and left little room for deploring Black's departure.

4.2.4. The development of propranolol

4.2.4.1. A "clean" drug

The chemists had already found a new range of analogous compounds with potency ratio's of 10-20 times greater than pronethalol, and with mixtures of properties that raised many biological questions. About twelve people at the chemical department - five Ph.D. research workers and their technical staff - worked on the project. A strong impetus came from patent-completion tasks and the chemists put their ingenuity into the exploration of the chemical characteristics of these bio-active compounds that made up "beta blockade". A stream of compounds flowed over the biologists laboratory benches. Many compounds with interesting activity were discovered and patented.

At the centre of research stood three classes of compounds (figure 4.1):

a. the benzodioxan-analogues

b. the naphthoxy-analogues: compound ICI 45520 (propranolol)

c. the phenoxy-analogues: compound ICI 45763

A.

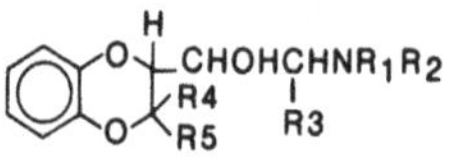

Benzodioxan-analogues,e.g. R1 = H;
R2 = C(CH3)3; R3,R4,R5 = H.(cf.compounds
15 and 16,Howe et.al (1970)).

B.

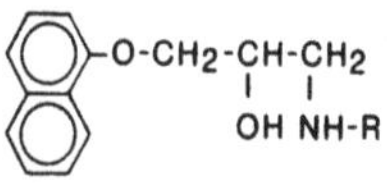

Naphthoxy-analogues: R = CH(CH3)2 (propranolol
ICI 45520)

C.

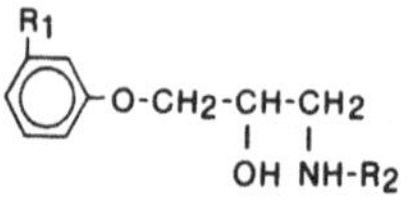

Phenoxy-analogues: R1 = CH3;R2 = CH(CH3)2 (toliprolol;
ICI 45763)

Figure 4.1
Three classes of potent new beta blocking compounds found at ICI in the early phase.

The benzodioxan-group contained the most potent compounds, many times more potent than predicted. There were, therefore, many potential compounds and the problem was "to pick the best".[41] Once the carcinogenic risk of pronethalol was acknowledged, the question arose to what extent this risk also affected propranolol and other look-alikes: "As it was not known if the "naphthalene" part of pronethalol was responsible for its carcinogenic action, it was decided that a phenoxy derivative should also undergo carcinogenicity testing in mice along with propranolol. If propranolol was carcinogenic and the phenoxy compound was not, the latter would have proceeded to clinical evaluation; but this did not occur as propranolol did not produce tumours".[42] It turned out that both compounds - ICI 45520 (propranolol) and ICI 45763 -did not produce tumours in mice.

Considering the reasons that led the ICI team to choose propranolol, Barrett suggested that propranolol *"was chosen on the grounds that the latter (ICI 45763, RV) possessed some degree of partial agonist activity, which was the reason for dropping DCI".*[43] The view that intrinsic activity represented an undesirable property was widely held in the laboratory.[44] This view was reflected in Black's objective to search for the purest representative of this new class of drugs, and Black had conditioned the people having a seat on the decision-making panel that selected propranolol for marketing.[45] Apparently having no purpose at all, intrinsic activity seemed to be rather disadvantageous: *"No, we thought that there was no benefit in intrinsic sympathomimetic activity because in angina it would increase resting heart rate and therefore you would not get the reduction in myocardial oxygen consumption that we thought was important".*[46] Therefore, as Shanks commented, there has been no real competition between the two compounds.

According to Fitzgerald, however, this aspect of the drug was of minor importance in decision taking. It was the lack of potency and the shorter duration of action in man that prohibited ICI 45763 from further development, *"not its intrinsic sympathomimetic activity, as much as people want you to believe that".*[47] Apparently Dornhorst and Robinson had advised the team to test both drugs in man but neither scientist was able to recall this point: *"It may be that I was asked. I don't have a clear recollection of it. And I certainly don't remember having any sort of formal conference. But it may well be that one of them called in and discussed it but there has been left no trace of that".* If there were any studies performed in man with ICI 45763 *"it certainly wasn't by Robinson and myself".*[48] Robinson adds that no one thought that total withdrawal of the sympathetic drive would be harmful.[49]

So, ever since DCI had been discovered, intrinsic activity was largely considered from a negative point of view: *"One was aware right from the beginning that there was a possibility of having the two effects (blockade and stimulation, RV) in the same molecule. And everyone thought how wonderful propranolol was that it had completely got rid of this stimulating effect".*[50] This fitted the idea of a clean beta blocker and explaining this Robinson touches upon an interesting aspect: *"Well, I think people always have an attraction to pure, simple action, I mean just as in mathematics, the elegance of a simple formulation is an attraction to mathematicians. And I think to a pharmacologist a drug which does one single thing is always more wonderful than a drug which...I mean, they talk of "clean" and "dirty" drugs. You speak of a dirty blocker if it also blocks five-hydroxytryptamine and histamine a bit. Things like phenoxybenzamine which block all sort of things as well as catecholamines, are regarded as dirty blockers. So a drug which is very specific for a single receptor and has no stimulating activity is like a very fine bullet. It appeals to people from an aesthetic point of view that a drug has a very pure action. That is pure esthetics and emotion".*[51]

So, from the very outset the ICI team followed the idea of searching for a nice, clean drug. Contributing to this fact was that the ICI scientists and their consultants were inspired by the idea of unravelling complex physiological mechanisms hitherto considered to be impossible. Indeed, the adage of the ICI team was *"If you want to block, you block".*[52]

Obviously, the issue of intrinsic activity revolved around questions that were raised in an ever-changing context. The academic field succeeded in developing more precise standards to evaluate this intrinsic activity.[53] It was Barrett who introduced the raised standards into the ICI project:

"Just prior to the departure of Dr. Black to the World Congress of Cardiology in Mexico City in 1962,

*he asked the author (Barrett, RV) to check whether this compound, now known as pronethalol, also
inhibited adrenaline-induced mobilization of free fatty acids. We chose to use an anesthetized dog and
to our surprise found no blockade but a marked increase in free fatty acid levels following pronethalol
injection. Thus it became evident that although partial agonist activity was greatly reduced by
comparison with DCI it had not been eliminated".*[54]

By that time it was suspected that patients during exercise might not be able to mobilize free
fatty acids and break down glycogen. Hence they might die in a shock-like state or strangle
when exercising or running for a taxi.[55] So, the initiative to evaluate intrinsic activity
positively, might have come from here but, though there was some discussion, it did not
became a clinical topic.

The clinical significance of intrinsic activity in the cardiovascular domain was far from clear.
Until new pharmacological tests appeared to assess this aspect with regard to cardiovascular
hemodynamics, it was largely neglected. Shanks commented that till late in 1963 pronethalol
was looked upon as a drug devoid of this property. In fact, the team was surprised when large
differences between pronethalol and propranolol were found. This occurred after
pronethalol had been withdrawn.[56] Furthermore, intrinsic activity was not a major topic and
it had no important influence on structure-activity research.[57] When testing propranolol and
ICI 45763 in man, marked differences in activity were observed which in themselves were
sufficient to encourage sticking to propranolol.[58]

So, while participants express different views, they in fact refer to different stages of the
project and to distinct issues. Moreover, there was no particular critical decision point:
*"Decision making was very fuzzy at that stage. I couldn't say who made the decision, singly or
collectively but we got propranolol (...) and we wished to continue with it".*[59] Indeed, there was no
real competition between propranolol and ICI 45763 but the decisions arose from the
successive stages of biological and clinical-pharmacological experiments with both drugs.

4.2.4.2. The rapid expansion of a successful drug

ICI was a newcomer in the cardiovascular area and the firm lacked an extensive network of
clinical centres such as powerful companies like Geigy possessed. This clinical vacuum was
rapidly filled because pronethalol found a fertile soil in British cardiology.[60] A major reason
seems to be that British doctors were very prone to use ganglion blocking drugs in
hypertension and they had learned to talk and to act in terms of sympathetic overactivity,
adrenergic discharge and the relationship between stress, sympathetic control and
cardiovascular disease. Pronethalol exhibited clear-cut effects on the sympathetic system. It
produced bradycardia, it reduced exercise tachycardia and it exhibited other clinical signs as
for example the effect on Valsalva's manoeuvre, a clinical procedure to assess the function of
cardiovascular sympathetic control.

Here was a drug with such impressive "clean" and clinically translatable effects on the
sympathetic system. This image was a powerful stimulus for many clinicians to persevere,
even when the drug seemed to run into difficulties.[61] And the same applies to its successor,
i.e. propranolol. Whereas ICI started with four clinical centres in 1961, in less than 4 years
it had attracted many more clinical investigators to study a variety of cardiovascular aspects

of beta blockade.[62] Dollery said: *"Because the beta blockers were discovered in England, they were investigated much more intensively here. There were an extraordinary number of cardiovascular groups in Britain who were working on different aspects of the beta blockers (...)".*[63]

The development of the beta blockers coincided with the rise of clinical pharmacology in British medicine. In the British context this discipline emerged from internal medicine whereas in other countries like Sweden it descended from pharmacology. The renowned cardiologists Rosenheim and McMichael encouraged Lawrence and Dollery to develop clinical pharmacology as a discipline. As Dollery stated: *"So it happened that the two people who were rooting for clinical pharmacology, were both in the cardiovascular area".* British clinical pharmacology began in the direction of cardiology and the first clinical pharmacologists like Prichard and Dollery happened to be interested in beta blockers: *"(..) and so the people we trained tended to go on and continued to be interested in beta blockers".*[64] Clinical pharmacologists had an exciting time because above all they wanted, and still want to measure drug action and fortunately beta blockers formed an interesting subject in this respect.

Clinical studies with propranolol started in the summer 1964 and in July 1965 the drug was marketed in the United Kingdom. Due to the close relationship with many British clinical centres, there was an enormous potential in reaching the therapeutic targets.[65] The rapidity with which clinicians used propranolol in a variety of clinical conditions, is most striking. This demonstrates an important aspect of the development of a new drug so nicely described by Black: *"When a drug with a new pharmacological action becomes available it is liable to be tried clinically in disorders which were not foreseen during its laboratory development. The umbilical connexion with the laboratory has been cut and we must rely on the vision of the clinician and be grateful for this. In this way, pronethalol was investigated in mitral stenosis (Stock and Dale, 1963), subaortic hypertrophic stenosis (Harrison et al., 1964) and hypertension (Prichard and Gillam, 1964)".*[66]

Other clinical indications soon followed: acute myocardial infarction; hypertrophic obstructive cardiomyopathy; hyperkinetic heart syndrome; and nervous-functional cardiovascular disorders. The field of cardiovascular research opened up.

4.2.4.3. Endangered drug

Whereas the therapeutic domain of propranolol's use continued to expand, it also became an endangered drug. Rapidly doubts were thrown upon the principle of beta blockade because many scientists and clinicians believed that the local anaesthetic activity underlied the anti-arrhythmic and anti-anginal effects of propranolol.

The ICI team undertook fierce efforts to defend their claims about propranolol and found support in the success of surgical sympathectomy. The study of Aphthorp and colleagues (1960) establishing the objective improvement of sympathectomy, was carried on by Chamberlain who in fact took the view that DCI might be a pharmacological substitute for surgical therapy. Despite several requests to Eli Lilly, initially in England and later in the United States, he did not receive supplies of DCI and was eventually surpassed by the publications about pronethalol. Subsequently, Chamberlain became involved in research on pronethalol and propranolol showing that the effects of these agents mimicked the beneficial effects of sympathectomy.

The ICI team drew upon the analogy between the surgical knife and the purity of chemical blockade exhibited by propranolol with the aim to convince the medical world; as Shanks comments: *"Yes, the studies that he (Chamberlain, RV) did with propranolol showing that the effect of propranolol on heart rate and exercise tolerance was very similar to that of stellate sympathectomy was very important for two reasons. One was it indicated the mode of action of propranolol in angina. And secondly, it dispelled or had to dispel the idea that it was the local anaesthetic effect of propranolol that was having an effect. (...) It was very important because many doctors believed that propranolol was working through its local anaesthetic effect in 1964 and 1965".*[67]

In addition, feverish activity at the laboratory bench took place. Stereochemistry produced the idea of separating the two isomers of propranolol, one with and the other without beta blocking action but both in possession of local anaesthetic effects. Mead Johnson provided ICI the key to the problem: *"And then along the way we heard about sotalol and then we thought it would be more realistic to get a beta-blocking drug that did not have local anaesthetic activity to compare it with propranolol. And so the plan was to develop ICI 50172, practolol, to compare it with propranolol".*[68]

In this context clinicians raised another problem initiated by the publication of Stock and Dale in 1963 about the occurrence of cardiac failure caused or aggravated by pronethalol. Rapidly, alarming reports about propranolol accumulated and brought the issue of cardiac failure to the fore. Before marketing approximately five thousand patients were treated with propranolol, two thousand in the United Kingdom, and three thousand abroad. In about five hundred patients treated in the United Kingdom, propranolol was administrated by the intravenous route. Twenty six patients died and fourteen deaths were attributed to the use of propranolol. In these deaths, unwanted effects such as bradycardia, bronchospasm and cardiac failure, were considered to be due to the basic action of the drug.[69]

The **radius of action** of damping the sympathetic drive of the heart became a clinical issue and clashed with the basic view of the ICI team that sympathetic (over)activity was detrimental to the patient's condition. It became clear that clinical conditions existed where, as Fitzgerald stated some years later, *"increased sympathetic activity is part of the necessary homeostatic response and its blockade leads to failure of homeostasis".*[70] Indeed, cardiovascular disease states presented a conflict between the benevolence of sympathetic adaptation at the one end and the malevolence of sympathetic (over)activity at the other end. The problem was of a **general** nature, e.g. how to determine the optimal balance in a variety of pathological conditions, as well as of a **particular** nature, e.g. how to apply the principle of beta blockade when faced with the pathological condition of the **individual** patient. In the latter case clinicians attempted to define the criteria for selecting the patients at risk. In the former case laboratory and clinical research workers attempted to elucidate the role of the sympathetic system in a variety of disease states.

However, the discussion about the application of beta blockers was complicated by the fact that the basic action of these drugs still formed a subject of scientific dispute. While it was well known that local anaesthetic drugs depressed the action of the heart, cardiac failure might be the result of this cardio-depressive action as well.

In particular, the intravenous administration of propranolol was acknowledged as very dangerous. As Goodwin stated: *"We have had five disastrous incidents following intravenous*

pronethalol or propranolol, one of which was fatal. (...) I would like to suggest that there is a sharp cleavage between the oral and intravenous use of these drugs and that the ampoule is a very dangerous weapon indeed that should be restricted to use in hospitals or places where immediate resuscitation is possible. (...) and I think perhaps the ampoule should not find its way into general practice at all".[71]
Oral administration, however, remained a problem as well, not only in anti-arrhythmic but also in anti-anginal treatment. Early clinical trials using fixed dose schemes and relatively low doses of propranolol - three times 20 mg. or one time 90 mg. daily - showed varying but not impressive rates of success. In 1965, however, Prichard and Gillam presented high rates of success when using high doses of propranolol, sometimes up to 4 gram per day.[72] Their approach consisted of individualizing dosages and using run-in periods. The clinician needed to take some time to search for the optimal dose, to achieve the best possible therapeutic result in each individual patient and to evaluate the adaptive mechanisms of the patient's body.
This in itself formed a clinical innovation introducing new experimental designs in therapeutic trials. But it raised two problems that were initially a set-back to propranolol's progress. First, this procedure demanded a different clinical approach which was unfamiliar to many doctors. Secondly, the dosage variance aggravated the scepticism and the doubts about the mechanism of action of propranolol and the risk of heart failure in cardiac therapy.[73] The high doses used exceeded by far the normal dose range required for producing beta blockade and supported the view that it was the local anaesthetic action rather than the beta blocking action that made propranolol an effective drug. Moreover, the cardio-depressive action - synonymous with local anaesthetic action - was believed to increase the risk of heart failure.
The view that beta blockade represented a simple and clear-cut therapeutic principle in cardiovascular treatment, so strongly held by the ICI scientists and presented to the medical world, struck back like a boomerang. Propranolol came to be perceived as a drug most difficult to handle in the clinical situation.
Barrett describes this general feeling very aptly: " (...) it *(propranolol, RV) gave consultant physicians, particularly cardiologists, a powerful new tool in the management of cardiovascular disease. But it was difficult to use for two reasons. It was difficult because not everybody understood the underlying physiology of autonomic control of the heart. Problems with its use came from a failure to anticipate dangerous levels of unopposed vagal inhibition. It was necessary to match the dose to individual patients quite carefully but further because of the, as then, undiscovered high first pass effect and the consequent variation in the rate of metabolism the dose required for different patients was very variable. They ranged from 10 milligrammes to 4 grammes! Those are the two things that stick in my mind... How could one drug work in the same way with a dose ranging from 10 milligram and 4 gram in one day for two different people? It was difficult to understand. I also believe that there was a mystique in the use of propranolol, in some ways it was a dangerous drug only to be used with great care by cardiac specialists".*[74]

This "mystique" of a difficult and dangerous drug frustrated propranolol's progress. In this context, a new compound, practolol, emerged as a possible solution.

4.2.5. The development of practolol.

4.2.5.1. Practolol: a tool in industrial research.

In April 1966 it was observed in anaesthetized dogs that practolol antagonized the effects of isoprenaline in the heart but not in the vessels. Subsequently, it was shown that practolol blocked beta-receptors in the heart more strongly than beta receptors in other tissues and the term 'selective blockade' was coined for this phenomenon.[75]
During 1964 - 1966 the ICI team was involved in a broad experimental program using several compounds as investigational tools.[76] The grid of properties of these beta blocking compounds is shown in table 4.1.

Table 4.1
Profiles of beta blocking compounds at ICI.

	Beta-blockade	ISA	MSA	"Selectivity"
d-Propranolol	+++	–	++	– –
l-Propranolol	– – –	–	++	– –
ICI 45763 (toliprolol)	++	+	+	– –
MJ 1999	+	–	– –	– –
ICI 50172 (practolol)	+	+	– –	+
ICI 50232	+++	–	– –	+

The ICI-team tested these drugs in animals and man. The first four compounds together with pronethalol became the subject of a research project. When pronethalol was replaced, propranolol became the target of research. The compounds, ICI 50172 and ICI 50232, entered the project later, in 1965.
From the very outset, the ICI scientists were puzzled by the effects of pronethalol on the peripheral blood vessels.[77] Then, an intriguing problem arose when marked differences between MJ 1999 and propranolol were observed. Since the major difference between the two compounds seemed to be the absence/presence of the local anaesthetic action, the separation of beta blocking and local anaesthetic properties with respect to the peripheral vasodilator effects became a central problem.[78]

This "vasodilator" project was carried out by Shanks and Dunlop at ICI and by Bricks and colleagues at the Departments of Physiology and Pharmacology at the Belfast University. Taking the new compounds into consideration, with sotalol as reference, it became clear that not local anaesthetic activity but another property could be the explanation for the differential effects. Table 4.2 shows the differences between propranolol and practolol.

Table 4.2
Differences between propranolol and practolol (ICI 50172).

Response	Propranolol	I.C.I. 50,172
Heart Rate	1	2.5
Cardiac Contractile Force	1	2.5
Plasma free fatty acids	1	3.0
Vasodepressor	1	370
Tracheal relaxation	1	150

Reproduced with permission from Barrett et al. (1967).

These differences are indeed great, and at first glance the above sequence of events seems to fit the classical pattern from laboratory to man: the discovery of the unexpected new property of practolol and its subsequent confirmation in man.
The pattern of discovery, however, is much more complex as the design of the project above indicates.[79] Furthermore, table 4.2 disguises the complexity of the physiological mechanisms involved. These mechanisms had to be unraveled in a whole series of experiments and in this respect the research program at Belfast was extremely important to the ICI project.[80] The Belfast group performed animal experiments as well as several human studies.[81]

4.2.5.2. Selectivity in industrial and academic research

Tissue-dependent variation in response was not an isolated phenomenon. Other industrial research teams also possessed a whole range of compounds that exhibited different responses in the various tissues. This was also the case in the field of beta stimulating drugs. The Glaxo scientists, Brittain and Jack, who were deeply involved in the search for bronchodilator drugs, already had highly selective compounds on the shelf. Their knowledge was kept confidential. The same applies to other industrial research teams.
Academic scientists were also familiar with highly selective compounds. The substance H 35/25, developed by AB Hässle, was such a compound.[82] Other compounds were N-isopropyl-methoxamine[83], N-tertiary butylmethoxamine and dimethylisopropylmethoxamine[84]. None of these compounds matched the **typical** beta blocking compounds in blocking the cardiac responses to catecholamines.[85] The following introductory remarks made by Levy (1965) are illustrative:

*"All of these parameters may be reduced by appropriate doses of a **typical** beta adrenergic receptor*

blocking agent such as dichloroisoproterenol. However, N-isopropylmethoxamine has been shown to be capable of blocking certain metabolic effects of catecholamines. (...) These metabolic blocking actions are shared by such **typical** *beta adrenergic receptor blocking agents as dichloroisoproterenol and pronethalol. Furthermore, like dichloroisoproterenol and pronethalol, N-isopropylmethoxamine produced a specific blockade of the inhibitory response to catecholamines in the spontaneously contracting isolated rat uterus. This is a structure which we have reported* **as possessing only** *beta inhibitory receptors. It is, therefore, apparent that N-isopropylmethoxamine does have* **certain** *beta adrenergic receptor blocking actions* **in common with** *other beta adrenergic receptor blocking agents. However, N-isopropylmethoxamine* **cannot be properly classified** *as a* **beta** *adrenergic blocking agent because of its much more restricted scope of blocking action".* [86]

The emphasis in this quotation is mine stressing the fact that terms such as "typical", "in common with" and "properly classified" attest to the process of profiling in which scientists create drug profiles and recognize compounds accordingly.[87] These compounds were investigated to delineate the profile of beta blocking compounds and to characterize beta receptors in various tissues.

Table 4.3 Lands' theory: selectivity in sympathomimetic effects.
Reproduced with permission from Lands et al. (1967).

OH
OH
CH(OH)CHR
NHR¹

Compound	R	Structure R¹	Lipolytic*	Relative activity Cardiac†	Bronchodilator‡	Vasodepressor§
l-Isoproterenol	H	CH(CH₃)₂	1,000 (2·1 μM)	1,000 (1·2 ng/heart)	1,000 (0·184 μg/lung)	1,000 (0·08 μg/kg, i.v.)
l-Norepinephrine	H	H	85	34	3	pressor ‖
Epinephrine	H	CH₃	61	48	230	82¶
1 (l-isomer)	H	C₂H₅	235	300	736	1,000
2	H	C(CH₃)₃	89	37	1,075	500
3	H	CH(CH₃)CH₂CH₃	262	160	250	228
4	H	CH(CH₃)CH.CH(CH₃)₂	165	100	230	200
5	H	H	214	208	350	200
6	H	CH(CH₃)CH₂CH.CH(CH₃)₂	510	171	173	145
l-Nordefrine	CH₃	H	143	80	7	pressor
7	CH₃	CH₃	45	21	120	266
8	CH₃	CH(CH₃)₂	28	12	112	133
9	CH₃	H	68	16	166	61
d,l-Isoetharine	C₂H₅	CH(CH₃)₂	4	3	115	67
10	C₂H₅	H	6	7	206	80

* Minced testicular adipose tissue of the rat. Glycerol determined by the method of van Handel and Zilversmit. See also Černohorsky et al.
† Rabbit isolated perfused heart (Brown and Lands).
‡ Guinea-pig perfused lung (Luduena et al.).
§ Vasodepressor action in anaesthetized dogs following rapid intravenous injection.
‖ Vasodepressor action after α-receptor blockade (Brown and Green).
¶ A value of 1·0 was assigned arbitrarily to l-norepinephrine and l-nordefrine.

Receptor system	n	Correlation coefficient
I. (β-1) Lipolysis/cardiac stimulation	15	0·950
II. (β-2) Bronchodilatation/vasodepression	15	0·957
Receptor I/II		
Lipolysis/bronchodilatation	15	0·206
Lipolysis/vasodepression	15	0·220
Cardiac stimulation/bronchodilatation	15	0·309
Cardiac stimulation/vasodepression	15	0·312
III. (α) Vas deferens/sm. intestine relaxation*	11	0·90

* Data from van Rossum.

Awareness grew that beta receptors were not a homogeneous group and might be divided into subgroups. Several hypotheses evolved and a topographical picture may be drawn between two extremes. At the one end was the receptor concept of Levy. According to Levy each tissue had its "own unique adrenergic receptor". This implies that there were 1..N receptors: heart, lung, blood vessel and so on.[88] Another hypothesis presupposed that next to an alpha and beta receptor there existed a gamma and a delta receptor.[89]

At the other end was the receptor concept which hypothesized the existence of one and the same universal "beta" receptor in all tissues. Differences in tissue responses were explained, for example, on the basis of kinetics, e.g. differences in approaching the receptor concerned in the various tissues; other explanations also appeared.[90]

Somewhere in this topographical landscape Lands was elaborating the concept of beta-$_1$ and beta-$_2$ receptors.[91] Lands proceeded in a similar way as Ahlquist, yet within the limits of present methodology.[92] By using a series of sympathomimetic agents he supported the hypothesis that two distinct receptor types were included within the single receptor population designated by Ahlquist as the beta-type. Innovatory to the Ahlquist' approach was that Lands compared the relative potency series of a number of compounds in four critical experimental systems: the heart, the lung, the vessels and adipose tissue, i.e. lipolysis: release of free fatty acids (see table 4.3).

Correlation of the results in these test-systems yielded a clear-cut pattern. The results obtained with adipose tissue (lipolysis) showed a high correlation with those obtained from the cardiac test. The same holds true for the correlation between the bronchodilator and vasodepressor actions of the investigated compounds.

Lands' classification set the stage for further research. Many accounts in the medical literature agree that starting with the work of Lands, it has become apparent that not all beta receptors are the same. Moreover, it is often stated that Lands' theory of beta-1 and beta-2 receptors was confirmed by the introduction of practolol, a beta-1 cardio-selective beta blocker, and salbutamol, a beta-2 bronchoselective beta stimulant.[93] This implies that first there was the theory, subsequently the compounds. Figures 4.2 and 4.3 suggest a more complex pattern.

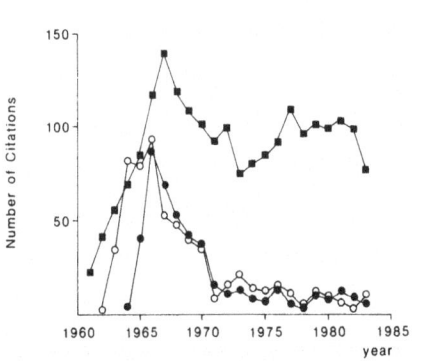

Figure 4.2
Number of citations per year from the Science Citation Index (SCI) to Ahlquist (1948) (■); Black and Stephenson (1962) (○); and Black et al. (1964) (●).

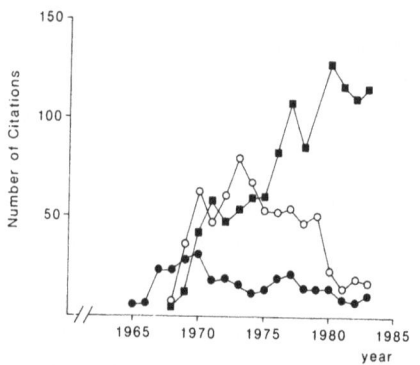

Figure 4.3
Number of citations per year
from the Science Citation
Index (SCI) to Levy (1964,
1966a, 1966b) 1967 (●);
Dunlop and Shanks (1968)
(○); and Lands et al.
(1967) (■).

Figure 4.2 shows a rapid increase in the number of citations referring to (Ahlquist's) theory as well as to the investigational tools, e.g., pronethalol and propranolol. Subsequently, the number of citations referring to the compounds rapidly declines. In contrast, the number of citations referring to the theory falls slightly and then remains at a fairly steady level. One could gain the impression that the compounds - pronethalol and propranolol - followed theoretical developments. This is not the case because the acceptance of Ahlquist's theory started with the discovery of DCI. A scientometric curve of dichloroisoprenaline could not be made because the Science Citation Index only starts in 1961.[94] I presume that the curve of DCI has a similar pattern as the one with respect to Ahlquist's theory.

Figure 4.3 differs slightly from figure 4.2, yet clearly shows the simultaneous rise in the number of quotations regarding the theory and practolol. The "practolol"-curve shows a biphasic character. There is a sharp decline in 1971 but this is compensated by an equally rapid increase in 1972. This is probably the case because of the practolol disaster. Practolol evoked serious side-effects which caused grave concern in the medical world.[95] The "practolol"-curve precedes the "Lands"-curve.

The "Levy"-curve represents the total number of citations referring to four experimental articles published by Levy. These articles were chosen because they represented the practical-experimental type of research in the academic field. The "Levy"- curve precedes the "Lands"-curve but never reaches a high citation score. Considering the narrow circles in which Levy's articles were cited, their impact was considerable. These scientometric figures are difficult to interpret because no qualitative analysis of the citations has been performed: what exactly has been cited, and was the quotation negative or positive?[96] Still, these curves show that the onset of this dramatic period in pharmacology and physiology was evoked simultaneously by both theoretical concepts and pharmaceutical compounds. The latter dropped out of the news but remained the subject of informal scientific communication.[97]

Mainstream thinking in academic pharmacology and physiology considered further differentiation of beta receptors unnecessary or even counter-productive.[98] Moran presented a paper at the 2nd Symposium on Catecholamines in which he discussed the state of the art regarding the pharmacological characterization of adrenergic receptors. He conceptualized the receptor as follows:

"First, it is assumed that there are constituents of cells, e.g., receptors, which react selectively with certain agonists. Secondly, it is assumed that the receptor-agonist interaction represents the first step

of a multistep sequential reaction which leads to the response of the cell. Such a sequential reaction can be viewed symbolically as

$$A \ + \ R \rightarrow AR \rightarrow a \rightarrow b \rightarrow c \rightarrow n \rightarrow Ef$$

where R is the receptor, AR the complex of agonist and receptor, a, b, c,n, the sequential steps subsequent to the receptor, and Ef the effect. Since the individual steps in most reactions are unknown, the receptor can be viewed most conveniently in an operational sense as the entire sequence from R to n,

$$A \ + \ \boxed{R \rightarrow AR \rightarrow a \rightarrow b \rightarrow c \rightarrow n} \rightarrow Ef$$

where all of the intermediate steps are unknown".[99]

The entire sequence from R to n was defined by Moran as **the operationally defined receptor.**[100] On the basis of this definition the variety of tissue responses could be explained by referring to divergent reaction sequences and blockade at separate sites in these sequences. For the time being no further differentiation of receptor subtypes seemed to be necessary: *"At present, the broad classification of two main adrenergic receptor types (∂and ß, RV) is the simplest and most convenient".*[101]

In contrast, pharmacologists and clinicians involved in therapeutic research in the beta blocker field, acknowledged that adrenergic receptors were by far more complex than originally envisaged. Braunwald, for example, stated that: *"(...) it should be evident that exploitation of the differences between beta adrenergic receptors in various tissues might make it possible to block selectively only certain beta adrenergic functions".* [102]

Furthermore, it is worth mentioning that at the time Lands elaborated his classification of $ß_1$- and $ß_2$-receptors he worked at the Sterling Winthrop Institute, i.e. in an industrial setting. Participants, involved in research on beta stimulating and blocking drugs during the 1960s, argued that Lands' theory came with the discovery of the selective compounds.

Jack commented: *"Our understanding of the theory came more with the discovery of salbutamol than before its discovery. It was only when the properties of that drug became clear that I was forced to ask why was it so different from the ones that went before. Lands had recently proposed the subdivision of beta-receptors into beta-1 and beta-2 subtypes but his evidence was thin since the selectivity ratio of his catecholamines was only about 20-fold. Salbutamol was the first vindication of Lands' hypothesis because we found it to be at least 1000 times more active on guinea pig tracheal muscle than on heart rate in isolated right atria and hundreds of time more active than on the force of contraction of left atria. Such differences were obviously real and consistent with the proposed subdivision of receptors".*[103]

Engelhardt, who worked at Boehringer Ingelheim and who was also involved in the search for bronchodilating drugs, commented in a similar way, yet added a typical industrial attitude towards Lands' theory: *"I have never had a high opinion of this rigid system of beta-1 and beta-2 since, in my experience, the changes from substance to substance are gradual and there really isn't such a sharp distinction. There is if you single out a few prototypes, but if you look at larger substance series, they merge smoothly. Therefore I have never really liked this idea or indication of this relatively* *inflexible classification into beta-1 and beta-2. But the differentiation, that is possible of course, we had already had that here in a model before Lands and the others appeared. For the fact is that we already had Berotec (fenoterol, RV), hadn`t we? That is from 1964 I think. That was the first agonist that clearly showed this differentiation".*[104]

In accordance with the accounts of Jack and Engelhardt, Carlsson wrote: *"I had the privilege of serving as a consultant at Hässle at that time, and, still maintaining this privilege, I have thus been able to follow the development of beta-adrenergic antagonists rather closely over the years. This area is a good example of the interaction between basic research and drug development. The new compounds serve as important research tools to define the receptors and to discover new receptor subtypes. The new knowledge thus obtained forms the basis for systematic work that aims at finding specific agents, acting selectively on one of the subtypes. In this way, the cardio-selective agents, the so-called second generation of beta-receptor antagonists, could be developed".*[105]

These accounts point in the same direction: the discovery of the selective compounds preceded theory, yet at the same time stress different aspects. Jack considers the compounds as evidence for the theory. Engelhardt points to the distance between theory and the wide range of compounds at the laboratory bench. Carlsson stresses the interaction between basic research and drug development.

However, it is worthwhile to be more specific about these events.

These compounds originated from industrial research programs with clear-cut therapeutic objectives. The compounds, studied by Levy, for example, were launched into the academic field by the Wellcome Research Laboratories.[106] Furthermore, the selective compounds were tested in experimental systems developed in order to classify compounds and receptors more precisely. These test-systems in their turn originated from specific therapeutic contexts: bronchodilation in the treatment of asthma, the relaxation of the womb to treat threatening abortion or premature delivery and the treatment of ocular, nasal or cardiovascular disorders. The compounds and the experimental systems were components of expanding therapeutic fields and of the divergence of pharmacological methodology into these areas. This two-tiered system of disciplinary expansion in pharmacology and a differentiation of therapeutic fields found crystallization at three levels[107].

1. **experimental**: specific test-systems became the targets of pharmacological research.

2. **technical**: specific compounds became the targets of comparative analysis of experimental results. At one time scientists in different fields used INPEA, MJ 1999, dichloroisoprenaline, pronethalol, Kö 592, isoprenaline and other compounds. Some time later they used propranolol, alprenolol, oxprenolol, pindolol, practolol, salbutamol, orciprenaline and terbutaline.

3. **theoretical and methodological**: theories (Ahlquist, Lands, drug-receptor theory) and methodologies (agonist-antagonist methodology) were created.

Each level had its own dynamics, yet interacted with the others and research at all levels was performed in both the industrial and academic context. Lands' theory was a creative contribution to pharmacological science but it was an ex-post-facto explanation as well. Not his theory but the creation of new compounds and experimental systems were the initiating events. Therapeutic constraints underlied his theory also and two examples attest to this point:

1. Lipolysis was but one metabolic effect of catecholamines, yet served as evidence while

showing a good correlation with the effects in the heart. In fact, metabolic effects raised much concern with respect to receptor classification and remained a major stumbling block to receptor theory.[108] The fact was that Lands' theory was projected upon the basic axis in the grid of pharmacological receptors: the heart and the lungs. This basic axis was also the result of therapeutic developments. From the viewpoint of beta blockade the undesired effects were in the lungs which raised much concern while the desired effects were in the heart. From the viewpoint of bronchodilator therapy the desired effector site was in the lungs while the undesired effects were in the heart.

2. Lands' classification - and the majority of the hypotheses of that time - rested upon an "one-organ one-receptor" assumption. Carlsson and Ablad were among the first to doubt this assumption and proposed the existence of both types of receptors in the various tissues.[109] Their doubts originated from their experiments on the receptors mediating the sinus rhythm in the heart. Thus, an experimental system that fell outside the scope of Lands, provided new theoretical insights. Moreover, their theory evolved through a comparative analysis of newly developed cardio-selective compounds with the non-selective standard drugs. When considering the interactions between the three levels described above, many different relationships may be noted. The development of the cardio-selective beta blockers reveals one particular pattern.[110]

The creation of Lands' theory has been described in detail because the development of the cardio-selective beta blockers is commonly considered within Lands' theoretical framework. The term "cardio-selectivity" as used nowadays arises from this framework.

This must not be confused with the term "(cardio)selective blockade" as used in th 1960s by the ICI team. Shanks and his colleagues did not refer to Lands' theory but largely drew upon the experimental work of Levy.[111] In fact, Lands' terminology was not applied to practolol until 1970 when during a symposium in London the term cardio-selectivity appeared.[112] According to Shanks Lands' theory had not much impact on the scientific world at that time.[113] Moreover, initially practolol did not attract much attention in pharmacology and physiology.[114] Robinson adds that beta receptors were still considered as hypothetical entities and theorizing about further differentiations of beta receptors was not taken very seriously.[115] According to the chemists, the ICI team exemplified a successful but also a very practical-empirical industrial research group.[116] Barrett stated: *"I don't think we paid very much attention to these developments (β_1-β_2 concepts of Lands, RV). This reflects the arrogance of a successful research team; the "who else is as good as we are" syndrome. Yes, we read the literature but I don't think we were very much influenced by it. As to the Lands classification I don't think we took it very seriously".*[117] Fitzgerald confirms the picture drawn by Barrett. According to him the nature of the group was responsible for selectively attuning to theoretical and practical developments in the experimental and clinical world: *"I mean, you have to understand the culture of the research department ... here have been very high calibre researchers. And that brings a certain security or arrogance which ever you want to call it. And so, yes, we had contacts but I think most people felt pretty secure in their own knowledge of the field. And so, we had six or seven absolutely outstanding people here in addition to Jim Black at that time".*[118] This is not to deny the fact that the ICI scientists tried to provide a theoretical basis for selective action but this project, started in 1968, was unsuccessful.[119]

The term selectivity therefore refers to a practical-experimental type of research and its origins must be sought in the use of specific test systems and compounds. To a large extent this type of research matched with Levy's experimental approach.[120] From this the search for selective drugs follows naturally.

4.2.5.3. The therapeutic interest

The selective action of practolol was but one aspect of the drug. It had become clear that practolol was a far less aggressive drug than propranolol. The general feeling was that practolol was an easy drug to administrate: it was non-toxic, its potency was one-third or one-fourth of propranolol, and it produced less cardiac depression than equi-active beta blocking doses of propranolol.[121] Yet, the drug had the same beneficial effects as propranolol. But practolol was also a puzzling compound. It reduced exercise tachycardia to the same extent as propranolol, but not isoprenaline tachycardia. Differing cardiovascular responses were observed when investigating the drug in animals pre-treated with various forms of anaesthesia, in conscious versus anaesthetized animals, and in animals versus man. And so, practolol was interesting for different reasons.

The drug seemed a logical candidate to be developed as the "intravenous" beta blocker. The issue was heavily debated in the narrow circle of consultants as well as in the cardiology community at large. Indeed, practolol was very, very mild on the heart, even when injected. As Robinson commented:

"My memories of practolol are that the most striking thing about it was how much safer it was when you gave it intravenously and all of us by that time had disastrous experiences with intravenous propranolol, usually in rhythm disturbances after infarction. (..) It quickly became apparent that whereas when you gave intravenous propranolol in that situation it always made the patients' circulation worse and sometimes it was disastrous, you could give practolol and usually the patient didn't mind having it at all. It was very obvious, the difference. Because we were dealing with a high-risk group of patients you didn't have to use it very often before it became apparent without formal trial that it was a lot safer than propranolol because propranolol always made them sicker".[122]

By that time, the competitive situation had changed. Oxprenolol was coming in and attracted much attention, particularly in the United Kingdom. Initially the ICI team did not worry too much:

"In 1964, when oxprenolol became a regular feature in European meetings and because of promotion of it by Ciba, we examined the compound in the laboratory. We found that it had some intrinsic sympathomimetic activity but were not very impressed by it. Perhaps it was a good example of British insularity: it was a foreign drug; it came from somewhere in Europe. Our colleagues in ICI, working in Europe, were more aware of its market potential because of the close relationship between physicians in continental Europe and Ciba, a trusted company".[123]

These warnings were not picked up but with the growing scepticism and negative experiences in the clinical world with propranolol, optimism at ICI waned. But not only at ICI. About 1967, Pfizer, for example, hesitated also in bringing pindolol on the market as an "intravenous beta blocker" and called off its attempt at that time since they felt there was no future for this type of drug.[124] Similar notes were struck at the managerial and marketing level: "Let's wait and see".[125] However, the research team exerted strong pressure to continue the project, and with success: profiling of the drugs was allowed to continue. Still, ICI struggled against the growing feeling in the medical world that its leading drug was too aggressive and too dangerous for ordinary use.

In this changing context, i.e. the rapidly growing clinical scepticism about propranolol, the discussion about an intravenous beta blocker within ICI and the industrial competition between Ciba and ICI, Barrett highlights the development of practolol as a cardio-selective beta blocker: *"Now when the oxprenolol issue began to be perceived by the UK marketing people of ICI, I believed they then saw that a new compound would be more advantageous than trying to defend the old compound. That was one thing which began to come from marketing. The other thing was a comment by Dr. Davey in one of our meetings that if we found that practolol did not have such an effective blockade of vasodepressant response, maybe it doesn't have so effective blockade of the bronchodilator response and we said, well perhaps.... but a search was organized of the research data (notwithstanding the scepticism of the investigating pharmacologists) and produced results which showed, to my surprise, that of all the compounds which had the best separation between blocking the heart rate and blocking the fall in blood pressure from the same dose of isoprenaline in anaesthetized cats, the best compound was our old friend ... practolol!"*.[126] Thus, Davey connected the aspect of selective action in beta blockade to a decreased risk of bronchospasm.[127]

The above reveals the particular context in which the term "cardio-selectivity" must be considered. This term implied the separation of hitherto indivisibly connected actions. But this term was beset with different interpretations which may be conveniently mapped out between two extremes: an **intra-cardiac** and an **extra-cardiac** meaning.

The intra-cardiac interpretation implied the differentiation of beta blocking effects in the heart, e.g. between chronotropic and inotropic actions of beta blocking compounds. These two actions were taken to be synonymous with beta blockade. In his introduction to the articles about propranolol in the American Journal of Cardiology, Braunwald speculated as follows:

"(...) it should be evident that exploitation of the differences between beta adrenergic receptors in various tissues might make it possible to block selectively only certain beta adrenergic functions. For example, if an agent were found which would block the beta adrenergic receptors in the sinoatrial node and specialized conduction tissue of the heart without affecting the beta receptors **in the ventricular myocardium** *(this author's emphasis, RV), then the anti-arrhythmic properties of such a drug which are exerted on these tissues might not be limited by its simultaneous removal of sympathetic support to the myocardium"*.[128]

The extra-cardiac interpretation implied differential effects between the heart and other tissues and organs. The effects on the peripheral vessels and on the lung were of interest for various therapeutic reasons.

The question arises if and how these interpretations influenced the ICI team. Fitzgerald emphasized the intra-cardiac interpretation: *"We were intrigued to find a drug that slows the heart with no effect on contractility. Practolol didn't change cardiac output. People were obsessed"*. [129]

In contrast, Shanks stressed the extra-cardiac interpretation of the differential effects of practolol on the heart and the blood vessels having motivated the team to capitalize upon the issue of selective blockade. Still, Shanks agreed that practolol attracted so much interest because it was a far less aggressive drug than propranolol.[130]

Indeed, the intriguing feature of practolol was that it was apparently such a safe drug, i.e. that it **seemed to affect the crucial hemodynamic parameters differently** to propranolol. Attempts were made to explain this in terms of specific properties of the drug but no satisfactory explanation could be given. In fact, practolol is still a mysterious drug.[131]

However, the context of the problem changed significantly in the ensuing years. As physicians gained experience with the beta blockers, they raised their standards to exclude patients with incipient and manifest heart failure from treatment with beta blockers. The issue was settled by restricting the use of propranolol. What remains of this dramatic period is the present disbelief that heart failure was once such a controversial issue. What also remains, is this unique selective action of practolol, so creatively unraveled by Shanks and his colleagues. But it was not merely pharmacological curiosity that motivated the team but also another therapeutic target, the risk of bronchial spasm, which formed a major impetus to develop this aspect of the drug.

4.3. The beta blocker project of Eli Lilly & Co.

In 1957 dichloroisoprenaline (DCI) was launched by the Lilly scientists, & Co. Powell and Slater.[132] The compound had been synthesized and screened in the mid 1950s for bronchodilator activity. The test-system used was the recovery of adrenaline-induced relaxation of tracheal tissue. Instead of the recovery expected, the compound produced the opposite effect, and further investigations revealed that all "inhibitory" actions of adrenaline were antagonized by the compound.

Moran attended the presentation of the paper by Slater in 1957 and "was struck by the fact that this compound might fit into Ahlquist's scheme of **alpha** and **beta** adrenergic receptors and that the heart was the crucial item".[133] Moran and Perkins went straight to the heart as the fundamental problem in the study of adrenergic mechanisms. From their results obtained with DCI they concluded that the compound confirmed Ahlquist's scheme of classification.[134] Powell and Slater readily agreed with this conclusion: "*In any event, the data* (those of Moran and Perkins, RV) *seems to add support for the Ahlquist concept of alpha and beta adrenergic receptors and suggests that this separation provides an useful frame of reference in discussions of sympathomimetic amines*".[135] Although the work of Moore and Swain and others on the beta blocking action of DCI is referred to, the authors were very cautious about the results.[136]

It is striking to see how DCI became the focal point of scientific attention and how it was used as an investigational tool: to tackle the separation of alpha and beta receptor mediated responses in various tissues; to re-evaluate the cardiac effects of the classic adrenergic blocking agents as phenoxybenzamine and phentolamine; to use as a key component in early structure-activity relationship (SAR) studies; and to establish the specificity of beta blockade.[137] This early work on DCI restrained chemical manipulation and helped to elucidate the basic issue of partial antagonism. According to Dresel (1960) who had shown that DCI exhibited considerable adrenaline-like activity - "high intrinsic activity" - this action of DCI decreased its value as an investigational tool.[138]

As described in Chapter 3 the profile of DCI as an anti-arrhythmic agent was created.[139] However, two problems emerged. On the one hand the theoretical problem: "Is it beta blockade or some non-specific action that inhibits the sensitivity of cardiac tissue to dysrythm?". On the other hand, the experimental techniques used became subject of discussion: "Do these experimental systems represent the ischemic state of the diseased heart?".[140] Both problems were fundamental to the course of academic research and evoked much caution in the field. Thus, academic pharmacologists posed at a very early stage the problem of specificity of beta blockade in cardiac arrhythmias. This problem was set aside by the ICI team because the therapeutic objective of the team had shifted from ventricular fibrillation to angina pectoris.

This clear-cut difference in therapeutic goal explains to a great extent the reserved attitude at Lilly. In an early phase Lilly's Cardiovascular Research Group had discussed the therapeutic potential of DCI but showed no further interest. As commented by Slater: *"We understood what we had found but underestimated the degree of intrinsic activity. We had few ideas for clinical utility and were not in a position to do detailed cardiovascular studies"*.[141] Caution in the academic world about the potential of DCI probably affected Lilly's decision taking but provided a therapeutic target: cardiac dysrythm. The compound was tried in patients with ventricular fibrillation and grave tachycardia but serious clinical problems arose that were attributed to the high degree of intrinsic activity.[142] The Lilly team returned to their laboratory bench trying to find a compound with less intrinsic activity. Amongst 100 compounds synthesized they found pronethalol and filed a patent but were too late.[143]

The Lilly story underlines the importance of the therapeutic target being connected to the main research program within a pharmaceutical company.

4.4. The beta blocker project of Mead Johnson

In the second half of the 1950s Mead Johnson Pharmaceutical Company became involved in the study of phenethanolamines, a class of drugs that were known to be very potent inhibitors of smooth muscle. A broad project was set up covering several therapeutic disorders: nasal decongestion, asthmatic attacks, and uterus relaxant action in threatened miscarriage. The pharmacological objective of this broad scope of therapeutic interest was to find antispasmodic drugs.

In 1960 the research group of Mead Johnson published their first results, e,g. a survey of the effects of isoxsuprine on non-vascular smooth muscle, and opens as follows: *"Among the phenethanolamines can be found the most potent of all known inhibitors of smooth muscle. Little practical use has been made of this property because of the concurrent existence of sympathomimetic, cardiovascular side-effects. Recently, however, a compound of this nature has been reported to produce pronounced relaxation of vascular smooth muscle with only minimal cardiac stimulation"*.[144]

Since isoxsuprine was credited with vasodilator properties, its potential in the treatment of peripheral vascular and coronary heart disease was rapidly acknowledged. The compound was developed by several companies in continental Europe and also developed by Mead

Johnson.[145] To the Mead Johnson scientists, the class of phenethanolamines seemed to be promising because the various analogues revealed marked differences in response, not yet exploited extensively by other companies. As it turned out, the phenethanolamines were the target for many industrial groups in the 1950s.[146]

During the search for bronchodilator compounds the Mead Johnson team also manipulated the chemical structure of isoprenaline. By introducing sulphonamide groups into the benzene ring the chemists discovered promising lead-compounds (table 4.4).[147]

Table 4.4
Structures of sulphonamidophenethanolamines at Mead Johnson.
Reproduced with permission from Larsen and Lish (1964).

Compound	R^1	R^2	R^3	R^4
MJ 1999	CH_3SO_2NH	H	H	$-CH(CH_3)_2$
MJ 1998	CH_3SO_2NH	H	CH_3	$-CH_3$
MJ 1996	H	CH_3SO_2NH	H	$-CH_3$
MJ 1995	H	CH_3SO_2NH	H	$-CH(CH_3)CH_2OC_6H_5$
MJ 1993	OH	CH_3SO_2NH	H	$-CH_3$
MJ 1992	OH	CH_3SO_2NH	H	$-CH(CH_3)_2$
MJ 1991	OH	CH_3SO_2NH	H	$-CH(CH_3)CH_2OC_6H_5$
Phenylephrine	H	OH	H	$-CH_3$
Epinephrine	OH	OH	H	$-CH_3$
Isoproterenol	OH	OH	H	$-CH(CH_3)_2$
Isoxsuprine	OH	H	CH_3	$-CH(CH_3)CH_2OC_6H_5$
Dichloroisoproterenol	Cl	Cl	H	$-CH(CH_3)_2$

The header structure above the table: $R^1 - \langle \text{benzene ring} \rangle - CHOHCHNHR^4$ with R^2 and R^3 substituents.

MJ 1999 (sotalol) and MJ 1998 are beta-receptor blocking agents.[148] MJ 1996 (amidephrine) is a potent alpha-receptor stimulant and pressor substance. Structural changes of this MJ 1996 molecule converts it into a depressor substance with beta-receptor stimulant action as is the case with MJ 1995. MJ 1993 is a potent pressor substance with slightly less beta-receptor stimulating activity than adrenaline. MJ 1992 is a depressor substance and a highly active beta-receptor stimulant, whereas MJ 1991 possesses in addition an alpha-receptor blocking activity of about 10% of phentanolamine, a potent alpha blocker. MJ 1996 was developed as a nasal decongestant, MJ 1992 as a selective bronchodilator while MJ 1998 and MJ 1999 were interesting for their beta blocking properties.

The beta blocking properties of MJ 1999 and MJ 1998 were revealed in test-systems using lung and uterus tissue. Both compounds were recognized because of their similarity of action with dichloroisoprenaline.[149] For some time there was no cardiovascular therapeutic orientation. Human studies were started for the nasal decongestant and the bronchodilator, not for the beta blocking compounds. From the ICI chemists it was learned that Mead Johnson had decided to leave the field after Black and Stephenson published their results with pronethalol.[150] However, the Mead Johnson team performed extensive cardiovascular and toxicological studies comparing MJ 1998, MJ 1999 and pronethalol[151]; and human studies with sotalol started around 1965. In 1965 a series of three articles was published covering the spectrum of actions of alpha and beta receptors in a variety of tissues. These articles were impressing because it appeared as though the Mead Johnson scientists had intellectually completed their work on the beta adrenoceptors antagonists and were launching their results into the academic and industrial world.

In summary, the beta blocker project at Mead Johnson project was contained within a broad research program searching for antispasmodic drugs for various therapeutic purposes. The compounds MJ 1998 and MJ 1999 were compared with pronethalol but there was no clear-cut cardiovascular objective.[152]

4.5. The beta blocker project of AB Hässle[153]

4.5.1. The early phase

AB Hässle is the oldest pharmaceutical company in Sweden, founded in 1904 and located in Hässleholm, a town in the south of Sweden. The little company was taken over by Astra in 1942. In 1953 the production of Hässle's products was transferred to Astra's factory in Södertalje close to Stockholm. The company's small group for drug development and the marketing department moved to Göteborg where a new medical school had been founded at the University of Göteborg providing the benefits of close collaboration.

The development of a modern R&D organisation gradually started based on collaboration with scientists at the University of Göteborg, especially the medical faculty, and the faculty of pharmacy, now in Uppsala but at that time in Stockholm. Trying to find meaningful objectives for drug development Östholm consulted several scientists in pre-clinical and clinical research. Folkow, professor in physiology, and Werkö, professor of cardiology, both underlined the need for better drugs for the treatment of cardiovascular disease. It was decided that Hässle should concentrate the company's limited resources for R&D in trying to develop cardiovascular drugs.

In 1958 Werkö recommended that Hässle start looking for anti-arrhythmic agents. At that time Hässle had no resources for chemical synthesis and biological testing. In co-operation with the faculty of pharmacy at Stockholm, Hässle had developed and patented a new principle to administer drugs in tablets giving controlled release of the active drug. This was the so-called Durules-principle. Werkö suggested that the Durules principle be tried to give a longer duration of action of the anti-arrhythmic drug quinidine so the drug could be given twice daily instead of three to four times daily. The aim of that project was also to reduce side-effects of the drug by cutting the peak of absorption. Since Werkö and his medical team were investigating quinidine as a treatment of ventricular fibrillation, a serious complication of myocardial infarction, and since blood plasma levels of this drug could be easily determined, a slow release preparation of quinidine was developed. Thus, the little company achieved a reasonable success; this slow release preparation still returns considerable profit.

In March 1959 Hässle started to build up a department for chemical synthesis of new compounds. The pharmacological screening during 1959 was performed by external labs but a pharmacological department was set up in 1960. Again Werkö recommended that anti-arrhythmic agents should be the priority project. He suggested that the chemical structure of quinidine should be used as a lead for the chemists. The aim of the "Anti-arrhythmic Agent Project" was to develop drugs with less side-effects than quinidine. Procainamide was also mentioned as a drug which could be looked upon as a lead.

In search of new screening methods for anti-arrhythmic drugs Hässle came in contact with Dr. Roberts at the Cornell University in New York.[154] He had studied a method, the "Vagus-amine dose test", for the in vivo evaluation of depressant drugs of the rhythmic function of the heart. The test system was based on the idea that amines like adrenaline and noradrenaline were important in the regulation of cardiac rhythm and were responsible for 'ectopic beats' in some pathological conditions. Adrenaline-induced arrhythmias formed a rather well-known experimental approach in pharmacology and physiology of cardiac rhythm. The "Vagus-amine dose test", however, was designed to determine potency curves of drugs that would depress the ectopic rhythm potential of amines. In this way quantitative measurements of depressant drugs in intact animals could be performed.[155]

This test-system was used as a primary screening test to search for "anti-adrenergic" drugs. Ahlquist's theory was not in the picture. In August 1960 Corrodi - *a chemist who could make literally every molecule*[156] - joined the team. It is interesting to note that at this stage the principle structure of pronethalol was one of the structures suggested by the leader of the project in february 1960, Dr. Corrodi; due to lack of resources these compounds were not synthesized.[157]

The project was not successful. In 1961 Östholm invited Dr. Arvid Carlsson, professor of pharmacology, to be a consultant of AB Hässle. Östholm comments:

"The most important result of the discussions with Arvid Carlsson was that he convinced me that screening of compounds using traditional pharmacological test methods were likely to lead to me-too drugs. Instead of aiming at defined clinical indications by screening for e.g. anti-arrhythmic agents he recommended us to start a new research project by looking at new biological concepts and elucidate the mechanism of e.g. agonists and antagonists on the adrenergic receptors in the heart. In doing so we might find anti-arrhythmic agents but also other drugs for treatment of cardiovascular diseases. He suggested that we should start from DCI as a chemical lead in synthesizing compounds for biological evaluation. At that time we at Hässle had never heard anything about the concept of adrenergic beta receptor blockade. It was introduced to us by Arvid Carlsson".[158]

Carlsson was mainly interested in the pharmacology of neurotransmitters and the central nervous system.[159] Since catecholamines were of importance to his work, he had visited the first Symposium on Catecholamines in Bethesda, Maryland in 1958. He was familiar with the field as a scientist and was interested in the Hässle project: *"I was not primarily interested in cardiac arrhythmias, I was interested by the concept. Blocking the sympathetic control of the heart. It seemed to me a reasonable thing".[160]*

Since dichloroisoprenaline was the basis of the concept of beta blockade, it was taken as lead-compound by the Hässle team. The project was re-named "Beta Adrenoceptor Blocking Agents". According to Carlsson this change of terminology reflected the conceptual shift, not a therapeutic re-orientation.[161] However, since beta blockade was a central theme of the project, the new territory of anginal attacks as put forward by the ICI-team in 1962, was easily assimilated. Hässle's main clinical interest was not only to develop anti-arrhythmic agents but drugs which could protect the heart from too much stimulation caused by emotional and physical stress: *"We talked about nervous heart disease"*. [162]

When the ICI team published their paper in 1962, it was realized that another, more powerful, group operated in the same area and was leading the way. At that time several compounds had been evaluated and one compound, H 29/50 (N-isopropyl-phenylethanolamine), selected for testing in man. Some other compounds, alpha-methyl derivatives of H 29/50 (figure 4.4(a)) exhibited unexpected effects: *"There were some drugs that had some funny differences in profile. That we found interesting"*. [163]

Since these compounds were very close to dichloroisoprenaline, they were sent to Moran in 1963 because of his great experience with that compound.[164] Hässle had contacts with Moran's Department; Dr. Ablad, who would become the leading scientist of the Hässle team, worked at the time in Moran's laboratory. Moran found interesting results that suggested *"a difference in cardiac and vasodilator adrenergic receptors and a need for further evaluation of the present beta-receptor classification"*.[165] In a very early stage the selective action of beta blockers was found due to Hässle's open communication with academic research but it remained a neglected area for some years. This academic orientation was reinforced by Ablad who had been trained both in animal and human pharmacology of the cardiovascular system. His arrival would turn out to be decisive in Hässle's success.

Initially, however, the project reached a deadlock. When the compound H 29/50 was tested in man, in Spring 1963, human volunteers responded with tachycardia and palpitations. These undesirable effects were attributed to the intrinsic activity of the compound. The same problem as with dichloroisoprenaline hindered further development.

In 1963 the Hässle team began to synthesize a new class of compounds: sympatholytic agents with a benzodioxane ring (figure 4.4(b)).

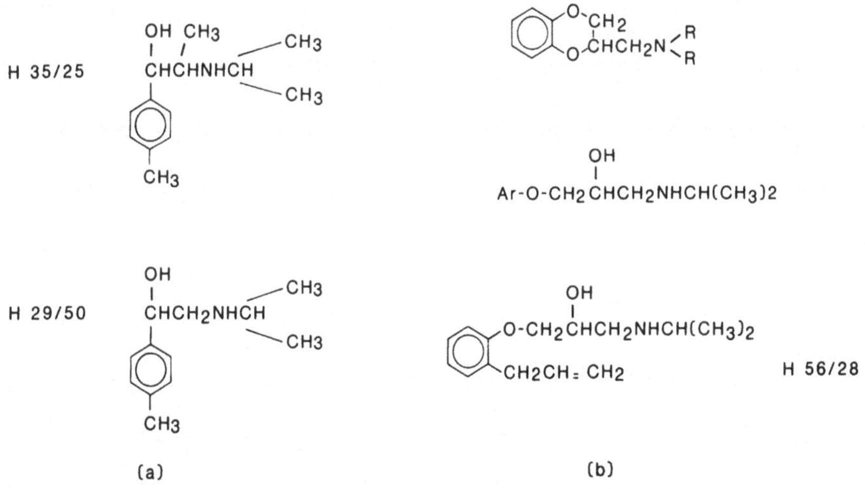

Figure 4.4
Chemical structures of beta blocking compounds found during the AB Hässle project:
(a) 1961-1962; (b) 1963-1964.

This class of substances originated from the work performed by Fourneau. The chemists opened the benzodioxane ring and replaced the tertiary amino group by an isopropylamino group. Almost 100 substances of this type were synthesized and tested. This class finally yielded a promising compound: H 56/28 (alprenolol). The Hässle team therefore claims to have arrived at alprenolol before propranolol was described, a claim supported also by Shanks.[166]

In contrast, Barrett and the chemists of ICI hold the position that alprenolol and oxprenolol as ring-opened propranolols were missed during testing at ICI.[167] Thus, competitors were able to enter the market with similar compounds after propranolol had been discovered. However much this may be true, and indeed this is the case with Ciba-Geigy, this position does not exclude the possibility that other firms arrived at such compounds before ICI.[168] In fact, Boehringer synthesized propranolol even before ICI did (chapter 7). At Hässle the first compound with the propranol-amino-side-chain as in propranolol was made in April 1964.[169] Berntsson comments: *"The first public disclosure of this kind of compound from ICI came in mid May 1964 and thus Hässle had started making this kind of compound before they knew about ICI's structures. H 56/28 later to become alprenolol was made on 27th of August 1964".*[170] During the period May - August 1964 the Hässle team feverishly attempted to find a suitable candidate. Since ICI patents formed an important set back for synthesizing new compounds, the feeling of a crisis evolved - *"Everything seemed hopeless"*[171] - until the line of research, started independently from ICI, yielded the success so eagerly strived for.[172]

The discovery of alprenolol as a patentable compound saved the project. Carlsson adds that Hässle was very lucky indeed.[173] In 1965, on January 2nd, a "crash program" started to bring alprenolol through toxicology, bio-availability study and animal and human pharmacology. Clinical studies started in June 1965 and in 1967 all the results were published.[174]

The design of the project was similar to that of other industrial firms. The various properties of alprenolol were obtained through an internal comparative research program using INPEA, MJ 1999, propranolol, alprenolol and some other compounds that originated from Hässle's laboratories. Swedish clinicians were very responsive to this type of drug and propranolol was investigated at several Swedish clinical centres.[175] From Hässle's point of view propranolol was the drug to compete with. The issue of intrinsic sympathomimetic activity of alprenolol came increasingly to the fore. Physiological, pharmacological and medical concepts about the sympathetic control of the cardiovascular system merged.

4.5.2. Intrinsic sympathomimetic activity of alprenolol

The "official history" of Hässle reports that the idea to ensure a physiological balance between adrenergic beta blockade and beta stimulation had been formulated at a very early stage: *"The project started early in 1960, being concerned with the development of a new anti-arrhythmic drug. At an early stage of the project the following goal was defined. Efforts should be made to develop a compound blocking the adrenergic beta-receptor, which should ensure a physiological balance between adrenergic beta-blockade and beta-stimulation".*[176] The accumulated influence of several events from different sources, however, seems to be more likely.

This idea emerged in the therapeutic context of cardiac arrhythmias. Excessive tachycardia and ectopic rhythm were the phenomena to be eliminated, but the body should be able to respond to various stimuli to the cardiovascular system, for example by enhancing cardiac activity through increasing frequency rate. From the medical point of view there is ample reason to suggest a balanced view between stimulation and blockade of adrenergic beta receptors in the heart. Beta blockade may give rise to bradycardia which is an undesired effect in a variety of cardiac arrhythmias, yet a desired action in other arrhythmic forms. Moreover, sympathomimetic agents were used in some types of cardiac arrhythmias but were contra-indicated in others. Thus, the adrenergic system as far as cardiac rhythmic function was concerned, was not an all-or-nothing system.

The idea of a physiological balance per se came in 1961 from Folkow.[177] Tracing this idea, Folkow and his team appeared to be involved in an extensive series of experiments during the 1950s and early 1960s concerning the sympathetic control of the cardiovascular system.[178] Folkow's ideas deviated from the classic view of Cannon about the all-or-nothing response of the adrenergic system, i.e. that it was merely involved in mass-activation responses during the defence reaction - the "emergency" responses of the organism in case of danger, emotional stress and fear. Therefore, Folkow investigated the functional differentiation of the sympathetic system at several levels and in several situations. He established that the direct sympathetic influence on the heart - using change of heart rate as an indicator of the effector response - was by far superior to the effects induced by the hormones from the adrenal medulla. This demonstrated a clear-cut functional differentiation between the two components of the sympathetic system: the hormonal and the nervous.[179]

In the same way he differentiated between the effects of the parasympathetic and sympathetic component of vegetative control of the cardiovascular system. Even so, Folkow established that within narrow margins of sympathetic stimulation a whole range of cardiovascular effector responses could be obtained. Folkow used physiological experimental procedures to measure the firing of sympathetic nerves in various physiological conditions. The results indicated that when animals are at rest, the average discharge rate in these nerves amounted to approximately 1 impulse/second. During emergency situations of excessive sympathetic activation the discharge rate merely increased to about 10 and maximally 20 impulses/second.[180]

Therefore, the concept of a balance - or in more modern terms "modulation" - with regard to the sympathetic control of the heart involves three aspects. Firstly, a balance between sympathetic and parasympathetic control of the heart. Secondly, the balance in sympathetic control through differentiated patterns of responses in various parts of the cardiovascular system. Thirdly, the balance between resting state - "endogenous sympathetic tone" - and the state of emergency - stress, anxiety, excitation and exercise. Particularly this latter aspect would turn out as crucial in signifying the pharmacological concept "intrinsic sympathomimetic activity".

However, the translation of this general idea of a balance into clear-cut pharmacological language has not followed a simple linear course. The intrinsic sympathomimetic activity did not play a major role in the early phase of the project. The negative clinical experiences with

DCI at Lilly were known to the Hässle team and strengthened the idea of reducing intrinsic sympathomimetic activity. The major problem was to find a suitable compound that would not give rise to tachycardia and other clinically undesirable effects. When H 29/50 failed at the clinical level and alprenolol turned out to be a promising compound though with some intrinsic activity, this aspect of the drug was related to the concept of balance.

4.5.3. The profiling of alprenolol

When heart failure became a central theme in the beta blocker field, awareness grew that sympathetic control was not merely detrimental to the patient's condition or that its sole function was to cope with emergency reactions. The Hässle team developed the view of beta blockade in terms of modulation, i.e. damping the sympathetic drive of the heart without disturbing the basal cardiac function.

The analogy of a room with a dimmer turning on light may help us to understand some basic concepts. A beta-receptor stimulating agent acts as the hand that touches the dimmer ("affinity for the receptor") and subsequently turns it until the room is brightly lit ("intrinsic activity" which is in this case maximal). A beta blocker acts like a lock, that is, it attaches to the dimmer but does not turn it ("no intrinsic activity", e.g. "complete beta blockade" as with propranolol) and prevents the hand from turning the dimmer. Alternatively, a beta blocker with intrinsic sympathomimetic activity (ISA) does touch the dimmer, turns it but never maximally ("partial agonist"). Now, it is easy to understand that compounds with varying degrees of ISA light up the room in varying shades and degrees. DCI, for example, which has an intrinsic activity of 0.73 compared to the maximal response of isoprenaline (= 1.00) lights up the room fairly well while alprenolol with an intrinsic activity of 0.16 provides a narrow shaft of light.

The patient with a heart which is abnormally dependent on an elevated sympathetic tone, e.g. in the case of heart failure, is analogous to the room at night. In order to walk around and to do things we need some light. If the light is turned out, we are helpless and we might hurt ourselves.

The question now arose as to whether the property of intrinsic activity afforded a significant therapeutic advantage. To elucidate this problem scientists need some artificial system in which the various states of the sympathetic system in the organism can be mimicked. That is to say they attempt to create a room with a switch that can be manipulated in a variety of conditions. Isoprenaline, acknowledged as the purest beta-1 receptor stimulant was used as the artificial hand to turn on light of different intensities.

The experimental model to investigate this issue became the vagotomized and adrenalectomized cat.[181] The basic idea of the test is that by cutting the nervus vagus (vagotomized cat) parasympathetic influences on the heart are eliminated. By removing the adrenals the hormonal part of the adrenergic system (adrenolectomy) is switched off. A 'clean' experimental system remains that can be manipulated in two principal ways. The first way is the reserpinized cat. The other is the non-reserpinized cat.

Injection of reserpine causes depletion of all the storage vesicles in the body that contain noradrenaline.[182] The reserpinized cat represents the organism deprived of any endogenous sympathetic activity and the various levels of sympathetic activity may be mimicked by administrating isoprenaline. Consequently, the non-reserpinized cat reflects the basal state of the sympathetic system.

In this way scientists hoped to obtain information about the direct effects of beta blockers on a heart devoid of vegetative control as well as the intrinsic activity of these compounds.

It falls outside the scope of this section to discuss the experiments that the Hässle team performed. Suffice to say that the test system described was used by the Hässle team to profile alprenolol with reference to other beta blocking compounds, to separate the various properties of these agents and to bring the contrasts between propranolol and alprenolol to the foreground.

Obviously, the (non-)reserpinized cat is a highly idealized test system. The system thus had to be interpreted both physiologically and clinically.

Figure 4.5 illustrates how Folkow's physiological work underlied the pharmacological experiments of the Hässle team to contrast alprenolol with propranolol.

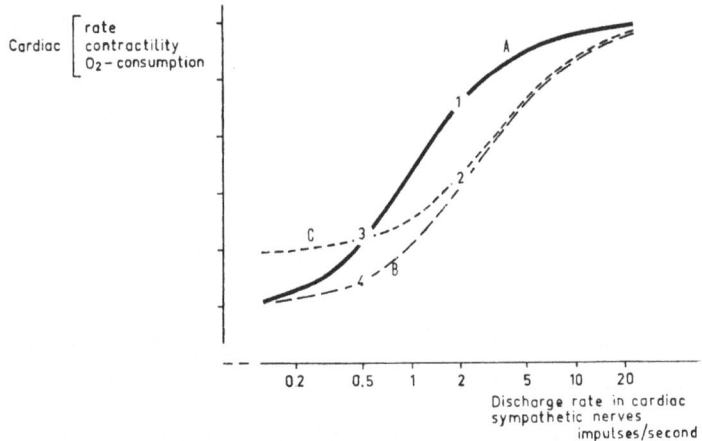

Figure 4.5
The influence of Folkow's physiological concept of balance on the pharmacological profiling of alprenolol and propranolol.
Reproduced with permission from Astra (1972).

The diagram depicts three curves in a conventionalized way which represent three types of relationships between sympathetic control and cardiac activity. Curve A represents the normal physiological situation. Curve B and C represent beta blockade without and with ISA, i.e. propranolol and alprenolol respectively.

The suggestion is clear. Propranolol completely blocks beta receptors and thus decreases the effects of sympathetic discharge rates over the whole range. Alprenolol leaves the adaptive potential of the sympathetic control of the heart intact over the range of the resting state whereas it cuts off this control at high(er) levels of sympathetic activity. Thus, physiology and pharmacology become deeply interrelated.

This interrelationship leads to medical concepts about angina pectoris and the role of the sympathetic control of the heart. Cardiologists agreed that blockade of high(er) levels of sympathetic activity was desirable in anti-anginal treatment whereas reduction of the basal state of the sympathetic drive was undesirable in angina patients with manifest or incipient heart failure. This agreement arose out of the view that the artificial hand, i.e. isoprenaline, had its analogy in the clinic. Isoprenaline and exercise induced hemodynamic patterns purportedly reflected the pattern of response of the sympathetic system both in normal human subjects and anginal patients. Both patterns underlined the clinical picture of angina of effort. Swedish doctors were responsive to this way of thinking, at an early stage. The relationship between angina of effort and the sympathetic system was extensively studied in Swedish cardiology.[183] Within this intellectual climate physiological and pharmacological concepts merged with the clinical view that the anginal state reflected an enhanced sympathetic drive of the heart.

Against this background the Hässle team profiled alprenolol in contrast with propranolol. Illustrative is the study of Forsberg and Johnsson assessing the effects of propranolol and alprenolol in five normal human subjects. Figure 4.6 represents the hemodynamic effects of propranolol and alprenolol (H56/28) as measured according to six hemodynamic parameters.

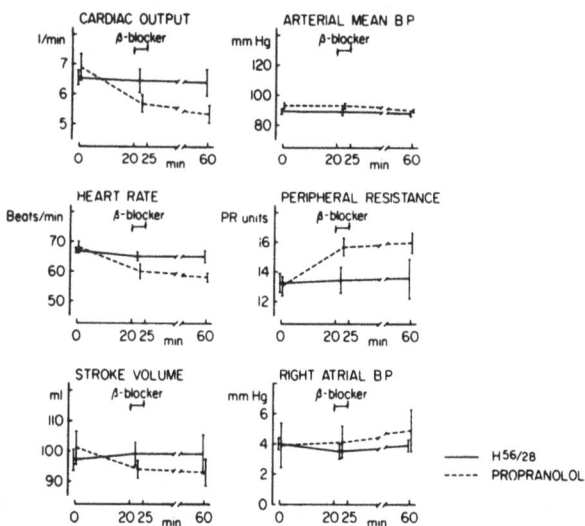

Figure 4.6
The profiles of alprenolol and propranolol according to six hemodynamic parameters.
Reproduced with permission from Forsberg and Johnsson (1967).

Propranolol markedly affected the six parameters while alprenolol does not alter them significantly. Though both compounds block the sympathetic drive to the heart to the same extent, e.g. the two compounds are equi-potent beta blockers, they influence basal hemodynamics differently. The hemodynamic effects of alprenolol are compensated by cardiac stimulation due to its intrinsic activity.[184]

4.5.4. Selective beta blockade

In 1964 the Hässle team had developed substances with different patterns of responses which included deviant actions on blood vessels. Some of these compounds were sent to Moran. The Hässle scientists were wondering about these unexpected response patterns: in particular they were curious about the clinical potential of compound H 35/25. This curiosity arose from the fact that Hässle possessed the distribution rights of some of Geigy's vasodilating agents such as apresoline. Since the team was fully engaged in the development of alprenolol during 1964-1966, and lacking sufficient financial and personnel resources, this remained a neglected area. During the crash program, somewhere in 1966, the Hässle team unexpectedly ran into the issue of selectivity. Ablad and coworkers were comparing some allyl-substituted phenoxypropranolamines (figure 4.7).

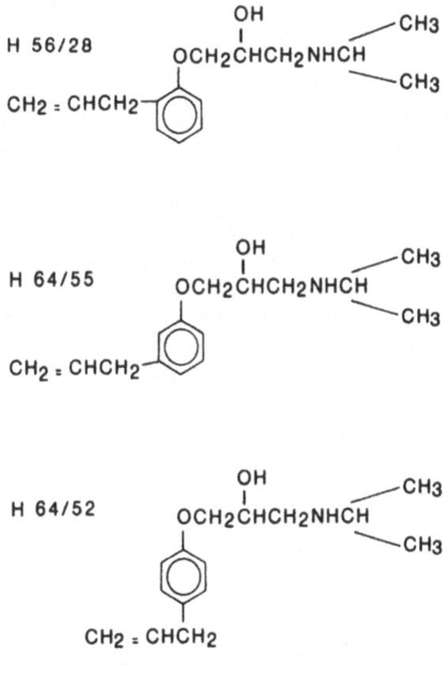

Figure 4.7
Selective beta blockers: allyl-substituted phenoxy-propranolamines in the Hässle project (1966).

Alprenolol (H 56/28) possesses an allyl-group in the ortho position whereas the compounds H 64/55 en H64/52 have the allyl group in the meta and para positions, respectively. The reason for this comparative analysis apparently originated from the processing in 1966 of the patent application of alprenolol in the USA. The US patent authorities requested comparative data on the pharmacological properties of the three allyl-substituted compounds. The test results revealed, unexpectedly, that the para-allyl-substituted compound (H64/52) is a cardio-selective beta blocker.[185] Thus, various compounds with an allyl-group were reconsidered and checked.[186]

Some preliminary studies seemed to reveal differences in cardiac, vascular and tracheal tissues. These results were discussed in the light of academic concepts about the differentiation of the beta receptor population. According to Werkö clinical experiences relating to side-effects in asthmatic patients, bradycardia and so forth entered these discussions. Of course, these problems were already acknowledged as a result of clinical experiences with propranolol. But as Werkö stated, these problems were also acknowledged in the small circle of clinical consultants that surrounded the Hässle project.[187] Werkö and his colleagues studied both propranolol and alprenolol in this respect. Their clinical experiences encouraged acceptance of the idea of developing more selective compounds. The Hässle team rapidly incorporated Lands' ideas in their framework because they fitted the typical experimental and clinical systems: heart, lungs and the vessels. Moreover, the experiences with H 35/25 that showed the opposite pattern of selective action, fitted the Lands' classification.[188]

Although the first incentive to study the allyl-substituted compounds was the issue of intrinsic activity, soon thereafter the differences in profiles were extended and yielded clear-cut differences in the actions in cardiac, bronchial and vascular tissues. Further development of the project was hampered by limited financial and personnel resources.

At that stage the project took a rather specific course. In 1967 ICI launched practolol. Thereafter more detailed studies with the allyl-substituted analogues yielded clear differences in profiles. Compound H 64/52 was 100 times weaker a beta blocker in the isolated trachea though it was also four times weaker than alprenolol as beta blocker in the isolated heart. With a ratio of 1 : 25, H 64/52 may be called a relatively selective beta-1 receptor blocking agent. Still, it was not good enough. It was not very potent and it possessed intrinsic activity and thus had no market potential in competition with practolol.

Subsequently, a series of new compounds were synthesized starting from the chemical structure of the para-substituted analogues.[189] Out of almost 100 compounds, two compounds were selected for further testing late in 1968: H 87/07 and H 93/26 (figure 4.8).

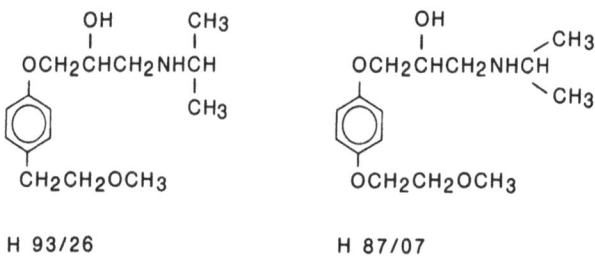

Figure 4.8 Two candidate compounds for bringing a cardio-selective beta blocker to the market by AB Hässle.

H 87/07 was about as potent as alprenolol. But it possessed a marked intrinsic activity, much stronger than alprenolol and practolol. Therefore it looked too much like pindolol. Yet, the compound was as cardio-selective as practolol and was considered a competitive antagonist.[190] In contrast, H 93/26 was less cardio-selective than practolol and H 87/07 and was not explicitly classified as a competitive antagonist.[191] The very reason for selecting H 93/26 for further development, was that the compound was devoid of intrinsic activity. This was considered an advantage compared with H 87/07. After all, the latter compound was too similar to pindolol in one respect and too much like practolol in another. Profiling of these two compounds during 1969 and 1970 took place in the context of hypertensive disease, and the lack of intrinsic activity received a new therapeutic meaning.[192]

It is interesting to see how an industrial team that had put so much energy into the discussion about intrinsic activity radically changed their minds by entering this new therapeutic area. But it is also striking that the research group again succeeded in creatively changing pharmacological theory. For, the early work at Hässle on the characterization of the pharmacological properties of metoprolol resulted in the modification of Lands classification of beta-1 and beta-2 receptors, i.e. the coexistence of β_1 and β_2 receptors in the heart and other tissues.[193]

The clinical and epidemiological studies on alprenolol in hypertension performed by Tiblin, Sannerstedt and Werkö, provided the Hässle team with the necessary backing to enter this new area at an early stage, about 1968. At the managerial and marketing level, this new course was resisted, just as at ICI. However, late in the 1960s the green light was given to move forwards. The aim was to restrict the use of alprenolol to the "common" indications angina pectoris and cardiac arrhythmias and to develop metoprolol as a cardio-selective beta blocker in hypertension.[194]

4.6. The beta blocker project at CIBA

The Biological Laboratories of CIBA (Basle, Switzerland) had a long research tradition in the cardiovascular field. During the 1950s CIBA scientists had found several important anti-hypertensive agents. The team entered the field of beta blockers after Black and Stephenson published their findings on pronethalol. The chemists of CIBA picked up this new possibility. They were already acquainted with the type of chemistry required in this respect because chemically pronethalol-like substances had been found as a result of searching for anti-hypertensive agents. Thus, several classes of catecholamine analogues were synthesized to isolate the effects of displacing noradrenaline. The natural course was to look for compounds that would inhibit, in some way, sympathetic function.

The pharmacologists started to investigate a series of pronethalol-like substances. Some compounds were recognized as a bradycardia producing substance, hence possessed pronethalol-like therapeutic potential for the relief of angina pectoris. Some 30 substances were synthesized and studied. In the middle of 1963 it became clear that pronethalol would lead nowhere as the compound turned out to be carcinogenic in mice and further studies were stopped. When propranolol appeared in the patent files, the team took up the synthesis of this new strain of beta blocking compounds. In August 1964 they synthesized the compound Ciba

39'089-Ba and whereas the ICI team had missed this possibility the compound, later known as oxprenolol (Trasicor) could be registered.

The clinical climate was very negative about this new class of compounds. Therefore the objective of Brunner and his colleagues was to find propranolol-like substances with much less cardio-depressive activity than propranolol. The negative attitude assumed by clinicians, in some way, was transferred to marketing and management. Some cardiologists outside the company, e.g. Rivier and Grandjean, supported the compound. Within Ciba, Imhoff and Gross (director) of the Medical Department backed up the claims of Brunner's research group.[195] It was agreed to bring oxprenolol to the clinic and just see what the drug would do. In 1968 was oxprenolol marketed but with a red package to warn physicians to be careful with this compound.[196]

Intrinsic activity was not important to the Ciba team in profiling their drug.[197] The major differences between propranolol and oxprenolol were the cardio-depressant effects. Somewhat later this issue was taken a step further: *"A very high degree of intrinsic stimulant activity is obviously a disadvantage and may even preclude the therapeutic use of a beta-blocking agent. In principle, however, it is possible that a slight intrinsic stimulant activity could diminish the intensity of certain side effects which result from the direct depressant effects of some beta-blockers. The results obtained up to now in clinical studies, however, do not furnish any evidence to support this assumption".* [198]

Whereas the Hässle team put full weight into this ancillory property of alprenolol, a sceptical attitude dominated Ciba's research group.[199] This scepticism, how paradoxical it may seem, reflected the fear in the German clinical world and oxprenolol would always be a constant source of medical anxiety.

In contrast, the Medical Department of Ciba in the United Kingdom took a different and obstinate course. Due to its strong position in the cardiovascular field, the department, first under the management of Rondel, then Burley, succeeded in attracting much attention in British medicine. But when asked whether support was coming from Basle, Burley commented: *"I must say: 'Almost not at all'. Well, again, it was a very interesting situation, and again it was probably rooted in this fear of heart failure and beta blockade. We found it extremely difficult to get any of the other parts of Ciba-Geiby interested in this program".* [200]

So, the further development of oxprenolol was a British affair. Particularly through the studies of Taylor and colleagues at Leeds, a two-sided view was developed. Firstly, some angina patients were in incipient heart failure and beta blocker treatment might trigger heart failure. Secondly, and more subtle, beta blockers without intrinsic activity produced in hemodynamic terms effects which indicated subliminal heart failure. In both cases beta blockers with ISA might be more beneficial. The latter viewpoint implied that there was a sort of continuum between the normal and failing heart.

According to Silk, a co-worker of Taylor, this viewpoint had not much impact then: *"The approach at that stage was fairly gross rather than subtle. (..) Originally, in the late sixties, early seventies, there was a feeling that there was heart failure and that there was normality, if you like, that was stable coronary heart disease. Provided you didn't treat your heart failure patients with beta blockers, well you were okay, but all the other patients...They didn't appreciate that there was a large grey area where you might potentially give treatment which was detrimental to the patient in hemodynamic terms but not actually force them into heart failure".* [201]

Whatever the precise impact of these views, and we are dealing here with marketing policies as well, the issue of heart failure occupied the minds of many physicians. Oxprenolol was forcefully presented as a "cardio-protective" beta blocker, a drug which because of its intrinsic activity, protected the heart against whatever stressful event including beta blocker treatment itself. Accordingly, oxprenolol would become a successful drug in the United Kingdom. Oxprenolol and practolol were almost simultaneously launched on the British market. When practolol had to be withdrawn, the market was open for oxprenolol. The drug would become the leading beta blocking drug in the United Kingdom.[202]

4.7. Conclusions

Industrial research on beta blocking compounds has had a tremendous impact, not only commercially but also in scientific and medical terms. Beta blockers became investigational tools in medical science and have helped to elucidate the role of the sympathetic system in the normal and pathological human condition.

It is striking to see how much the creation of compounds has a life of its own. This creative activity is largely an affair of industrial scientists and the role of medical chemistry is pivotal to scientific progress. The compounds developed and the activity of creating profiles become a focal point of scientific attention.

The crucial role of experimental systems in therapeutic innovation has been described. These test systems, which are the result of expanding therapeutic fields, help scientists to elucidate new aspects of drugs and diseases, to perform more precise measurements, and to transform basic and clinical concepts.

In chapter 3 it was shown that Ahlquist's theory was a prime force in the field but that its further development was entangled in the interaction between both activities, i.e. the creation of compounds and test systems. In this chapter it was shown that Lands' theory followed the developments regarding compounds and experimental systems. While receptor concepts were translated into biochemical terms, as exemplified by Moran's definition of the operational receptor, pressure came from industrial and therapeutic research to provide a theoretical basis for the highly selective compounds needed. In the late sixties and early seventies Lands' theory was generally accepted.

The industrial projects described were developed within their particular contexts, and were dependant on the therapeutic targets, the laboratory style, equipment and scientific expertise. Still, in each case the interactions with the wider scientific and medical environment were evident. The initial therapeutic target was ventricular fibrillation and other forms of cardiac dysrythm. At AB Hässle the development of anti-arrhythmic drugs had its own course. In addition, the projects at Eli Lilly and, in particular, Mead Johnson emerged from a classical tradition in pharmaceutical research: the search for anti-spasmodic drugs for a variety of clinical conditions including lung disease. The shift to the cardiovascular domain, the key to the development of the beta blockers, was beset by many difficulties.

The ICI project took a different course which, in its creative phase, was a one-man-affair. Black moved forwards with force, and despite the scepticism, he put his ideas to the test, supported by his charismatic personality and enthusiastic leadership. Due to the emphasis of this thesis in elucidating the cognitive structure of the body of scientific and medical knowledge, the role of Black, a "true innovator", has been pushed into the background. The same applies to other individual scientists as well as the policies and social organizations of the individual companies. However, it has become clear that Black's ingenuity prospered when he moved into the vacuum of anti-anginal treatment. This vacuum was created because the medical views about angina pectoris and classic therapy had shifted. This will be further discussed in subsequent chapters. A remarkable feature of the ICI project is how powerful the initiative was to develop the beta blocking drugs. The interaction between various disciplines was intensive and enthusiastic co-operation was readily forthcoming from many clinical centres in the United Kingdom.

While the area of application of propranolol continued to expand, the drug also ran into trouble. The present prejudices and preconceived opinions about the development of the beta blockers arise from this period. For example, the role of surgical sympathotectomy was minor in the early phase but very important when the question of local anaesthetic activity began to arise. Other questions revolving around stereochemistry, intrinsic activity, cardio-depression, and cardiac failure were central to a complex and at times fuzzy discussion which started in the early 1960s but lasted for many years.

The substantial shift that the Hässle team made with respect to intrinsic activity is evidence of the dramatic changes in perspective that can occur in therapeutic research. Although this is subject to marketing policies, important scientific and medical issues were also at stake. Moreover, the intellectual context in which the Hässle project developed, clearly differed from that of the ICI project.

The powerful consultant group of the Hässle team which attracted another outstanding scientist, Ablad, provided the theoretical concepts and experimental methods to profile alprenolol in contrast to propranolol. The open communication with academia and clinicians, which characterized the Hässle team from the very outset, markedly influenced the course of the Hässle project.[203]

The Hässle project was not so important from a marketing perspective, and as far as the ICI team was concerned, the Hässle group was no threat at all; in fact, its work was not even noticed for a long time. However, the Hässle group had an indirect effect on propranolol. Firstly, the knowledge the Hässle team produced concerning alprenolol was applied to oxprenolol, another beta blocker with intrinsic activity. Secondly, the second-generation beta blocker, metoprolol, became a joint activity of Hässle and Ciba-Geigy.

From this point the enormous competition between ICI and Ciba in the United Kingdom comes to be seen in another light.

The course of the Ciba project was most interesting. The German medical climate hampered the project at Basle and created the gap between Ciba's medical department in the United Kingdom and Switzerland. Thus, the life of oxprenolol became largely a British affair and developed its course on the basis of the excellent contacts of Ciba with British cardiological centres.

The clash between ICI and Ciba affected the internal development of the beta blocker project at ICI. The scene of battle between ICI and Ciba was formed by the supposed cardio-depressant actions of propranolol, and had two fronts. The first one was courting the favour of the opinion leaders in cardiologists' circles. There the dangers of the intravenous route - "some patients died on the needle" - were spelled out. This was a major threat to propranolol's progress because, especially in cardiology, an intravenous drug is preferred. Such a drug attracts cardiologists to do research into a wide range of problems. It is a conditio sine qua non for profiling any new drug.

The second front, probably the most important from a long term point of view, was the competition to win over the "ordinary doctor". Since Ciba was stressing oxprenolol as a less aggressive drug than propranolol, with a beneficial mild intrinsic sympathomimetic activity on the heart and thus "cardio-protective", ICI was urged to counteract this strategy. Practolol became the weapon. Practolol, thus, would be the drug for common practice. The objective was to crack the mystique about propranolol as a difficult drug, a dangerous drug, only for the use of specialists.

Barrett states: *"I believe that the introduction of practolol showed ordinary doctors that beta blockade could be used in a way that did not make them worried. It was a much less aggressive drug in that its intrinsic sympathomimetic activity, its lack of membrane stabilizing action or whatever did not make it have so much dramatic effect on cardiac output, did not precipitate cardiac failure, did not produce acute bronchospasm which you couldn't reverse. It gave ordinary doctors a measure of confidence. And I believe that the introduction of oxprenolol, more or less contemporaneously, - and it did not have the adverse side-effects - was similarly benefited by the recognition that here was a drug that ordinary doctors could use with patient benefit without doctor anxiety".* [204]

This episode touches upon an essential character of innovation. As Shaw once wrote: *"The reasonable man adapts himself to the world: the unreasonable one persists in trying to adapt the world to himself. Therefore all progress depends on the unreasonable man".* [205]

Both aspects were pertinent to the ICI team. Propranolol was considered a good drug, the consequence of creative thinking. After all, it embodied "innovation" itself. Indeed, as if it were the unreasonable man, the ICI team tried to adapt the medical world to propranolol. Fitzgerald stated that it was a matter of selecting the right patients for the right drug. Doctors failed to do so through their lack of knowledge of the physiology underlying the drug.[206] Barrett added to this that the less gifted the doctor was, the more problems he raised; doctors who understand the drug, never complained. [207] This attitude was reinforced by the view that propranolol was not only the best therapy but also the best tool a scientist could wish for.

However, such a change does not occur instantaneously. Various routes were followed including new theoretical and methodological approaches which were not only applied to angina pectoris but also the field of heart failure, another field of intricate scientific concepts and innovating medical therapies. Indeed, the problem of heart failure was not resolved instantaneously; and in fact it never has been, at least not theoretically. The major advance of the time was that clinical practice raised its standards for identifying the patients at risk. In this way clinical practice paved the way for using beta blockers in the right patient at the right time and in the right way.

While this "unreasonable" attitude became perceived as a rational behaviour in clinical practice, the ICI team became "reasonable". The team was urged to adapt their profile of the ideal beta blocker. Consequently, practolol most perfectly matched this ideal profile.

The practolol story, thus, leads to the conclusion that medical perceptions, directly mediated by the consultants or indirectly mediated by opinion leaders of the medical profession and the strategies of competitors, were heavily imposed on the experimental work in the ICI laboratories. Similarly, other stages of the ICI project as well as other industrial projects contribute to this conclusion.

Chapter 5. Verapamil: dying drug or sleeping beauty?

5.1 Introduction

The past decade verapamil (Isoptin) has attracted great interest in the scientific and cardiological community. This interest is due to the fact that the compound represents the prototype of an entirely new class of compounds with a novel therapeutic principle, e.g. the calcium antagonists. Furthermore, verapamil has become a tool in physiological and biochemical research of cardiovascular disease and serves to extend calcium channel research to the molecular level.

This new family of drugs is steadily growing and the same applies to the range of clinical applications. Some of the areas in which these drugs are being used or investigated include angina pectoris, myocardial infarction, arrhythmias, cardiomyopathy, hypertension, peripheral vascular disease, migraine, cerebral ischemia, esophageal spasm, asthma , epilepsy and atherosclerosis.

The calcium antagonists, also variably referred to as calcium channel modulators, calcium channel inhibitors or slow channel inhibitors, have been identified as one class of drugs. Fleckenstein and co-workers paved the way for this novel therapeutic classification and classified this family of drugs as acting on the transmembrane flux of calcium. The complex and intricate actions of calcium in the electrical and mechanical processes in the heart are beyond the scope of this thesis. It suffices to say that calcium has been recognized as playing a central role in the translation of the electrical processes in the muscle cell membrane into the mechanical result, namely muscle contraction.[1]

Unlike the beta blockers, the calcium antagonists are chemically entirely different compounds from one another. Though despite these differences they share common properties, it has become clear that there are three, perhaps four, distinct types or subtypes. A recent World Health Organization Committee has decided to subdivide the antagonists into at least three distinct classes: **dihydropyridine** or **N** type, **phenylalkylamine** or **V** type, and **benzothiazepine** or **D** type. The N, V, and D type refer to nifedipine, verapamil, and diltiazem, respectively.[2] Verapamil became available in Europe in 1962 while nifedipine was synthesized in 1967 and marketed in the early 1970s; diltiazem was developed at a much later date.

Verapamil has a remarkable history. Although developed as a coronary vasodilator, verapamil was soon acknowledged as a compound with beta blocking activity. Subsequently, a heated discussion developed resulting in the late 1960s, in verapamil being rejected as a beta blocking compound. In due course however, verapamil became recognized as a calcium antagonist, a new pharmacological category that elicited much scientific and clinical interest.

Therefore it is interesting to examine how these three therapeutic principles were developed by scientists and clinicians. Emphasis will be placed on verapamil's development as an anti-anginal drug. This severely restricts an historical description because the enthusiastic recognition of the anti-arrhythmic actions of the drug by one way thinking has markedly inhibited the development of verapamil as an anti-anginal agent and in total the development of the therapeutic principle of calcium antagonism. Therefore, the concepts about the anti-arrhythmic actions of verapamil will be briefly included. After a short overview of its early history (5.2), the therapeutic principles of coronary vasodilation (5.3) and beta blockade (5.4) with respect to verapamil will be discussed. This is followed by an account of the discovery of its calcium antagonistic action. Much of the credit for developing the principle of calcium antagonism is due to Fleckenstein and his work during the 1960s will be described (5.5). It is not intended to provide a comprehensive picture of his thoughts and his experiments nor of the local and the wider scientific context in which he worked. In contrast, how verapamil and related drugs were identified as a separate class of drugs will be discussed. Additionally, the important role of drugs as tools in experimental and clinical research will be substantiated. Subsequently, the way Fleckenstein's concept of calcium antagonism was accepted is assessed with the help of a scientometric analysis with the objective of finding out how calcium antagonism became a therapeutic principle in medicine (5.6). Finally, the theory of drug and disease profiles is applied to mark the development of verapamil (5.7).

5.2 The early history of verapamil

Around 1960 the German firm of Knoll AG, located in Ludwigshafen, entered the field of cardiovascular drugs with the development of a new coronary vasodilating agent. From a series of analogues of papaverine, widely acknowledged as a powerful smooth muscle relaxant and coronary vasodilator, the substance D 365 (iproveratril, verapamil) was selected. Early pharmacological studies established that verapamil was a potent coronary vasodilator, a hundred times more effective than papaverine in producing coronary dilatation. In 1963 the drug was introduced onto the German market. Shortly before verapamil was developed Boehringer, Hoechst and Cassella-Riedel had introduced dipyridamole (Persantin, 1959), prenylamine (Segontin, 1960) and carbochromen (Intensain, 1963), respectively, as coronary vasodilators. According to Pfennigsdorf this constellation and the diminished belief in coronary dilation as an effective therapeutic principle has hampered a rapid initial develop-ment of verapamil in Germany.[3]
In due time Pfizer showed interest in the compound. However, clinical trials in the United States were stopped when toxicological studies showed that verapamil, when administered in large doses to beagle dogs, could cause cataract, a serious eye disease. Though this discovery prohibited clinical research in the United States, verapamil was available in many countries. Still, this toxicological reaction affected further clinical research as Knoll advised clinicians to use doses not exceeding 480 mg daily.[4]

5.3 Verapamil: a coronary vasodilator?

According to Haas (1962), head of pharmacology at Knoll, verapamil fulfilled all the criteria, set by the scientific and clinical community, defining coronary vasodilation.[5]
Despite the strong competition verapamil attracted considerable clinical attention. Based on

a literature list provided by Knoll, 42 clinical articles were published during the period 1962 - 1969 in German journals whereas over the same period merely 7 articles were published in Anglo-American journals. Charlier discusses in his textbook **Antianginal Agents** 32 clinical articles about verapamil of which 15 were published in Anglo-Saxon journals, 12 in German journals and 5 in other journals (Brasilian, Italian, etc.). Charlier's sample contains fewer German and more English clinical articles than Knoll's literature list. If Charlier's sample is examined according to the clinical judgment of the anti-anginal effect of verapamil the following pattern is seen (table 5.1).[6]

Table 5.1

Therapeutic judgment of verapamil in clinical articles published
in the Anglo-American and German context from 1962-1969,
as discussed by Charlier (1971).

	Anglo-American			German		
Clinical judgment	+	-	E	+	-	E
Number of articles	4	3	8	10	0	2

+ = positive; - = negative; E = exploratory.

Almost all the German articles referred to by Charlier report positive results with verapamil in anti-anginal treatment. Some even stressed extraordinary results with regard to treatment success in almost 95% of all patients.[7] As was usual in clinical trials in the early sixties there was no double blind controlled trial performed in Germany. Two articles discuss other features of the drug. In contrast, Anglo-American clinicians were not unanimous about the therapeutic benefits of verapamil. In some cases these clinicians reported beneficial effects; the majority was much more reserved or reported negative results.[8]

However, the major difference in clinical judgment in both medical contexts was related to the mechanism of action. From the very outset German clinicians agreed to classifying verapamil as a coronary vasodilator. However, from the beginning Anglo-American physicians doubted the coronary vasodilator action as the proposed mechanism of action of verapamil.Mignault (1966), for example, stated: *"It is possible that Isoptin's effect on blood flow is not responsible for the improvement of the clinical symptoms in patients with coronary heart disease"*.[9] Luebs and his co-workers wrote that *"...Isoptin...failed to raise coronary blood flow in patients with coronary artery disease. (..) The results indicate, therefore, that the improvement of angina pectoris need not depend on an increase in coronary blood flow".* [10] The American investigators Neumann and Luisada (1966) probably represent the most extreme example of the Anglo-American position. In their study patients from a geriatric home were selected. Since the structural changes of the coronary arteries in elderly people must be the cause of anginal attacks the authors claimed that *"...any improvement would not be due to "vasodilation" of the coronary vessels but to a different and more complex mechanism".* [11]

5.4 Verapamil: a beta blocker?

At an early stage, late 1962 and early 1963, it was noticed that verapamil differed from the well-known coronary vasodilators in two respects. Firstly, a negative inotropic activity in the isolated perfused heart was established that clearly differed from dipyridamole.[12] The second aspect was some similarity of action with pronethalol. This was an exciting discovery.[13] After all, Knoll would be the second firm after ICI to have a beta blocker.[14]

Since these two features of verapamil differed from the known coronary vasodilators, Knoll asked Fleckenstein to investigate the mechanism of action of verapamil. In 1964 Fleckenstein published his results considering verapamil as the most potent beta blocking agent known at the time. In due course, when propranolol and MJ 1999 became available, he succeeded in differentiating these 'specific beta blockers' from verapamil. Verapamil became known as a *"coronary vasodilator with β-adrenolytic properties".* [15] Because of its additional coronary dilating action it was suggested that the therapeutic value of verapamil exceeded that of the pure beta blockers. German scientists and clinicians took this 'mixed' profile of verapamil for granted. Because it was admitted that verapamil - and also prenylamine - did not exhibit all the effects of beta blockers, it was called a "sympatholytic" agent. When discussing the therapeutic approach to coronary heart disease at the Freiburg Hospital, Gebhardt and Büchner recommended starting first with dipyridamole and, when no improvement occurred, to switch to verapamil (or prenylamine) since it combined beta blocking properties with coronary vasodilating action that "pure" beta blockers did not exhibit.[16]

In British and American medicine a different therapeutic course was followed. Since the concept of coronary vasodilation was rejected, clinicians attributed beta blockade to verapamil as the mechanism of action. Melville (1964), for example, stated: *"It would therefore appear that Iproveratril may exert its effect on the heart by blocking β-receptor adrenergic (sympathetic) mechanisms".* [17] Thus, the dominant view in the middle of the 1960s was that verapamil was a beta blocking compound. With the advent of more specific compounds verapamil's deviant pattern of action became increasingly clear. Subsequently, a heated debate started as to whether verapamil was a beta blocker or not!

On August 5th, 1967, the ICI scientists Fitzgerald and Barrett took the offensive in a letter to the Lancet entitled "What is a ß-blocker?".[18]

Since the characteristic feature of ß-blockers is their high degree of specificity, claims about any new agent exhibiting beta blocking properties should be scrutinized carefully: *"By definition", for a drug to be classed as a β-receptor antagonist it must be shown that: (a) it competitively antagonizes the chronotropic and inotropic effects of exogenous adrenaline and isoprenaline as well as antagonising stimulation of the sympathetic nerves; and (b) it does not antagonise the positive inotropic effects of digitalis, calcium, and aminophylline".* [19] Propranolol obviously met these two criteria. Compounds which block both catecholamine and non-catecholamine-induced positive inotropic effects do so by direct **non-specific** depression of myocardial contractility. According to Fitzgerald and Barrett an example of such a compound was verapamil!

This was criticized by Bateman, Director of Medical Services of Pfizer in the Lancet, August 19, 1967.[20] In the United Kingdom Pfizer was the license holder of verapamil which was marketed under the name 'Cordilox'. Bateman's comment on the claims of Fitzgerald and Barrett was as follows: *"Yet it has been shown that this drug (propranolol, RV) possesses other properties, notably a quinidine-like effect and local analgesic effects. Which of these are responsible for the effectiveness of propranolol in angina pectoris? At a recent symposium on adrenergic-blocking drugs held by the New York Academy of Sciences the consensus was that the effect was due to the quinidine-like action of propranolol, and not to the β-blockade it produces".*[21] Thus, Batterman rejected the suggestion that propranolol represented pure beta blockade; it was a 'dirty' drug as well. Moreover, he argued that there was still uncertainty about the purity of beta blockade because, quoting Shanks, *"there was still not sufficient information to indicate if fulfillment of these criteria (as enumerated by Shanks, RV) is adequate for classification of a compound as a β-receptor antagonist".*[22] In his letter Shanks replied that *Bateman should have stated "that 'these criteria' referred only to blockade of cardiac β-receptors and the isoprenaline depressor response. The studies of Dr. Fitzgerald and Dr. Barrett were much more extensive than any which had been completed when my paper was given (September, 1965)".* [23] Indeed, the profile of pure beta blockade encompassed various properties to be assessed in animals and man. According to the ICI scientists these properties could not be attributed to verapamil.

When profiling a new class of drugs there is always a need for "clean" drugs.[24] This idea of a nice, clean tool governed the strategy of ICI's scientists but they were also worried because propranolol was an endangered drug. Fitzgerald and Barrett explicitly referred to this threatening situation when stating: *"...the most widely studied β-blocking drug, propranolol, is known to be effective in angina pectoris. However, it is by no means certain that these beneficial effects are due entirely to β-receptor blockade, since propranolol has actions other than simple β-blockade".* [25] Thus, a situation developed where verapamil was accused of its "dirty" beta blocking action while at the same time propranolol was discussed for its actions other than beta blockade.

The central questions were whether beta blockade or local anaesthetic activity underlay the therapeutic effects in angina and whether it precipitated cardiac failure. To answer this one should be sure of having compounds that exhibit, next to their other actions, a simple and clear beta blocking action. Propranolol possessed such an action and verapamil did not. So, the heart of the matter lay in the therapeutic controversy over propranolol.

Emphasizing the therapeutic side of the debate Bateman stated: *"I believe that Dr. Fitzgerald and Dr. Barrett have made out a good case for propranolol as a research tool, and for the investigation of the sympathetic nervous system it is undoubtedly of great value. We must, however, be careful not to extrapolate too uncritically pharmacological findings established in the healthy cardiovascular system of young animals to the conditions obtaining in the ischaemic hearts of middle-aged human beings, and we are, after all, concerned with the day-to-day management of myocardial sclerosis in man".* [26]

The suggestion is clear. Propranolol might be the cleanest β-blocker and the nicest tool but this is purely from the scientific point of view, not from the therapeutic viewpoint. According to Bateman verapamil was associated with additional characteristics that annulled the negative secondary effects of pure beta blockade. Therefore, verapamil might be given to patients with bronchospasm and cardiac insufficiency for whom propranolol is contraindicated.

It may be argued that we are dealing here simply with a clash between ICI and Pfizer while both firms were offering commercially inspired arguments to defend their position. True, the stakes were high because despite the controversy about propranolol, beta blockade was experienced as a promising new approach in cardiac therapy. Pfizer armed with verapamil entered into the controversy about propranolol attempting to profit from the promising future of beta blocking drugs. The ICI scientists exerted great effort to repel this new competitor. But it would be too easy to consider the controversy as a mere marketing battle. Bateman's letter set off a chain-reaction of letters to the Lancet and the discussion spread to other journals. In due course, criteria were defined for assessing pure beta blockade and evaluating the purity of action of verapamil.

The two tracked line of reasoning which Bateman followed is clear. The first was to define verapamil as a beta blocker but leaving enough room to account for its different pattern of action. The second was to hit the weak spot of propranolol, e.g. its pure beta blockade and strong cardio-depressive action which so many clinicians considered as the cause of trouble with patients suffering from imminent or manifest heart failure. Both lines had to be reconciled. It was the clinic that had to settle the matter: *"The most valuable evidence for verapamil therefore comes from the bedside, and many clinical papers testify to its beneficial effect in patients with angina and with cardiac arrhythmias of various etiologies".* [27]

However, Bateman fought a losing battle. British and American clinicians had defined the boundaries within which evidence coming from the bedside was assessed. Clinicians acknowledged that angina of effort was the disease of major concern and that the adrenergic hemodynamic disturbances bringing on anginal attacks could be easily pinpointed by antagonism to isoprenaline or exercise induced tachycardia. The majority of Anglo-American clinicians assessed beta blockade in accordance with the criteria put forward by the ICI team. Several clinical studies repudiated an antagonizing effect of verapamil on the critical parameters. In 1968 the column "Today's Drugs" in the British Medical Journal commented: *"A characteristic property of beta-receptor blockers is the competitive inhibition of the cardiac action of isoprenaline in doses that do not depress the heart. Verapamil in therapeutic doses (80 mg thrice daily) has no significant effect on isoprenaline-induced tachycardia in man, nor does it cause any reduction in the tachycardia provoked by physical exercise in healthy volunteers. This is in marked contrast to the effects of propranolol and is evidence that verapamil is not a beta-receptor blocker".* [28] The Drugs and Therapeutics Bulletin stated: *"Recent correspondence in the Lancet has strongly criticized the claim that verapamil is a beta blocking agent; an attempt to justify and uphold the claim induced careful quotations from articles of workers who consider that verapamil is not a beta-blocking drug".* [29]

Moreover, clinical experience showed that verapamil could precipitate or aggravate cardiac insufficiency thus rejecting the suggestion of Bateman that verapamil could be beneficial in those situations where ß-blocking agents were contra-indicated. An editorial comment in the British Medical Journal (1968) stated that British clinicians therefore could not recommend the compound for the treatment of the angina pectoris patient.[30] The Drugs and Therapeutics Bulletin arrived at the same conclusion in 1967.[31] Two years later the same journal, in assessing new experimental and clinical material, still maintained its view.[32]

It was admitted, however, that verapamil had some effect in angina. Several German clinical reports were referred to but these were carried out under uncontrolled conditions and were therefore not taken as being conclusive. Still, there were controlled clinical trials that reported beneficial effects. However, some were negative such as the double-blind trial of Phear who concluded that "no significant relief of angina by verapamil was found". Sandler who reported a significant beneficial effect from verapamil at a high daily dose of 360 mg, comparable to that yielded by propranolol in the same type of angina patients concluded: *"Provided verapamil has no deleterious effects on the heart or other organs then the exact mechanism of action in angina, whether this involves beta-receptor blockade or direct depression of myocardial contractility, is of less importance than whether the drug is an effective agent in angina pectoris".* [33] This minority point of view could not reverse clinical scepticism. The efficacy of propranolol or verapamil was not of prime importance in the discussion. It was precisely their presumed mechanism of action that ruled the debate.

Verapamil was rejected as a beta blocker. But even if it was such a drug, the same drawback as given for propranolol, would also apply to verapamil. Moreover, its additional coronary vasodilating activity evoked scepticism in the English speaking medical world. Furthermore, the sheer fact that Sandler reported beneficial effects for verapamil, when administrating **high** doses, did not speak in favour of the drug. This fact was merely seen as evidence of its direct cardio-depressant action, and verapamil came to be considered primarily as an direct cardio-depressant drug. Thus, verapamil became involved in the discussion about the quinidine-like action of propranolol: *"It was originally assumed that the undoubted beneficial effects of propranolol in angina of effort were due to its established action on blockade of beta-receptors. However, the dose required to control angina sometimes far exceeds that needed to effect complete beta-receptor blockade. Propranolol must therefore exert other actions which contribute to its beneficial effect in this disease, and one of these is a quinidine-like depressant action on the myocardium. It is this effect of propranolol that is shared by verapamil".* [34] Indeed, as Shanks formulated, *"There is considerable evidence to show that verapamil is primarily a myocardial depressant in animals and without pharmacological effect in man".* [35] The rubric 'Today's Drugs' concluded: *"Verapamil is not an alternative to propranolol as an antagonist to cardiac adrenergic beta-receptor stimulation. It has, however, been shown in controlled trials to benefit some patients with angina. Verapamil is a cardiac depressant and may produce or aggravate cardiac failure".* [36]

So, the majority point of view was that verapamil was not a beta blocker. Despite the doubt that remained about this fact it was generally considered that verapamil was no **alternative** for propranolol, because it could not claim any therapeutic advantage. This general appreciation may be best illustrated by Wilkinson's statement in his letter to the Lancet of 1967: *"It seems to me that Dr. Bateman should decide whether verapamil is a ß-blocker, and accept that it has all the advantages and drawbacks which he has ascribed to ß-blockade, or place verapamil in some other pharmacological category".* [37]

5.5. Verapamil: a calcium antagonist! - The elucidation of verapamil's mechanism of action by Fleckenstein.

When Fleckenstein was asked by Knoll and Hoechst to investigate verapamil and prenylamine, he was already involved in a research program aimed at investigating the energy expenditure of the beating heart. In particular, phosphates as the source of energy for the heart were studied by Fleckenstein and his colleagues in an extensive series of experiments during the 1950s.[38]

In this study it was observed that during relaxation the hypoxic heart expanded dramatically and it markedly exceeded the degree of dilation of the normal resting heart. This observation was an eye-opener to Fleckenstein. Hitherto dilation was considered a mere passive process of relaxation following the active contraction of the heart. Now it appeared that even during rest the heart had to maintain its muscle tone at the expense of energy. During the second half of the 1950s techniques were developed to measure the degree of dilation of the heart during rest and contraction.[39] These measurements of tone and contractility of the heart were correlated with the energy state of the heart. Concentrations of adenosinetriphosphate (ATP) and creatinine phosphate (CP), representing the energy source of the heart, and inorganic phosphate (Pi) as well as other metabolic end products of creatinine phosphate, were measured to determine the energy state of the heart.

The heart was tested in a variety of experimental situations: during hypoxia, ischemia, carbon monoxide and nitrogen respiration as well as during the administration of a series of toxic agents such as barbiturates, Co^{2+} and Ni^{2+} ions, local anaesthetics, cyanide, fluoroacetate and 2,4-dinitrophenol.

Two types of cardiac failure were established. Some agents induced a situation of contractile failure with low concentrations of ATP and CP versus high concentrations of Pi indicating that high-energy phosphates were broken down. This type was called **deficiency-insufficiency** ("Mangelinsuffizienz"). The second type referred to states of cardiac insufficiency associated with high concentrations of ATP and CP versus a low level of Pi. Somehow the use of these high-energy phosphates was inhibited. This second type was called **utilization-insufficiency** ("Utilisationsinsuffizienz"). The latter type was particularly induced by the administration of Co^{2+} and Ni^{2+} ions, barbiturates and local anaesthetics. The contractile function of the heart could be restored when administrating Ca^{2+} ions, sympathomimetic amines and cardiac glycosides.

At several times Fleckenstein discussed the relevance of his experimental models to the clinical pictures of cardiac failure. Though the clinical situation was more complex than the experimental, his distinction between two types of cardiac failure seemed to be clinically relevant in one very important respect. It was known that heart failure due to cardiac valvular disease was very responsive to cardiac glycosides. Heart failure as a consequence of hypoxia was not. The analogy with Fleckenstein's experimentally induced heart failure was that utilization-insufficiency was very responsive to cardiac glycosides whereas the other type was not. The therapeutic success of the cardiac glycosides served as the standard to correlate experimental and clinical forms of cardiac failure.[40]

Fleckenstein's research program was interfered with by the development of the beta blocking agents. Soon it was acknowledged that both compounds just like DCI and pronethalol induced utilization-insufficiency.[41] On the basis of these experiments verapamil and prenylamine were classified as beta blocking agents, verapamil being the most potent known at that time (1964) since it was five to six times more active than pronethalol.[42] Thus, four groups of compounds were used as tools by Fleckenstein to study the energy state of the failing heart: 1. nickel- and cobalt-ions; 2. barbiturates; 3. beta blocking agents; and 4. local anaesthetics. The CP/Pi ratio was used to differentiate between the two forms of heart failure and to classify the detrimental effects of the various agents. Figure 5.1 is illustrative.[43]

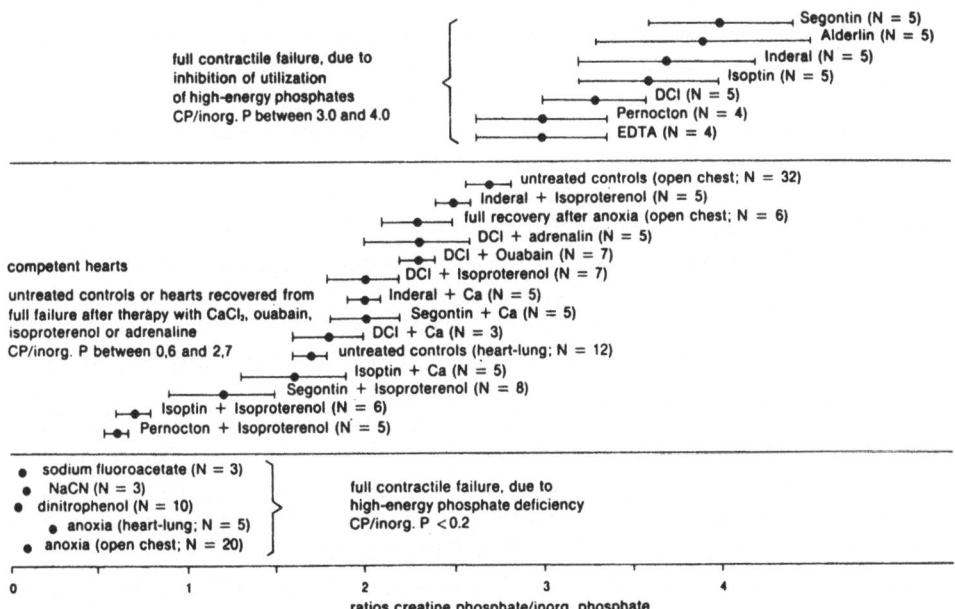

Figure 5.1
The classification of inhibitors and promoters of the calcium action in excitation-contraction coupling - ratios of creatine phosphate/inorganic phosphate in the myocardium of the left ventricle guinea pig hearts in a state of normal competence, during severe contractile failure of different types, and after recovery.
Reproduced with permission from Fleckenstein et al. (1968a).

The bottom of this figure represents the experimental conditions in which the CP/Pi ratio decreases below 0.2. This indicates deficiency-insufficiency. The top reflects utilization-insufficiency in which the ratio exceeds 3.0. The middle plan represents the competent hearts of untreated animals or of animals who have recovered after the administration of sympathomimetic compounds, cardiac glycosides, calcium or after a period of anoxia. This shows a characteristic feature of Fleckenstein's work. While working in the particular context of cardiac insufficiency, he started to elaborate a general concept of the mechanism of cardiac contractility and the factors that could disturb that process.

Pivotal to Fleckenstein's experimental work was that he was committed to both the concepts of beta blockade and coronary vasodilation.[44] Verapamil and prenylamine formed an interesting merger of both concepts. In 1967 he published two large articles in the German Journal for Cardiovascular Research ("Zeitschrift für Kreislaufforschung") encompassing about 50 pages. The titles testified to his committment to both concepts: *"About the mechanism of action of new coronary vasodilators with simultaneous oxygen saving myocardial effects, prenylamine and iproveratril (verapamil, RV)"*. [45] Newly developed beta blockers as well as several coronary vasodilating agents were used to unravel the properties of verapamil and prenylamine. A new element in Fleckenstein's work was the acceptance of the criteria of beta blocking activity.[46] This enabled him to differentiate between "beta blocking doses" and "cardiac insufficiency inducing doses" of the various compounds.[47] Pronethalol and propranolol exhibited beta blocking action at doses that were three to ten times smaller than the doses producing loss of contractile function. In contrast, verapamil and prenylamine produced both effects in a dose range that partially overlapped. Moreover, it appeared to be easier to restore normal heart function with the help of sympathomimetic compounds in the case of heart failure induced by verapamil and prenylamine than when propranolol was used.

The crucial point is that Fleckenstein started to **separate** negative inotropic and beta blocking effects in the heart. This change of view was reported by Fleckenstein's group in the following: *"It is a most natural thought that the inhibition of contractility and frequency by beta receptor blockers, Segontin and Isoptin could be based on an elimination of the sympathetic drive as a consequence of a specific blocking of sympathetic transmitters which are amassed in the myocardium and which attach to the myocard. Initially we ourselves were inclined to accept this simple explanation as well"*. [48] The question *"Is the inhibition of contractility and frequency by β-receptor blockers, Segontin and Isoptin a result of sympatholysis in the heart?"* which the author themselves posed was answered accordingly: *"Consequently, the extent of the reduction of the force of contraction and the heart rate in situ is not strictly correlated with the degree of the beta receptor blockade"*. [49] In another passage a similar answer was given: *"It may be concluded from all these results that a beta receptor blockade need not necessarily be associated by a strong cardio-inhibition and conversely that a strong cardio-inhibition need not necessarily be associated by a beta receptor blockade"*. [50]

These quotations illustrate the attempts to separate beta blocking and negative inotropic effects. Fleckenstein and co-workers also refer to the discovery of MJ 1999, a beta blocker with very little negative inotropic activity.[51] Yet the quotations show ambiguity as well. The ambiguity of both answers is reflected in the term "..need not necessarily be associated by..".[52] What this term exactly means is far from clear. This ambiguity is repeated in the naming of segontin and verapamil. Pronethalol and propranolol were called by Fleckenstein "specific" beta blockers. Verapamil and prenylamine, however, were not labelled "aspecific beta blocker" nor were they repudiated as beta blocking compounds. Throughout his articles the names verapamil and prenylamine were used separately to the term "beta blockers"; the quotation that marked the change of view as well as the question described above, illustrates this separation in terminology. Still, both compounds were also qualified with the phrase "with beta blocking properties".[53] Moreover, both compounds were described in terms of "insufficiency-doses" and "beta blocking doses". By this time he had already distanced himself from his earlier statement that verapamil and prenylamine were potent beta blocking agents.

Beta blocking and negative inotropic action were separated at the molecular level as well. At the molecular level the relationship between the bio-electrical and mechanical processes in the heart became increasingly a central part of Fleckenstein's work. This relationship was conceptualised as the phenomenon of **excitation-contraction coupling**. Excitation-contraction coupling was intensively studied in basic physiology of muscle action and gradually invaded cardiovascular physiology. Whereas during the 1950s the role of Na^+ and K^+ ions in the excitability of cardiac membranes was discussed, it was the electrophysiological significance of the Ca^{2+} ions that started to evoke interest in the late 1950s.[54] Calcium ions as potential mediators between the electrical stimuli at the surface of the cell and the mechanical processes inside the cell became increasingly appreciated as a fruitful working hypothesis. Calcium became therefore a key messenger in the cascade of biochemical events initiated at the membrane and resulting in an activation of the enzymes that transform phosphate bound energy into mechanical work. The exact site in the cascade of biochemical events with which the beta blocking compounds, prenylamine and verapamil interfere, however, was far from clear. Fleckenstein et al. proposed two mechanisms:

a. the blockade of calcium movements from the membrane to the contractile system or competition with the enzymes that transform chemical energy into mechanical energy;

b. the blockade of sympathomimetic amines. These amines act as synergists of calcium with respect to the phosphate splitting enzymes, i.e. they act in a "co-catalytic" way, or as stimulators of calcium diffusion into the contractile system.[55]

Since the exact site of action was not known, ambiguity at the molecular level remained. The following two quotations are characteristic:

"In the end, much more decisive for the checking of the mechanical myocardial functions is the interference with the "electromechanical coupling" in which specific beta blockers as well as Segontin and Isoptin work particularly as a calcium antagonist, in that they diminish the physiological intermediate function of the calcium ions between the bio-electrical excitation process and the contractile activity" [56]

"All these findings indicate that the negative inotropic myocardial effects of beta receptor blockers as well as of Segontin and Isoptin are based on a complex inhibition of the myofibrils-ATPase, because both (a) the aspecific calcium-displacement and (b) the specific elimination of the endogenous catecholamines resulting from a beta receptor blockade ultimately always coincide" [57]

Thus, the term "calcium antagonist" has two meanings. Firstly, it denotes the **general** phenomenon of interfering with the excitation-contraction coupling, a concept on which Fleckenstein's group comments: *"that well-defined reactions are hidden behind the none too precise concept of 'electromechanical coupling' (...)"* [58] Secondly, it denotes the **particular** site in the cascade of biochemical reactions which are interfered with. It is intriguing that the beta blocking effect was coined with the term **"specific"** whereas competition with or antagonism to calcium is connected with the term **"aspecific"**. This ambiguity continues when the authors discuss the exact mechanism of action of verapamil and segontin. Evidence for this point is their conclusion: *"Apparently Segontin and Isoptin are in the first place active as calcium antagonists on the myofibrils-ATPase, and only in the second place as agents which displace* *catecholamines from the beta receptors".* [59] This quotation comes from the German summary and for the first time the term "calcium antagonists" appears in connection with verapamil and prenylamine alone; the English summary does not mention the term. Instead it says:*"The negative inotropic effects of Segontin and Isoptin seem to be due to the first mechanism (a)"* , i.e. the mechanism as described above.

The difference between "beta blocking doses" and "insufficiency inducing doses" seen in the separation of beta blocking and negative inotropic effects was of therapeutic interest according to Fleckenstein and his colleagues. In the case of pronethalol and propranolol the beta receptors were almost completely blocked before the negative inotropic effects became manifest. In the presence of verapamil and prenylamine these oxygen saving effects are accomplished while the heart is still capable of responding to the sympathetic drive. This was therapeutically important because the application of the beta blockers consisted according to Fleckenstein of the art of manoeuvering between the Scylla of non-effective doses and the Charybdis of an immanent insufficiency of the heart.[60] For this reason, the risk of cardiac insufficiency was much less in the case of verapamil and prenylamine than with the application of specific beta receptor blocking agents.[61]

Thus, the basic physiology of muscle action and biochemistry of the energy state of the heart enabled Fleckenstein to differentiate between the actions of the various compounds on the mechanical activity of the heart. A variety of compounds served as tools to elucidate the basic mechanisms whereas the latter in their turn served to characterize these compounds. However, the **specificity** of the observed phenomena had to be established.

The distinction between the "electrical" and the "mechanical" processes in the heart served to establish the specificity of the observed phenomena. For example, compounds might interfere with bio-electrical processes in the heart - the process of impulse generation and conduction - which could induce secondary changes which result in contractile failure.[62] This separation of the bio-electrical process from the mechanical activity in the heart remained a continuous thread in Fleckenstein's studies.

However, the emphasis lay on establishing the effects of verapamil on cardiac contractility. Fleckenstein was not strongly interested at the beginning of his work, in the explanation of negative chronotropic and dromotropic effects in terms of antagonism. But later he succeeded in characterizing these effects too, as representing an interference with Ca-dependent phenomena.

The reason to focus on cardiac contractility, and not on the inhibitory effects of verapamil on nomotopic (sinus node, atrio-ventricular node) and on ectopic pacemaker activity, was rather simple as Fleckenstein commented. At a very early stage, in the beginning of the sixties, it was recognized that calcium plays a crucial role in the electrical processes in the heart. Further observations on the role of calcium in bio-electrical processes in various biological systems accumulated. However, Fleckenstein decided not to enter immediately a new battlefield before the new concept of calcium antagonism had gained more solid grounds in pharmacology and physiology because of the widely held view that electrical processes were based on sodium/potassium exchange.[63]

This battlefield was also pointed out by Vaughan Williams. There was great resistance to the idea that next to a fast inward depolarizing current in cardiac muscle tissue, carried by sodium, and depressed by quinidine, there existed a second, slower, current carried by ions other than sodium, e.g. possibly by calcium ions. This was suggested by Vaughan Williams in his 1958' paper on the mechanism of action of quinidine but it was ignored until in the late 1960s, particularly through the work of Reuter, it was established that there existed a second "slow" inward calcium current in the heart. Subsequently, verapamil was classified as an anti-arrhythmic agent restricting the slow inward calcium current in the heart.[64]

Due to the selective attention to the development of verapamil as an antianginal drug, this aspect of the drug's history requires further investigation.

Regarding the specificity of the observed phenomena another issue had to be settled, i.e. that the negative inotropic effects of verapamil and prenylamine were unrelated to their coronary vasodilator properties.[65] This was done through an extensive series of comparative studies of verapamil/prenylamine, beta blockers and coronary vasodilating compounds - classic (nitro-glycerine) and new (dipyridamole). Accordingly, verapamil and prenylamine were attributed a potent, and what is more important, also a therapeutically beneficial effect with respect to the coronary circulation. In this respect Fleckenstein remained committed to the coronary vasodilator concept.[66]

Fleckenstein therefore attributed verapamil and prenylamine a **special** place in the treatment of coronary insufficiency and angina pectoris for two reasons. The first reason was that both compounds were coronary vasodilating agents. Verapamil and prenylamine occupied a therapeutically advantageous position with which a beta blocker could not compete.[67] Secondly, both compounds left the cardiovascular responses to the sympathetic system reasonably intact. Without doubt verapamil and prenylamine were preferable because there was no danger of a sudden cardiovascular breakdown such as latent cardiac failure, peripheral collapse, and acute loss of blood.[68] This was a clear-cut advantage in comparison to the beta blockers.

This latter aspect underlines the new therapeutic principle of "non-specific calcium antago-nism" that was elaborated within the context of cardiac failure. In this state it was essential to leave the sympathetic system unaffected and this is precisely what verapamil and prenylamine were able to do. For both reasons Fleckenstein stated: *"in the case of Segontin and Isoptin, the combination of two important therapeutic principles seems to be rather unique and particularly useful in the treatment of angina"*. [69]

In subsequent studies this intermediate position of verapamil and prenylamine between the "classic" and "new" approach in anti-anginal treatment, however, was converted into the new pharmacodynamic principle of calcium antagonism. In 1968 Dr. F. Dengel, the chemist of the Knoll company in Ludwigshafen, who had synthesized verapamil, came to Freiburg bringing with him a new derivative of verapamil, D600 (Gallopamil), a compound much stronger than verapamil, and asked Fleckenstein to test it. In some short communications the compounds verapamil, D600 and prenylamine were now presented as a new **class** of compounds. Whereas in foregoing years terms like "calcium antagonistic effects" were used, now this class was denoted as "calcium antagonists".[70] A year later, Dr. Kronenberg, the leading pharmacologist of Bayer, came to Fleckenstein with two other compounds, one labeled "Bay a 1040", the other "Bay a 7168". The chemical structure of both compounds was kept secret. Fleckenstein was asked to investigate them because these very potent coronary vasodilators also exhibited unexplained strong negative cardio-depressant actions. Subsequently, these drugs were put in a separate category classified as calcium antagonists.

New techniques in electrophysiology enabled scientists to separate the ion fluxes at the level of the cardiac cell membrane. Accordingly, it was shown that separate holes in these membranes existed, one being the "fast channel" for the sodium ions, the other being the "slow channel" through which the transmembrane flux of calcium took place. Moreover, the cascade of further biochemical reactions that lead to the transition of electrical into chemical and subsequently mechanical energy was clarified. The specific site of action of the calcium antagonists could then be established. By accepting these new concepts and methods Fleckenstein was able to delineate calcium antagonism as a new pharmacodynamic principle. A characteristic of Fleckenstein's work remained his committment to the close relationship between pathology and biochemistry. Emphasis shifted towards the pathological consequences of biochemical derailments concerning the energy state of the heart. The central question became in which circumstances was calcium necessary for the structural integrity of the heart and which pathological conditions caused a calcium-overload in the heart such that destruction and necrosis occurred.

Fleckenstein's studies expanded into more extensive profiling of the various compounds, into the elucidation of their mechanisms of action and their role in various ischemic heart disorders.

5.6. Citation analysis of the concept of calcium antagonism elaborated by Fleckenstein.

In 1971 Fleckenstein summarized his concepts and experimental results in a large review article published in what would become a very influential book in the field, **Calcium and the Heart.**[71] The total number of 644 citations from 1971 till 1985 indicates the widespread acknowledgment of Fleckenstein's work.

To assess the way his ideas were accepted by the scientific and medical community a scientometric analysis was performed. The methodology used is explained in appendix II. Figure 5.2 shows citation curves with respect to three articles (Fleckenstein (1971), curve A; Fleckenstein (1977), curve B; and Fleckenstein (1983), curve C respectively) and to a set of articles consisting of the 'top 11' of his quoted work, i.e. curve D.[72]

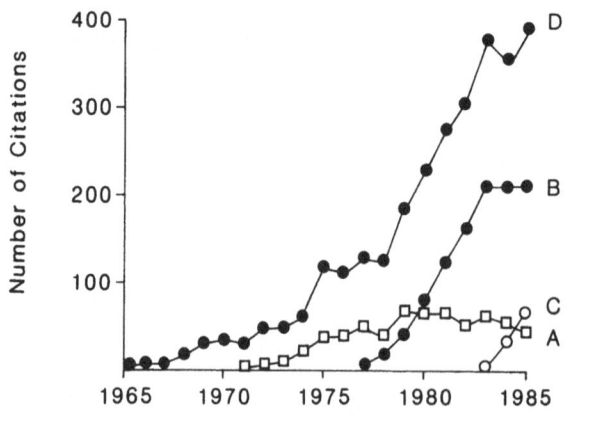

Figure 5.2
Number of citations per year, from the SCI, of Fleckenstein: A = (1971); B = (1977); C = (1983); and D = ("top 11").

The rapid increase in quotations represented by Curve B and C neutralize the displacement of curves A and B respectively indicating that colleague scientists identify the subsequent articles as defining the framework of ideas within which further research is to proceed.[73] Since all three articles are review articles, the increase of citations probably reflects the expansion of the concept of calcium antagonism to neighbouring fields. Curve D approximates the sigmoid curve of typical growth of science networks and specialties that may be divided in stage 1 (exploration), stage 2 (unification) and stage 3 (Decline/Displacement).[74] It may be expected that the framework developed in stage 2 and 3 provides a suitable basis for practical application.

To see how scientists and clinicians recognize and quote Fleckenstein's work, a citation-context analysis was performed (see for methodology appendix II).[75]

Table 5.2
Context analysis of citing articles to Fleckenstein.

1973	Citation-context			
	Exp	Conc	Ther	Total
Type of article				
Animal-exp	20	8	0	28
Human-exp	1	0	0	1
Clin-ther	1	0	0	1
Total	22	8	0	30

1975	Citation-context			
	Exp	Conc	Ther	Total
Type of article				
Animal-exp	35	35	1	71
Human-exp	1	2	0	3
Clin-ther	2	2	2	6
Total	38	39	3	80

1977	Citation-context			
	Exp	Conc	Ther	Total
Type of article				
Animal-exp	26	35	2	63
Human-exp	9	1	0	10
Clin-ther	3	0	1	4
Total	38	36	3	77

Table 5.2 shows three matrices for each mark year, namely 1973, 1975 and 1977 respectively. In 1973 the majority of the quotations are of experimental nature the number of which increases in 1975. The slight number of quotations which belong to the category "conceptual" in 1973 markedly increases in 1975 and remains almost the same in 1977. This indicates that the concept of calcium antagonism was sufficiently elaborated to be recognized and to credit Fleckenstein as its creator. There is a slight increase in the number of citations compared to the categories "human-experimental" and "clinical-therapeutic" but this shift is marginal.

The results suggest that until 1977 Fleckenstein's work has been cited mainly within an experimental context, and that clinicians did not connect the concept of calcium antagonism as elaborated by Fleckenstein to the activity of the compounds they used. It is of course possible that clinicians referred to other articles of Fleckenstein not contained in this sample. In this case a reasonable assumption would be that these are articles outside the scope of this analysis in which Fleckenstein discussed the therapeutic implications of his concept. Since Fleckenstein discussed therapeutic aspects throughout his entire work and never published an article merely indicating therapeutic aspects, this seems highly improbable. However, it may be possible that clinicians, as opposed to Fleckenstein's colleague scientists, referred to a great variety of articles due to their ignorance of the field of calcium research. Another possibility is that the concept of calcium antagonism was too abstract and too new to be acknowledged by clinicians who were at the time, generally, not well acquainted with developments in biochemistry. This possibility was suggested by Fleckenstein himself, to the author.[76] Other interviewed scientists and clinicians supported this suggestion.[77] Clinicians probably referred to medical opinion leaders up to date with biochemical developments and convinced by Fleckenstein's ideas at a very early stage. Closer examination of the passages of the articles in the human-experimental or human-clinical category which referred to Fleckenstein, confirms this suggestion, but reveals also a more specific mechanism. The following two passages are characteristic:

"Verapamil, which has also been classified as a calcium-antagonist (Fleckenstein et al. 1967), has been used successfully in the treatment of patients with paroxysmal supraventricular tachycardia and in reducing heart rate in atrial flutter and fibrillation (Bender 1967; Schamroth et al. 1972)" [78]

"Verapamil has been used clinically for therapy of cardiac arrhythmias and angina (Melville et al., 1964; Schamroth et al., 1972). There is considerable evidence that the drug exerts its effects by altering the movement of calcium across the external cell membrane (Fleckenstein, 1971; Haeusler, 1972)" [79]

These passages credit Fleckenstein in having classified verapamil as a calcium antagonist or having elucidated its basic mechanism of action. Yet with regard to the therapeutic activity of verapamil these passages refer to the clinicians who were involved in therapeutic research with the compound early on and who related the beneficial effects to the concept of calcium antagonism. Subsequently, clinicians keep on referring to this early clinical work, not citing Fleckenstein's articles directly.

The clinical articles of Sandler et al. (1968), Schamroth et al. (1972) and Livesley et al. (1973) were most frequently cited. The article of Schamroth and co-workers concerns the anti-arrhythmic properties of verapamil, the other two to the anti-anginal effects of the drug. Figure 5.3 shows the citation curves of the articles published by Sandler et al. and Livesly et al.

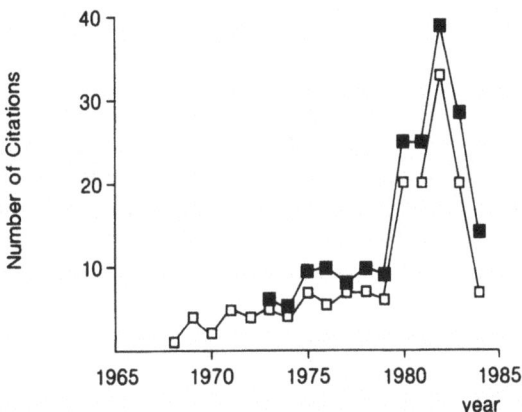

`Figure 5.3
Number of citations, from the SCI, to Sandler et al. (1968) (□); and Livesly et al. (1973) (■).

Both curves show a continuous though variable flow of citations at a rather low level during the 1970s and a marked increase from 1980 onwards. This suggests that both articles reached a relatively small circle of clinicians till about 1980. The aim was to establish the therapeutic effectiveness of verapamil in angina pectoris, particularly so during the first half of the 1970s. The target disease was angina of effort. Some clinicians tacitly accepted Fleckenstein's concept; others criticized it or elucidated other aspects of the mechanism of action.[80] In general, research efforts were very small.[81] The total number of articles about verapamil with regard to angina pectoris over the period 1971 - 1975 amounts to merely 28. Of course, it might be argued that new developments are made primarily within an informal research network. This possibility seems very unlikely. Around 1970 verapamil was considered as a "dying drug".[82] The German industry Knoll was comparably small and had not performed a national and/or international widely spread clinical research program. The major area that first attracted clinical interest in Anglo-American and German medicine was the anti-arrhythmic effect of verapamil. In this context several contacts were ready at hand, and Knoll gratefully acknowledged the willingness of renowned Anglo-American cardiologists to develop the drug as a first step for use in anti-arrhythmic therapy.[83]

Thus, in physiology and medicine in the English speaking world the mechanism of action of verapamil was elaborated within the context of cardiac arrhythmias. The 1960s were dominated by the attempt to explain the fundamental actions of anti-arrhythmic drugs solely in terms of their depressant effects on the rate of depolarization of action potential. This action could be correlated with the local anaesthetic potencies of the known anti-arrhythmic compounds.[84] We need only to recall the fact that the observed anti-arrhythmic actions of the beta blockers were also ascribed to their local anaesthetic actions. Similarly, the anti-arrhythmic action of verapamil was attributed to its "quinidine-like" properties. Further investigations using quinidine, propranolol and verapamil and other compounds as reference drugs, suggested novel archetypes of anti-arrhythmic actions. Accordingly, terms like "calcium entry blockers" and "slow channel blockers" denoting the effect of verapamil and related compounds on the calcium-mediated "slow channel" in the heart, bear witness to the origin of these concepts in the context of cardiac arrhythmias.[85]

To understand the dynamics of calcium antagonism in the field of angina pectoris, another compound, nifedipine, seems to be more important. As described earlier, nifedipine was synthesized in 1967 and was developed as a coronary vasodilator. In late 1969 Fleckenstein was contacted by Kronenberg, director of Pharma Research and Development of Bayer, to investigate nifedipine. The pharmacological and medical departments of Bayer, however, remained very sceptical about Fleckenstein's concepts.[86] Still, a consensus emerged that the mechanism of this drug was different to that of both beta blockers and nitrates. Lichtlen describes the relevant developments as follows:

"In order to gain more knowledge on this topic (the mechanism of action of nifedipine, RV), it was mandatory to bring physiologists, pharmacologists and cardiologists together to exchange ideas. This occurred, on a small scale, at a meeting in Wuppertal in 1970 and, on a large scale, during the 1st Adalat Symposium in Tokyo in November 1973. Tokyo was chosen because a number of Japanese researchers, notably Hashimoto, Kimura, Taira, Endoh and Hosoda, had also been working with nifedipine since the late 1960s and had made some extremely interesting and important observations. At the clinical level, these observations especially concerned **angina at rest**. *At that time, this variant form of angina was a relatively frequent cardiac disease in Japan. These patients were treated with nitroglycerin; however, the results were not always satisfactory. At the first Adalat Symposium, Mabuchi reported that half of these cases were refractory to long-acting nitroglycerin. In contrast, according to Mabuchi, nifedipine was able to completely interrupt and prevent resting angina due to spasm. Hosoda et al. stated that nifedipine had 'a marked preventing effect on attacks at rest or during sleep in 87% of these patients'. According to Hosoda, 'the variant form of angina pectoris responded particularly well to nifedipine', an observation which had already been made by Kimura in 1972".*[87]

Thus, two developments were crucial. Firstly, the profile of nifedipine was differentiated from beta blockers and nitrates at the experimental and clinical level. With respect to clinical research this implied that the mechanism of action was linked to typical angina of effort. Secondly, nifedipine was related to other forms of angina pectoris which had raised little interest from European and Anglo-American cardiologists but attracted considerable attention from Japanese cardiologists. However, in Europe Maseri and co-workers drew the attention of Western cardiologists to the occurrence of coronary artery spasm in angina patients and reported in 1979 on the efficacy of verapamil in those patients.[88]
The first symposium on nifedipine was held in Tokyo, november 1973 which was preceded by some smaller conferences in Japan and in Germany. This symposium was the first in a series of subsequent symposia specifically devoted to nifedipine.[89]
It shows that as far as nifedipine is concerned its clinical development is a particularly German-Japanese achievement. Important contacts were made between German and Japa-

nese scientists among which some renowned cardiologists, and these formed the fertile soil for the further development of the concept of calcium antagonism. In due course verapamil entered the angina field on the wave of success of nifedipine. In this respect table 5.3 shows an interesting pattern.

Table 5.3
Number of clinical articles about verapamil
and nifedipine, and the proportion (%) of
clinical articles relating to angina pectoris.[90]

	Verapamil		Nifedipine	
Period				
1966 - 1970	56	46%	0	- -
1971 - 1975	196	13%	28	64%
1976 - 1980	388	18%	258	48%
1981 - 1985	964	22%	1188	27%

The table shows that nifedipine has been investigated particularly as an anti-anginal agent. The small number of articles during the period 1971 - 1975 is due to the fact that it was registered in 1973 and that reports of clinical trials appeared in the medical literature somewhat later. This contrasts sharp with the pattern related to verapamil. During the period 1966 - 1970 about half of the clinical articles concerned angina but evaluated the drug as a coronary vasodilating or beta blocking agent. Whereas clinical attention to verapamil increases after 1970, the proportion of clinical articles devoted to angina pectoris becomes considerably lower. This indicates that during the period 1971 - 1975 verapamil has been investigated for indications other than angina, particularly as an anti-arrhythmic drug. A large number of these studies were initiated independently of the company reflecting the cardiologists special interest.[91]

The scientometric analysis of Fleckenstein's concept of calcium antagonism, shows some unexpected results. Clinicians did not refer to the concept during the years 1973, 1975 and 1977, at least not extensively. The scientometric curve regarding Fleckenstein's work therefore represents to a great extent the "diffusion" of the concept of calcium antagonism in the experimental sciences. Instead, citation-context analysis revealed a particular mechanism through which basic concepts and therapeutic actions were connected, i.e. the separate reference made by clinicians to those clinical articles that established the therapeutic efficacy of the calcium antagonists and the concepts elaborated by Fleckenstein. Subsequently, attention was given to the informal research networks in which these connections were made.

It was shown that as far as anti-anginal therapy is concerned, nifedipine seems to have been far more important than verapamil in the further development of the concept of calcium antagonism. During the first half of the 1970s the profiles of verapamil and in particular nifedipine were disentangled from those of the nitrites and beta blockers while the category of angina pectoris became subdivided. These developments will be analyzed in the next section.

5.7. The application of the theory of drug and disease profiles.

In this section the theory of drug and disease profiles will be applied to the historical material presented in the preceding sections. Firstly, the changing concepts about the basic action of verapamil - i.e. coronary vasodilation, beta blockade and calcium antagonism - will be discussed (5.7.1). This is followed by a discussion of its cardio-depressive effects (5.7.2).

5.7.1. Changing views on the basic action of verapamil

The nitrites and dipyridamole make a good case for illustrating the changing views about coronary vasodilation which also influenced the views on the mechanism of action of verapamil. For British and American clinicians accepted the fact that the nitrites were a beneficial therapy and dipyridamole was not. While both drugs dilated coronary vessels, the importance of coronary vasodilation in relieving angina pectoris was doubted. On this basis, both drugs were used as a tool to investigate the disease mechanism.

The role of the various parts of the coronary vessel system was investigated, i.e. the role of large and medium coronary arterial vessels, the collateral vessels and the coronary stenoses. New concepts such as that of "steal-phenomenon" originated from this research. The steal-phenomenon postulated that a drug dilated coronary vessels with the result that blood supply to 'healthy' areas in the heart is **stolen** from the ischemic areas, i.e. those areas which are badly in need of blood and oxygen supply.[92] In due course intra-cardial perfusion was distinguished from coronary blood flow. On the basis of these new distinctions the effects of the nitrites and dipyridamole were determined. For some time, these effects on the coronary vessels were discussed, yet their significance in altering the course of the disease remained doubtful.

During the 1960s other aspects of the nitrites came to the fore to explain their beneficial effects. Awareness grew that the generalized vasodilation of the nitrites was the key action. Systemic venodilation (decreased pre-load) caused a decreased mechanical load on the heart, hence decreased demand. Systemic arterial vasodilation (decreased after-load) did the same. Accordingly, the mechanism of action of the nitrites could be interpreted in terms of supply and demand.

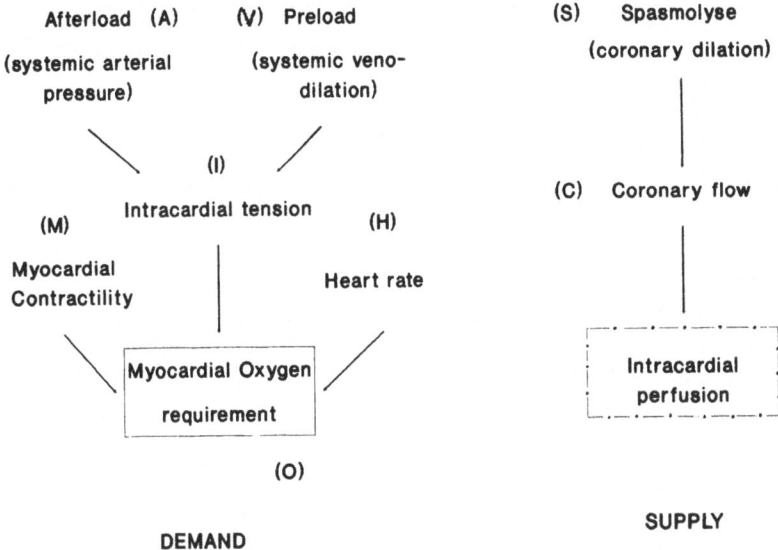

Figure 5.4
The interplay of major hemodynamically related factors leading to the disturbance of the supply-demand balance.

Figure 5.4 shows the view about the mechanism of angina pectoris as it emerged in the late 1960s and prevailed during the period 1970 - 1975. This representation reasonably approximates the principle variables directly or indirectly modulating myocardial oxygen requirements and supply, yet simplifies the existing body of knowledge in this field in several respects. (1) Interrelationships between variables of the left column (concerning demand) and those of the right column (supply) are deliberately left out. The same applies to the variables within the right or left column, that is with respect to inter-relationships other than depicted, for example, between (A) – (V). Particularly from the viewpoint of recent knowledge this may be confusing. Nowadays scientists are able to take these interrelationships into account, hence calculate the net effects more precisely.[93] However, in the early 1970s this simplification was of less significance.
(2) The box containing the variable intra-cardial perfusion is depicted with dotted lines. It is not taken up in the analysis because it was not a first-line concept.
(3) The major determinants of myocardial demand and supply are depicted, not the minor determinants.[94]
(4) The characters between the brackets denote the variables but obviously these variables possess values as well. Henceforth, the capitals will denote disease characteristics, and the lower case letters the characteristics of drugs. The removal of values yields an artificial

terminology. In reality (H), for example, will denote an increased heart rate in a particular disease (but a decreased rate in another disease) while (h) denotes a decreased heart rate caused by a particular drug (but an increased rate in another case).

(5) Between the variables causal relations are depicted. However, the principal variables are ranked independently from their supposed pathogenetic role. To some extent this is related into the distinction between major and minor determinants. However, within the sequence of major processes, hence within the set of major variables, a ranking may occur as well.

(6) The causal relations can be included as elements into the profiles but will be left out of consideration.

Thus, the simplifications are of a threefold nature. Firstly, the degree of precision with which the body of knowledge is represented. Secondly, the elimination of values and priorities of elements of the profiles. Thirdly, the exclusion of the causal relations. The major reason for these simplifications is to keep the analysis simple and instructive. Figure 5.5 represents the knowledge of the disease mechanism of angina and of the mechanism of action of anti-anginal drugs.

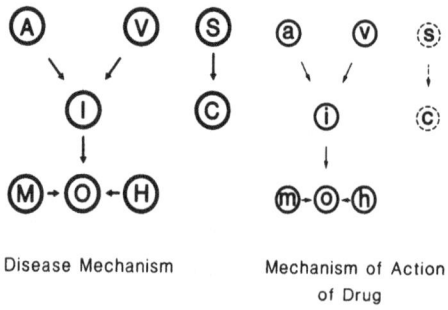

Disease Mechanism

Mechanism of Action
of Drug

Figure 5.5
Representation of the knowledge of angina pectoris and anti-anginal drugs reduced to the first aspect of the concept of profile: membership; the causal relationships between the characteristics are depicted (arrows) but not included into the analysis.

These structures can be translated into the language of profiles. Firstly, there is the disease profile of angina pectoris (= P):

$$P = \{A, V, I, M, H, O, S, C\}.$$

Secondly, we have the wished for (functional) drug profile (wf) with respect to P.

$$wf = \{a, v, i, m, h, o\}.$$

The wished for profile lacks elements s and c according to the view that emerged during the 1960s that ischemia itself caused vasodilation because of the production of metabolic products that acted as powerful vasodilating agents. Hence, it was considered very unlikely that any drug could evoke an additional dilation.

But what is the operational drug profile of(x)?

The set of(x) contains characteristics, ascribed to drug x, which belong to the domain of functional characteristics (F). However, suppose of(x) might have a, v, i, m, h, o, s or c as elements. Then, excluding the empty set, 255 sets (= $(2^n - 1)$; n = 8) are possible, for example:

drug x :   of(x) = {a,v}
drug y :   of(y) = {h,m}
drug z :   of(z) = {o,h,m,i,v,a}

Drug z   would be a clinician's dream because drug z perfectly matches wf. This is an utopian ideal and drug x and y are more realistic.[95] When comparing drug x and y in view of wf, then by definition:

$$| \, of(x) \, \Delta \, wf | \; = \; | \, of(y) \, \Delta \, wf | \, .$$

We see that drug x is as good or as bad as drug y with respect to wf. The profiles (of) of the nitrites, verapamil, nifedipine and propranolol around 1970 can be formulated - including values - as follows (table 5.4).

Table 5.4
Profiles of anti-anginal drugs.

	(Nit)	(Ver)	(Nif)	(Pro)
(a)	↓↓	↓	↓↓↓↓	↑/↔
(v)	↓↓	↔	↔	↓/↔
(i)	↓↓	↓	↓↓↓	↔/↓
(m)	↔	↓↓	↔	↓↓
(o)	↓↓↓	↓↓	↓↓↓	↓↓↓
(h)	↑	↓↓	↑/↔	↓↓↓↓
(s)	↑	↑↑	↑↑↑	↓/↑
(c)	↔	↑↑	↑↑↑	↓/↑

(Nit) = nitrates; (Ver) = verapamil; (Vif) = nifedipine;(Pro) = propranolol; (↓) to (↓↓↓↓) = moderately to very strongly decreased; (↑) to (↑↑↑↑) = moderately to very strongly increased; (↔) = no change.

It is presumed that the profiles listed above are 'realistic' enough to represent the knowledge about the drugs concerned. The values have to be excluded in order to deal with the first aspect, i.e. membership, of the "logic of profiles" only, and table 5.5 is obtained.

Table 5.5
Reconstructed profiles of nitrites (Nit), verapamil (Ver),
nifedipine (Nif) and propranolol (Pro) on the basis
of the presence/absence (+/-) of characteristics.

	(Nit)	(Ver)	(Nif)	(Pro)
(a)	+	-	+	-
(v)	+	-	-	-
(i)	+	+	+	-
(m)	-	+	-	+
(o)	+	+	+	+
(h)	-	+	-	+
(s)	+	+	+	-
(c)	-	+	+	-

As a result, the operational functional drug profiles are:

of(nit) = {a,v,i,o,s}[96],
of(ver) = {i,m,o,h,s,c},
of(nif) = {a,i,o,s,c},
of(pro) = {m,o,h}

Now we are able to make some remarks about the relationships between these profiles and some historical developments described above.

When verapamil was introduced as a coronary vasodilator, its operational therapeutic profile differed from the one depicted above, e.g. of(ver) = {s,c}. Once, its additional properties were found, and suppose these were "i", "m", "o" and "h", verapamil was considered as a drug with beta blocker properties. For, of(ver) ∩ of(pro) = {m,o,h}.

Several arguments accumulated during the second half of the 1960s leading to the rejection of verapamil as a beta blocker.

One was that more elements than depicted here were added to the set of(pro), relating to features which verapamil did not possess. For example, characteristics related to blockade of the sympathetic drive such as blockade of isoprenaline and exercise induced tachycardia. The discussion between the ICI scientists and Bateman illustrates this.

Another argument was that, in order to classify a compound as a beta blocker, its effects on various established indications had to be estimated. A compound might mimic the effects of propranolol in angina pectoris, but when it doesn't in other diseases with the established effectiveness of propranolol, then the compound is probably not a beta blocker.[97]

The third argument was the conflicting results in clinical trials. All beta blockers had been found very effective in angina pectoris in contrast to verapamil.

The fourth argument was that of(ver) contained the characteristics "s" and "c" which beta blockers did not possess.

Once rejected as a beta blocker, verapamil was a mere coronary vasodilator (of(ver) = {s,c}). But the views about this type of action had changed. This latter point brings us to the development concerning the nitrites. In the early 1960s it was the case that of(nit'') = {s,c} while in the late 1960s of(nit) = {a,v,i,o,s}. The following sequence emerges (figure 5.6).

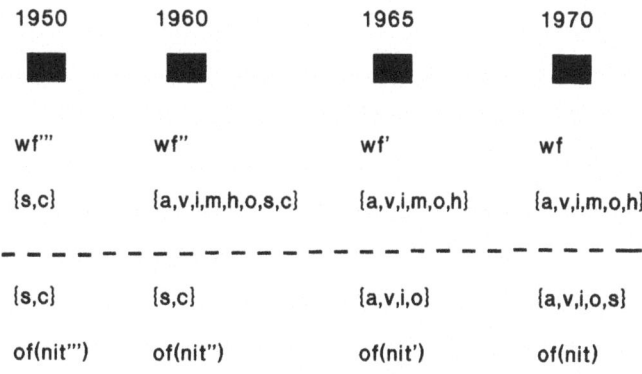

Figure 5.6
Sequence of events regarding wf(angina pectoris) and of(nit) from 1950 to 1970.

Since the changing sets representing the action of the nitrites kept on intersecting the wished for functional profile of angina pectoris, the nitrites remained worthwhile drugs throughout the 1960s. For despite the changes with respect to the nitrites (of(nit''') - of(nit)), these were paralleled with changes regarding wf - from wf'' to wf. Verapamil was indeed a dying drug, because it was inferior both to propranolol and the nitrites (l of(ver) ∆ wf l > l of(nit) ∆ wf l ; l of(ver) ∆ wf l > l of(pro) ∆ wf l).

However, a new feature in the history of verapamil was seen during the first half of the 1970s, when the syndrome of angina pectoris was split into two categories, classic (exertional) angina and vasospastic angina, hence the situation represented in figure 5.7.

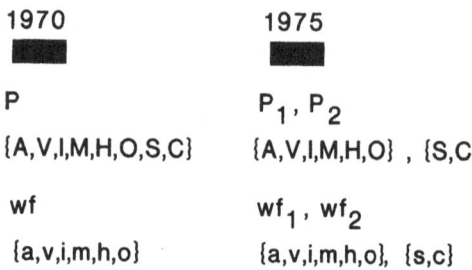

Figure 5.7
Differentiation of the profiles of angina pectoris and the wished for functional drug profiles from 1970 to 1975.

As a result of this sub-division we can understand how verapamil came to be established as a useful drug in both forms of angina pectoris (P_2 as well P_1). The intriguing point is that nifedipine was responsible for this process of subdivision, the result of which was transferred to verapamil. Firstly, nifedipine was clearly distinguished from the beta blockers. Secondly, its nitrite-like action was established, yet it was differentiated from the nitrites as well. Thirdly, its potential efficacy with respect to distinct sets of angina patients was proposed, particularly its effect in variant angina. Fourthly, nifedipine was increasingly acknowledged as a calcium antagonist.

Using the operation of symmetric difference it becomes apparent why it was easier to distinguish nifedipine than verapamil from the beta blockers:

(1) $| \text{of(nif)} \vartriangle \text{of(pro)} | > | \text{of(ver)} \vartriangle \text{of(pro)} |$

With respect to the distinction from the nitrites, the situation is as follows:

(2) $| \text{of(nif)} \vartriangle \text{of(nit)} | < | \text{of(ver)} \vartriangle \text{of(nit)} |$

Indeed, it was hard to believe that nifedipine did not have a nitrite-like action. In fact, the Bayer scientists and some other participants of the 1st Nifedipine symposium considered nifedipine as a nitrite-like compound. Although its complex profile was readily identified, the "direct" effects of nifedipine were very different from its "indirect" effects. Considering its direct effects (in-vitro studies), nifedipine appeared to be a coronary vasodilating, negative inotropic and chronotropic agent which was much stronger than verapamil. To unravel its complex actions all sorts of concepts were put forward but the concept of calcium antagonism was not very helpful. For clinicians and scientists involved in nifedipine-research this concept only explained the basic mechanism of nifedipine on the vessels.

This situation changed for three reasons. Firstly, the spasmolytic effect on the coronary vessels became a therapeutic target in itself when coronary vasospasm was recognized as a cause of (several forms of) angina pectoris. Secondly, a new therapeutic target, i.e. the prevention and counteraction of myocardial ischemia, emerged. Then, the direct effects of nifedipine on myocardial contractility and coronary perfusion became important. These effects were part of of(nif) and were the immediate result of calcium antagonism. Thirdly, but not related to nifedipine, the negative chronotropic effects of verapamil, which are direct effects as well, were also explained in terms of calcium antagonism.

As a result, Fleckenstein's claim regarding the direct effects of the calcium antagonists, e.g. their oxygen-saving effect, their negative inotropic effects, their preventive effect on calcium overload and cardiac necrosis, became acceptable. In addition, the similarity of the direct action of nifedipine and verapamil, although different in their overall action, strengthened Fleckenstein's argument for classifying both compounds as calcium antagonists, separate from the nitrites and the beta blockers. However, the dissimilarities between verapamil and nifedipine would eventually lead to the recognition of different subtypes in the class of calcium antagonists.

To estimate Fleckenstein's contribution to the field, the distinction between experimental and clinical characteristics (chapter 2) is useful.
Accordingly, we have:

(1) PE= the experimental profile of a particular disease;
(2) PC= the clinical profile of a particular disease;
(3) P= PE ∪ PC;

(4) ofe(x)= operational functional-experimental profile of drug x;
(5) ofc(x)= operational functional-clinical profile of drug x;
(6) of= ofe ∪ ofc;

(7) wfe= wished for functional-experimental profile in view of PE;
(8) wfc= wished for functional-clinical profile in view of PC;
(9) wf= wfe ∪ wfc.

Fleckenstein worked to establish the effects of verapamil and related compounds on the energy expenditure of the heart, the release of calcium from sarcoplasmatic and mitochondrial stores, on calcium and sodium channels, on cell membrane permeability and on the architecture of cardiac tissue. That is, he attempted to delineate elements belonging to ofe(ver) and ofe(nif). These processes were also being investigated in basic (experimental) research into disease mechanisms. This knowledge of experimental disease characteristics, i.e. PE, affected the wfe profile.

Scientists may use different sorts of heuristic principles to connect the various profiles. One simple heuristic principle (HP) is:

HP1 =: ofe(x) Δ ofe(y) ⊂ ofe(x) Δ ofe(z)   →   ofc(x) Δ ofc(y) ⊂ ofc(x) Δ ofc(z).

This principle says that if drug x and y are more similar in experimental respect than x and z, then x and y are also clinically more similar than x and z. So, when Fleckenstein classified verapamil (x) and nifedipine (y) as calcium antagonists experimentally and distinguished both from the nitrites or beta blockers (z), he claimed that their respective functional-clinical profiles were also more similar than with respect to the nitrites or beta blockers. But in fact, Fleckenstein claimed even more, as illustrated by the next heuristic principle:

HP2 =: ofe(x) ∆ wfe ⊂ ofe(y) ∆ wfe → ofc(x) ∆ wfc ⊂ ofc(y) ∆ wfc.

This principle says that the (dis)similarities between x and y with respect to the wished for functional-experimental profile apply also to the (dis)similarities between x and y regarding the wished for functional-clinical profile. By reversing these heuristic principles, we get:

HP3 =: ofc(x) ∆ ofc(y) ⊂ ofc(x) ∆ ofc(z) → ofe(x) ∆ ofe(y) ⊂ ofe(x) ∆ ofe(z).

HP4 =: ofc(x) ∆ wfc ⊂ ofc(y) ∆ wfc → ofe(x) ∆ wfe ⊂ ofe(y) ∆ wfe.

The list of heuristic principles may be extended, e.g. by replacing the qualitative relations for the quantitative relations, by substituting other drugs for x, y and z, and by introducing a time dimension, i.e. a sequence of events in which the various profiles are changing - for example: ofe(x) → ofe(x') → ofe(x'') → ofe(x'''). In this way a fairly precise picture may be obtained of the way knowledge is transferred from one domain to the other, in a repetitive process. This is partly what happened when Fleckenstein elucidated the actions of verapamil, D600, pren-ylamine and nifedipine and differentiated them from the beta blockers and the nitrites. Obviously, different strands of knowledge contribute to this process.

5.7.2. The cardio-depressive effects of verapamil.

When the local anaesthetic or cardio-depressive actions of verapamil were discussed, scientists tried to sort out which actions it possessed. Was it a local anaesthetic, that is, a cardio-depressive agent, or was it a beta blocker? Did verapamil exert either type of action? If so, it should be classified accordingly. If not, the profile had to be re-constructed. Most importantly, the "quinidine-like" action was discussed from the therapeutic viewpoint. Thus, of(ver) with respect to of(qui) and similarly of(pro), where "ver" denotes verapamil, "qui" quinidine, and "pro" propranolol. Four therapeutic cases were pivotal to the discussion:

a. the relief of arrhythmias;	wf(ar)
b. the relief of anginal pain;	wf(ap)
c. the reduction of work load of the heart.	wf(ap)
d. the precipitation\aggravation of heart failure;	wf(ar), wf(ap)

Following each of the cases (first column), their "nature" in terms of the theory being presented in this study, is listed (second column). The first case refers to cardiac arrhythmias

(= P(AR), hence to wf(ar)). The second and third to angina pectoris (= P(AP), hence wf(ap)). The fourth case, which is more complex, refers to an undesired effect (with respect to both diseases).

The first two cases are rather simple to illustrate following the same kind of reasoning in the foregoing section. An example is two events, dated 1964 and 1968, relating to arrhythmias (figure 5.8).

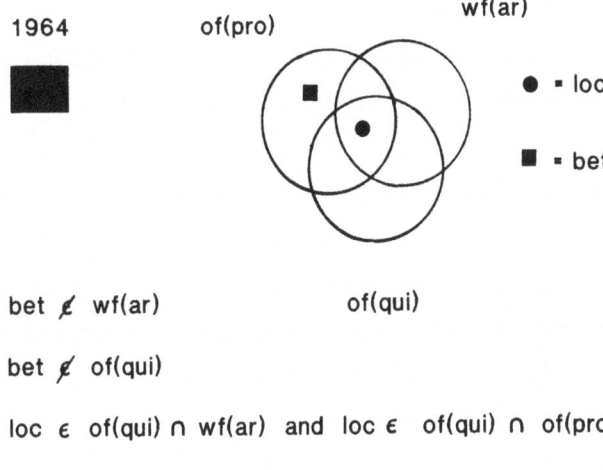

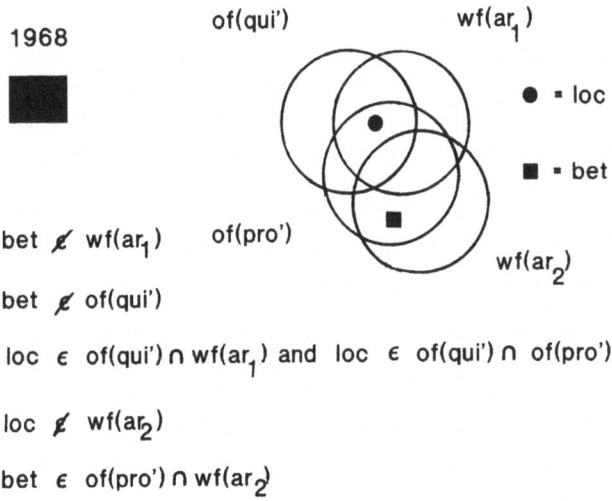

Figure 5.8
Shift in profiles of anti-arrhythmic drugs: local anaesthetic (quinidine-like) and beta blocking activity in cardiac dysrythm.

The crucial issue centered around beta blockade and quinidine like action. Now, suppose the former is represented by "bet" and the latter by "loc" - the term "loc" denotes "local anaesthetic (or quinidine-like) activity" and contrasts with "qui" which denotes the compound quinidine. Note that bet and loc may represent a set itself containing therapeutic characteristics with respect to cardiac arrhythmias. Furthermore, suppose bet $\in$ of(pro) and bet $\in$ of(pro'); loc $\in$ of(qui) and loc $\in$ of(qui'); as well as loc $\in$ of(pro) and loc $\in$ of(pro'). Then figure 5.8 is obtained.

Figure 5.8, including the formal statements, expresses a particular shift between 1964 and 1968. Initially the quinidine-like/local anaesthetic action of propranolol instead of its beta blocking action was ascribed to its anti-arrhythmic effect. Then, two forms of cardiac arrhythmias were differentiated.[98] The quinidine-like action (denoted by loc) appeared to be crucial to the first form, whereas beta blockade action (represented by bet) was crucial to the second form.

The reasoning which applies to the quinidine-like action of propranolol in cardiac arrhythmias can also be applied to verapamil. Once verapamil was rejected as a beta blocker, its quinidine-like action remained - in addition to its coronary vasodilator action. In the course of the 1960s the drug was coming to represent a completely novel type of anti-arrhythmic action.

The second therapeutic issue was whether the relief of anginal pain was due to a direct local anaesthetic effect or to beta blockade. One strategy for settling this issue was to compare the stereoisomers, i.e. the laevo and dextro isomers, of propranolol which appeared to be equally active in producing direct cardiac depression while their beta blocking activities were quite different. Another strategy emerged when sotalol came available, i.e. a beta blocker without local anaesthetic activity.

These strategies distinguish between structural and functional characteristics of drugs as described in chapter 2. Accordingly, the exchange of knowledge between these two domains can be described as in the case of experimental and clinical functional characteristics described above.

The third and fourth therapeutic issues are much more complex, particularly so because they are interrelated. Since their clarification requires introducing values into the analysis, and this will be discussed in chapter 7, only the prevailing views are summarized here.

Main stream thinking is characterized by five routes (figure 5.9a). The routes Fleckenstein attempted to elaborate, fell outside the scope of the field (figure 5.9b).

The routes 1 - 5 defined the boundaries within which basic scientists and clinical scientists were allowed to introduce new mechanisms of action. Fleckenstein's attempts, for example, to segregate verapamil and related compounds such as prenylamine (Segontin) from the beta blocking compounds by their action on Ca^{2+}, was disregarded by workers in the beta blocker field. Vaughan-Williams commented: *"If you go back to the early literature..say, Fleckenstein. He didn't make a distinction between beta blockers and calcium antagonists. He published about, could be in 1968, a sort of spectrum, it was all to do with calcium, and there were agents which increased the calcium activation and those which decreased the activation. Beta blockers were just on this scale, part of the scale" .*[99]

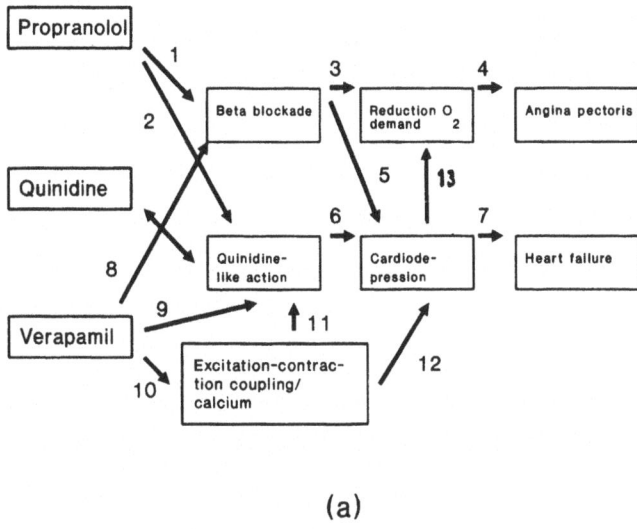

(a)

General view

1.   1 → 3 → 4 (yes)
2.   1 → 5 → 7 (yes)
3.   2 → 6 → 7 (possibly)
4.   8 → 3 → 4 (no)
5.   9 → 6 → 7 (probably)

Fleckenstein's view

6.   10 → 12 → 13 → 4 (yes)
7.   8 → 3 → 4 (no)
8.   8 → 5 → 7 (no)
9.   10 → 12 → 7 (yes)

(b)

Figure 5.9

So, when Fleckenstein used the beta blockers as tools, he used these in a way which was neither recognized nor accepted. Fleckenstein's procedure was to use high doses and the value of unravelling the basic mechanisms of the contractile function of the heart while operating at the toxic level of the various compounds, raised scepticism. Particularly so, because the issue of cardiac failure aroused much controversy. How then, could a compound which obviously possessed such a strong cardio-depressant action, possibly be good in angina pectoris? Indeed, Fleckenstein did put beta blocking and cardio-depressive action on a par while considering them as different ways to the same objective: reduction of the oxygen demand of the heart. Such a thought was unheard of at the time.

5.8. Conclusions

The majority of British and American cardiologists rejected verapamil as a beta blocker, and beta blocker or not, it was no alternative to propranolol in anti-anginal treatment. Therefore, the decline of the coronary vasodilation concept, and the therapeutic claims about beta blockade, affected verapamil's viability such that it became a "dying drug" in late 1960s.[100] But behind the scenes research continued and verapamil pointed the way to new perspectives in the cardiovascular area. This undercurrent of scientific creativity demonstrated itself when the novel type of anti-arrhythmic action of verapamil was unraveled and the little company of Knoll was pleasantly surprised when this aspect of the drug attracted so much attention. Simultaneously, the field of anti-anginal therapy was revolutionized. Nifedipine formed the focus of new perspectives which were transferred to verapamil as well. This aspect of the history of verapamil, a drug waiting to be re-discovered, elicited the expression of "a sleeping beauty".[101]

It is striking to see how "old" concepts and drugs at the same time provide the basis for unraveling new aspects of drugs and diseases. This applies to dipyridamole, nitrites and other coronary vasodilators, and also to quinidine and the beta blockers. The same may be said about the way Fleckenstein approached the new principle of calcium antagonism. Working on the biochemistry and physiology of myocardial excitability and contraction his research moved within the limits of the developing views of drug action and disease mechanisms. Yet simultaneously, by applying the new concepts and techniques and relating them to clinically defined targets, Fleckenstein broke through these boundaries. In this study several examples of differential relationships between experimental research and clinical investigations have been touched upon in an inductivist way. Some were mentioned in describing the history of verapamil and Fleckenstein's research project including the scientometric analysis performed, and others were illustrated when applying the theory of drug and disease profiles, which also highlighted some landmarks in the historical description.

Finally, the question arises: "Why did it take so long before the calcium antagonists were accepted as worthwhile anti-anginal drugs?". Some interesting points may be noted.

The first refers to the decline of the coronary vasodilator concept. After such a dramatic defeat much effort is needed to reverse the scepticism about compounds once conceived of as coronary vasodilators.

Secondly, the beta blockers caused a great stir in cardiology and formed a rapidly expanding field, particularly so, once they were recognized as anti-hypertensive agents. This fact certainly contributed to the continuing interest in this class of compounds. Where the money flows, there scientific progress goes and this was certainly true for the beta blockers. Pharmaceutical companies world-wide provided cardiological centres with the money to perform clinical research.

Thirdly, and very importantly, the major issue that formed such a stumbling-block with respect to the beta blockers, i.e. their cardio-depressive effects, became settled. The claim of Fleckenstein that verapamil and related compounds did the same as beta blockers but left the sympathetic drive intact was no longer a feature for promoting a new compound. Moreover, clinical experience showed that verapamil caused or aggravated heart failure.

Fourthly, it wasn't easy to say that verapamil and nifedipine were 'similar' compounds because their spectrum of activities differed markedly. To say that these compounds are 'calcium antagonists' is open to different interpretations. The opinion of fundamental scientists that these agents block 'slow channels' in cardiac cell membranes is but one aspect. It was recognized that throughout the organism calcium played an important role as the mediator of communicative biochemical events. But more importantly, therapeutically complex patterns of action had to be separated. In fact, this implied the further differentiation of calcium antagonists on the one hand, e.g. to profile verapamil with regard to nifedipine and other compounds, and to differentiate its activities from other drugs, notably of the nitrites, on the other.

Fifthly, shifts in medical views of angina pectoris took place in the first half of the 1970s and accelerated in the late 1970s. The dominant view of angina of effort decayed and new subsets of angina patients were created. Within this spectrum of various forms of angina pectoris, the efficacy of verapamil and nifedipine could be reconsidered. Subsequently, these compounds, once burdened with the unpopular label "coronary vasodilators" were shown to be equally effective in the treatment of angina pectoris when compared in double blind tests with beta blockers.

Chapter 6. Metamorphosis of a disease
Profiles of angina pectoris in Anglo-American medicine

6.1. Introduction

This chapter covers the development of views about angina pectoris in Anglo-American medicine. The historical description roughly covers the period 1950 - 1980 but emphasis is given to shifts in the late 1950s and early 1970s. The aim is to show that changing views on disease can be described adequately in terms of the language of disease profiles.

However, this chapter serves two other purposes as well. One is to discuss the changing perspectives of angina pectoris that set the stage for the development of the beta blockers and the calcium antagonists which has been described in chapter 4 and 5. For this reason, the rise and decline of the syndrome of "angina of effort", the revival of the theory of coronary spasm and the increasing differentiation of the disease entity of angina pectoris will be described in considerable detail. The other purpose is to provide a basis for highlighting the differences with the medical views in German speaking countries. These differences will be the topic of the next chapter when providing the medical background of the beta blocker project at Boehringer Ingelheim.

Firstly, an historical account of Anglo-American medical views of angina pectoris will be given (6.2). Then, through cognitive maps (6.3) and social maps (6.4) of the profiles of angina pectoris the body of knowledge over the period 1950 - 1960, 1960 - 1970 and 1970 - 1980 will be discussed.

6.2. Anglo-American medical views of angina pectoris

Angina of effort: a typical form of angina pectoris

"There is a disorder of the breast, marked with strong and peculiar symptoms, considerable for the kind of danger belonging to it, and not extremely rare, of which I do not recollect any mention among medical authors. The seat of it and sense of strangling pain and anxiety with which it is attended may make it not improper to be called angina pectoris.

Those who are affected with it are seized, while they are walking, and more particularly when they walk soon after eating, with a painful and most disagreeable sensation in the breast which seems as if it would take their life away if it were to increase or to continue: the moment they stand still, all this uneasiness vanishes. In all other respects patients who are at the beginning of this disorder are perfectly well, and in particular have no shortness of breath, from which it is totally different". [1]

In this way Heberden described the syndrome angina pectoris in his lecture to the Royal College of Physicians of London in 1768. Heberden's description of the picture is what became later known as the **typical** form of angina pectoris. English language medical literature of the 1950s and 1960s understates this typical condition of angina pectoris, so perfectly described by Heberden.

What sort of elements make up typical angina pectoris? To be sure, angina pectoris is but a symptom. It is rather unusual to recognize only a symptom in order to label a nosologic entity, but with angina pectoris this is the case. If the symptom is genuine, the diagnosis is accurate. The patient has pain in the chest, very often paroxysmal of nature. The pain is not perceived as originating in the heart but appears to be localized in the surface area of the chest wall. Complex nervous pathways through which pain from the heart is conducted and finally projected in the chest wall area, are responsible for site and character of the pain. Theories of pain, for example those of MacKenzie and Head have influenced the observation of patterns of anginal pain at the bedside or in the consulting-room.

Many other conditions may cause pain in the chest as well and at a symposium devoted to thoracic pains in 1956, seventy-eight clinical conditions were enumerated as capable of causing pain in the chest.[2] Despite this complexity English medical literature is characterized by the great trust and sheer confidence with which the physician is able to make the diagnosis through careful history-taking.

The diagnosis of typical angina pain involves many factors but the most important feature was its relationship to exertion. Friedberg declared in his influential textbook in 1956 that physical exercise was *"by far the most frequent and most significant precipitating cause of angina pectoris"*.[3] Other conditions such as digestion, cold, emotion and pathological circumstances such as tachycardia could evoke anginal pain too but it was bodily exertion that was the most typical feature of anginal pain. Moreover, precisely this relationship to exertion differentiated anginal pain from other chest pains. According to Friedberg, who listed twenty clinical conditions that had to be differentiated from angina pectoris, pain in these conditions *"is chiefly distinguished from angina pectoris by being unrelated to general bodily exertion, especially walking rapidly or uphill"*.[4]

This relationship between pain and exertion vividly illuminates the specific name that has been given to typical angina pectoris, e.g. angina of effort. Whenever other precipitating factors seemed to be more important than exertion, this was considered atypical. Emotion is a precipitating factor and may be involved as often as exertion. On the other hand, the symptom is disregarded particularly because it reveals functional disorders without organic, hence without clinical significance. This ambiguity appears several times. When discussing emotion, Friedberg stated: *"While intense emotional states may provoke in neurotic persons various forms of pain in the cardiac area which are distinct from angina pectoris, they may also and often do cause definite attacks of angina pectoris, whether or not there is an associated neurosis"*.[5] According to Wood in his classic textbook **Diseases of the Heart and Circulation** of 1952, probably the most influential[6] textbook of British cardiology in the period 1950 - 1965: *"Pain may also be induced by emotion..but this is perhaps less typical, emotionally produced pain being more often innocent and associated with anxiety states"*.[7]

Emotional stress like anger, fear, worry and excitement was well-known to the physician as precipitating events in chest pain. Evidence of this point was the popularity of tranquilizers and the recommendation of a less emotionally stressful life style. However, the clinical significance was determined by the similarity of the behaviour of anginal pain in case of exertion.[8] Friedberg had this comment: *"The prompt occurrence of transient chest pain with emotion and its prompt subsidence when the emotional stimulus abates are strongly suggestive of angina pectoris".* [9] Emotion was considered a genuine symptom when it mimicked the pattern seen in exertion. Exertion was considered as the most frequent and significant symptom. To quote Wood: *"Attacks are brought on especially by walking uphill, or against the wind, by hurrying after meals, or by any unaccustomed exercise".* [10]

Undoubtedly angina of effort - also termed "exertional angina" - represented the major clinical pattern of angina pectoris in Anglo-American medicine, and this was especially so in the 1950s. During the 1960s this picture reached its zenith.

The characteristic features of angina pectoris and the certainty of its diagnosis are striking features of English medical textbooks. Wood stated that if chest pain is consistent regarding site, quality, duration and relation to cardiac work, *"the diagnosis must stand under any conditions except malingering".* [11] Friedberg's textbook radiates the same confidence: *"A great variety of conditions associated with chest pain are sometimes mentioned as requiring differentiation from angina pectoris. However, when the distinctive clinical character of angina pectoris is clearly understood, its confusion with other diseases causing pain in the chest and upper extremity should be rare. Almost always the typical clinical history suffices to make the differentiation".* [12]

Symptoms: voice of nature?

If so much trust and confidence is laid in the outstanding features of angina pectoris and in the clarity and power of history-taking as a clinical tool, why then were cardiovascular techniques coming to dominate the field during the late 1940s and 1950s? Sophisticated techniques such as electrocardiography and cardiac catheterization became applied clinically on a wide scale. According to Dexter this period *"was characterized by such progress in cardiology as the world had never seen before".* [13] Cardiology entered a new era. Clinicians started to integrate their technical experiences and expertise with their clinical observations.

The introductory remarks in Wood's textbook refer to this potentially conflicting situation: *"The more conservative physicians may have witnessed these and many other less important technical developments with some misgiving, but relatively few have expressed reactionary views. Yet there is already plenty of evidence to show that we are in danger of losing our clinical heritage and of pinning too much faith in figures thrown up by machines. Medicine must suffer if this tendency is not checked. In presenting this book I have attempted to maintain a proper balance between man and his instruments, between experienced opinion and statistics, between traditional views and the heterodox, between bed-side medicine and special tests, between the practical and the academic, and so to link the past with the present".* [14]

This balance has been upset throughout the history of angina pectoris. Despite the apparent power of history taking physicians came to rely on technical evidence. An editorial in Circulation noticed with bitterness: *"The failure of some physicians to obtain a thorough history in patients with angina pectoris is of great concern. They seem to rely mainly on electrocardiographic data recorded after exercise tests of varying degrees of exertion in order to determine whether or not a patient has the anginal syndrome".* [15]

The bitterness originated from the view that *"an exercise electrocardiogram is indicated in only a few patients, since an accurate diagnosis of angina pectoris can practically always be made by means of a careful interrogation".* [16]

The emphasis on technical measurement and the decreasing diagnostic skills raised much concern in the medical profession. Presenting an address on **Cardiac Symptoms** at the 1951 meeting of the American College of Physicians, Sir John Parkinson, commented:

"The subject of symptomatology will always retain its importance in medicine because symptoms form the first contact between patient and doctor. It is the voice of nature, and when a patient complains he enters our world and we recognize a human need. For convenience I shall apply the term 'symptoms' to subjective sensations of which the patient complains. While everyone agrees on their value in approaching a diagnosis, symptoms have been moved to the background by current interest in signs and in scientific technique. But if we apportion too little time for eliciting symptoms, we shall suffer in our diagnosis". [17]

If there is a disease that illustrates Parkinson's remarks, then probably the best candidate is angina pectoris. While there seemed to be no need for technology at all, diagnosis of angina pectoris became increasingly technical.

The simple question "Why did physicians need so much technology when the diagnosis of angina pectoris can be made with the help of history-taking?" requires a complex answer which falls outside the context of this chapter. Without doubt this trend reflected the scientific and technical upheaval in general medicine after the Second World War. Three issues, however, are worth mentioning: 1. the symbiotic but strained relationship between cardiology and cardiac surgery; 2. the striving for objectivity in therapeutic evaluation; and 3. the "physiological or hemodynamic movement" in cardiology.

The symbiotic relationship between cardiology and cardiac surgery

When the rapid advance in cardiology took place during the late 1940s and 1950s, *"surgeons have invaded what was once forbidden territory and are rapidly turning miraculous operations on the heart into the commonplace (...) It is, perhaps, not really a coincidence that more precise methods of diagnosis became available just when surgery demanded them".*

In this way Wood sketched the early beginnings of the symbiotic relationship of cardiology with cardiac surgery.[18] Professional conflict certainly underlies this need for differentiation and precision in diagnosis. The use of new methods for accurate diagnosis of surgically correctable heart diseases affected clinical taxonomy. The 1940s and 1950s witnessed the pioneering of coronary artery surgery based upon the rapidly growing view in the 1950s, *"that coronary artery surgery should be physiologic, i.e., the operation should increase the blood supply to the myocardium".* [19]

The pioneering of these techniques took place in patients with severe forms of angina pectoris, such as severe angina at rest or angina decubitus which are refractory to therapy. Commenting on the impressive results of his procedure, Vineberg wrote: *"When a bed-chair invalid of the angina decubitus type, using 300 nitroglycerin tablets per week, after internal mammary artery implantation becomes pain-free and returns to work, it suggests that the implanted artery has contributed fresh blood to the ischemic myocardium".* [20] By and large disabled patients were the subject of pioneering in cardiac surgery. These patients were easily distinguished from those with angina of effort or myocardial infarction.

Though cardiac surgery took a fresh start in the 1950s, also in the anti-anginal field, it is particularly the method of coronary artery bypass grafting introduced by Favorolo in 1968 that caused a great stir in cardiac surgery and cardiology.[21] This therapeutic achievement merged with the application of coronary angiography according to the method introduced by Sones in 1959 and widely applied during the 1960s.[22] Coronary angiography enabled the visualization of the coronary vessels in the patient and subsequently it became a major breakthrough in the diagnosis of coronary heart disease. This was not merely confined to the domain of heart diseases in need of surgical correction. It also affected clinical taxonomy of heart disease in general. But in angina pectoris in particular this took place during the late 1960s and 1970s with the rise of coronary bypass surgery.[23]

The bypass operation grew rapidly in popularity. Some 22.000 operations were done in the United States in 1971, approximately 45.000 in 1973 and about 57.000 in 1975. Preston (1977) estimated that the total monetary cost associated with this operation amounted to about 1% of the annual national health expenditure.[24]

Another aspect, related to the symbiotic relationship between cardiology and cardiac surgery, underlies the differentiation of the various forms of angina pectoris. Diagnostic terms such as "typical" or "atypical" angina weren't the only true criteria anymore. Prognostic and therapeutic criteria to assess the patients at risk and to determine benefits and costs of therapy, be it pharmaceutical or surgical, appeared on the diagnostic scene. These criteria were expressed in terms such as "intractable angina", "angina resistant, refractory or unresponsive to therapy" or "unstable angina". These terms entered cardiology late in the 1960s. Until this time this particular conflict between pharmaceutical and surgical therapy affected clinical taxonomy of angina pectoris only in a limited way.

The need for objectivity in therapeutic evaluation

The second issue lies at the centre of anti-anginal treatment and is confined to the question of therapeutic evaluation. There are few areas in medicine in which the placebo-effect and the flimsy evidence of uncontrolled observation in the claims of therapeutic effectiveness have been argued so eagerly and heatedly as in the field of angina pectoris.

Anti-anginal treatment became a test-case for the controlled study of therapeutic effectiveness. As Silber and Katz (1953) stated: *"It is apparent, from even a casual survey of the literature dealing with the medical treatment of angina, that confusion and conflicting reports surround the use of each of the coronary drugs currently in favour. Such discrepancy in results has as its basis the poorly designed clinical experiment. In this regard, several factors are of major importance; some concern the object of the study, others the investigator".* [25]

But largely the bias on the part of the investigator originated from his or her **object**! Beecher pointed out that: *"Observation is difficult enough when objective signs are under consideration; it is more difficult when subjective responses are examined. Then not only is the patient's sending station of doubtful accuracy but the observer's reception of the signals is confused by extraneous noises produced* *by tradition, by confusion derived from his own more or less acute perception, by his failure to seek patiently for the truth, but most all by bias".* [26]

Obviously Beecher touched upon the contrasts between symptoms and signs, the subjective and the objective, and the title of his own editorial comment was "clinical impression and clinical investigation". Indeed, two opposing trends declared themselves and were evidence of the profound differences of opinion as to what should be the aim of therapeutic evaluation. One stream of cardiologists focussed on anginal pain which is after all why the patient entered the world of the clinician. The other stream focussed on the measurement of objective parameters which, rightly or wrongly, were considered to be the expression, if not of the pain, in any case of the natural course of the disease.[27]

Despite the heated debate, the general consensus was that carefully designed clinical experiments were capable of eliminating the investigator's bias. One was then left with the object of study. In this respect it is striking to see how amongst clinicians involved in therapeutic evaluation, be they proponents of the "subjective" or the "objective" approach, **the obscure character of the syndrome angina pectoris, i.e. the object of the study**, was spelled out. Two quotations illustrate this point. One comes from Silber and Katz who relied solely upon the relief of pain as a criterion of the efficacy of any anginal drug and who rejected exercise or other 'objective' tests. The other comes from Russek et al. who strongly supported the use of objective therapeutic goals.

"One must first appreciate the marked variability in the incidence and severity of pain that occurs in patients with angina who are receiving no therapy whatever. These vagaries occur not only under the influence of season, climate, disease in other organ systems, and emotional disturbances but also under apparently unchanging conditions. (..) Because of such variability, the conviction has grown in our department that observations (...) should be made for a minimum of one year in a large group of patients. (...) Second, in choosing patients for study, only those with severe angina should comprise the group. By severe, we refer to patients experiencing a minimum of several attacks of angina a day" [28]

"...if pain represented a definite entity and reflected a fairly constant degree of coronary insufficiency in each patient. Obviously, this is not the case. Pain is of infinite variability and to date has not been accurately quantitated in man either subjectively or objectively. Furthermore, even if such precise measurements were possible, pain could not reliably reflect the status of the coronary circulation or the degree of myocardial ischemia" [29]

True, both quotations, though in different terms, discuss the value of pain as therapeutic endpoint and as marker of the disease but they also touch upon the variability and multiplicity of anginal pain as well. Whereas, the characteristic features of anginal pain was stressed when discussing clinical diagnosis, the irregularity of the same pain was emphasized when the question was therapeutic evaluation. Indeed, the precision of the diagnosis of angina pectoris constituted an indispensable premise to every clinical therapeutic investigation.

In this atmosphere, the difficulties of the history-taking of angina of effort, such a clear and genuine diagnosis, were stressed. Not history but technical evidence, not symptoms but signs should form the bottom line of therapeutic evaluation. Accordingly, it was not the voice of nature that spoke to the clinician but the hand-made manipulation of nature to serve the purpose of accurate diagnosis.

The "hemodynamic movement" in cardiology

During the course of this technical invasion in cardiology, various types of clinical examination have been used to assist the physician in his diagnosis. Their significance lies in the bridge these techniques were supposed to build between angina pectoris as a symptom complex and angina as a patho-physiological entity.

By the 1950s the combined method of electrocardiography and the standard exercise test was widely accepted as the index of the pathological state of the myocardium in angina. As Wood stated: *"the only reliable test, however, is to obtain an electrocardiogram immediately after maximum effort, when characteristic depression of the RS-T segment, with or without inversion of the U wave, clinches the diagnosis"*. [30] Friedberg is somewhat more reserved in this respect because this test might not actually simulate the conditions which produce pain in any given patient.[31] Both Friedberg and Wood declared the standard exercise to be of accessory value in diagnosis.[32] However, the crucial point to be noted here is that this standardized test played an enormous role in therapeutic evaluation. On the one hand to guarantee the clinical diagnosis of the patients selected for the treatment test: "27 patients with typical angina were selected..." is the kind of statement that one regularly encounters in clinical articles about angina pectoris during the late 1950s and 1960s.[33] On the other hand these tests provided the critical parameters to be assessed with regard to therapeutic effectiveness. When in the late 1950s and early 1960s the standard exercise electrocardiographical test came to be criticized for its validity, specificity and sensitivity, this critique did not alter the dominant role of exercise tests in clinical research and therapeutic evaluation. Since the test embodied the category angina of effort it strengthened its already dominant position in clinical taxonomy.

Concomitantly with the development of exercise testing, the 1950s witnessed the rapid invasion of cardiac catheterization with which it was possible to measure intra-cardiac pressures and volumes. These hemodynamic parameters represented **internal cardiac work** in contrast with exercise tests that measured **external cardiac work**. But both were linked by the idea that it was the increase of cardiac work that evoked the anginal attack. And cardiac work was essentially a hemodynamic concept. Outstanding journals at that time, such as Circulation and Circulation Research, reinforced this hemodynamic approach. The preponderance of acute and short-term exercise and hemodynamic tests testify to the overwhelming influence this approach.

Together with this hemodynamic movement, mechanistic thinking dominated experimental medicine and cardiology. As Robinson stated: *"At that time, I think the pendulum is swinging back now, at that time there was an extremely mechanistic approach to medicine. The heart and circulation lent itself to a sort of engineering approach better than any other system. So it was very much in tune with the mood of the time. People were keen to see just how far you could go in analyzing the heart and circulation in mechanical terms. They were busy doing Fourier's analysis, pulse waves, rates of shortening, dp/dt, the rates of pressure rise in the ventricle (..)"*. [34]

The term mechanistic did not bear a negative meaning at that time. Cardiologists were intrigued by the sort of experiments that the new techniques enabled them to perform. Some

of this fascination is expressed by Chamberlain when he describes the preference of British cardiologists with respect to Circulation in comparison to the British Heart Journal: *"Circulation was an exciting journal in the 1960s. If you go back and look at them now, they're exciting. They were full of wonderful articles by super people. And British Heart Journal, nobody believed that it was in the same class as Circulation. That was the journal. It was way, way, way ahead of any other cardiac journal (..) Everything was miles behind. So, Circulation was where the progress was".* [35]
Circulation and also Circulation Research marked the frontier of Anglo-American cardiology in the 1950s and 1960s. The new techniques created a new brand of cardiology which had considerable impact in Britain. In fact, the interviewed clinicians all declared Paul Wood's textbook as the standard reference work which formed the living evidence of this new stream in cardiology. As Chamberlain stated: *"Really, he (Paul Wood, RV) came to cardiology virtually saying that I don't believe a thing. And he started from scratch. His textbook was based entirely on his own observations and with the new scientific cardiology, cardiac catheterization and so on. He started with nothing as it were. He didn't believe anything that anybody else had written. It wasn't to say that he denied it. It is just that he thought that it was better to wipe the slate clean. (..) And his teaching had enormous influence in the late 1950s and early 1960s (...) And his book was the Bible, for all British cardiologists".* [36]

What has been said is not to deny the cleavage between fundamental research in cardiology and general medical practice. This cleavage originates in opposing traditions in British medicine which in fact have a long history, and could be termed "naturalist" versus "scientist". The "scientific" tradition is characterized by its emphasis on the study of physiological mechanisms, its orientation towards clinical science and pure research, and its attempts to bring the clinic closer to the laboratory. In contrast, the "naturalistic" tradition was confined to communication and personal contact between doctor and patient, to clinical observation and the natural history of the disease.
These traditions have fought it out on rhetorical battleground, but there seem to be genuine grounds to distinguish both streams in British medicine. Swales, from whom the terms "naturalist" and "scientist" are borrowed, describes this long-lasting struggle in British medicine to explain that otherwise the Platt-Pickering-debate never could have taken place on British soil.[37] This famous debate during the 1950s and early 1960s about the nature of hypertension was shaped by this undercurrent of conflict in British medicine. Two quotations illustrate the differences between both traditions. One quotation comes from Lewis when defining the position of the scientific tradition in 1930 at the founding of the British Medical Research Society. The other one is from Ryle, a Guy's physician, appointed to the Regius Chair of Physic at Cambridge and finally to the Chair of Social Medicine at Oxford, advocating the naturalistic approach:

(Lewis): "This science seeks by observation and otherwise to define diseases as they occur in man: it attempts to understand the diseases and their many manifestations and here especially makes frequent use of the experimental method. It makes definite experiments upon disease or watches the effects of experiments conducted by injuries however these arise: it culls or actually creates and uses physiological and pathological knowledge immediately related and applicable to the diseases studied" [38]

(Ryle): *"There is a similarity between the approach of the great naturalists who owed their achievements to careful observation, recording and analysis and that of the famous names of medicine. If we exclude for the moment (although they too were essentially naturalists) the great discoverers in physiology like Harvey and the great discoverers in the realm of public health like Jenner, both of whom on the basis of close observation performed a historical experiment, we find that the ranks of the famous physicians are chiefly filled with men belonging to the observational school. These made no such great revelations in thought or practice as did Harvey and Jenner, but they provided by degrees the chapters of a great uncompleted 'Compendium of the Natural History of Disease'"* [39]

Both traditions have affected cardiology just as much as they have influenced other disciplines in British medicine. The scientific tradition has produced the renowned British clinicians like Lewis and MacKenzie who built up British cardiology in the 1920s and 1930s, and Pickering, Wood and McMichael who framed British cardiology in the Post-Second-World-War period.[40]

However, the aims of this tradition were not, and never have been dominant considerations for the majority of the British cardiologists outside the university clinics.[41] When asked what the reference journal for practicing cardiologists was, Silk commented on the situation in British cardiology:

"For the British cardiologists this has always been the British Heart Journal. But that was 'botanical'. In a sense, it was just describing interesting conditions, not actually whether you were going to do anything. But you know, if you had a rare fellow or some type of rare anatomical thing, you described the findings. It is more or less like 'Oh, I found another new plant! Isn't this interesting?'. That is, why we describe this as botanical. And the problem was that the British Cardiac Society was more or less like that. The Heart Journal reflected that way of thinking. And that was if you like classical cardiology. So, it was didactic and it was heavily organized or orientated toward structure, not actually to do anything, not necessarily to therapy. And that meant that...another stream developed of people like Dr. Taylor who were interested in drug therapy. But drug therapy in British cardiology was never really interesting which meant that these people were pushed out and they went to allied fields" [42]

In this sense British cardiology has been markedly naturalistic. Yet, implicitly other aspects are addressed as well, in particular the orientation towards drug therapy.[43] In the research for this thesis gaps were encountered in the empirical material needed for characterizing more precisely the groups in British cardiology and general medicine who formed the basis of the hemodynamic way of thinking about angina pectoris and anti-anginal treatment.

This apparent conflict in British cardiology is reflected in the opposing terms used by Wood to strike the right tone in the introduction to his famous textbook, which Chamberlain called the "Bible" and Silk a "classic, a work of Homer-type of thing".[44]

However carefully the formation of the new type of cardiology, created by Wood, has to be considered against the background of opposing traditions in British medicine, it incorporated the new concepts of physiology and hemodynamics.

The beta blockers very much profited from this physiological thinking in cardiology. *"And the beta blockers"*, Dollery stated, *"were really a group of drugs where you could do that relatively easily and make rather precise measurements. You could measure exercise tachycardia, you could do isoprenaline dose-response curves. If you wanted to measure the action of a benzodiazepine or a tricyclic antidepressant or a penicillin or something like that, that was extremely difficult. It was the simplicity of fairly precise measurements".* [45]

In similar terms Robinson recalled: *"All these very mechanical approaches were very fashionable and of course beta blockers altered a lot of these things. So it was possible to put actual figures on what they did (..) You put a beta blocker in and the heart rate comes down, the rate of rise of pressure fell and the end-diastolic pressure went and all these things you could measure, they were altered by beta blockers".* [46]

Atypical forms of angina pectoris

Whenever there is a typical disease pattern, a variety of atypical pictures emerge and such was the case for angina pectoris. In the course of lifting out angina of effort from daily medical practice, the category of coronary insufficiency lost its dominant position in the clinic during the 1950s. This term was a popular clinico-pathological concept that emerged during the 1930s and early 1940s as the result of pathological observations of sudden death in patients who at post mortem examination were found to have coronary disease without coronary thrombosis or occlusion. Thus, pathology linked the nosologic entities angina pectoris and myocardial infarction together in a new way, 'acute coronary insufficiency' being the intermediate between these two syndromes. [47]

During the 1950s this pathological link was joined by the physiological concept of coronary insufficiency. Opponents of this concept readily recognized the straight-jacket into which angina pectoris was being pushed. Raab, for example, noticed:

*"It is generally agreed that the typical anginal symptoms are provoked by **a paroxysmal state of hypoxia of the heart muscle** for which **two coinciding factors** are usually made responsible: (1) a static one, namely coronary sclerosis with resulting **narrowness of the coronary bed**, and (2) a dynamic one, namely an **acute increase of myocardial oxygen consumption** which exceeds the diminished 'coronary reserve' (dilatability) of the coronary vessels. It is widely taken for granted that the latter factor is attributable solely to an augmentation of cardiac work"* .[48] Obviously, the anginal attack originates under conditions which are associated with an increase of cardiac work, i.e. 'angina of effort', but Raab refers to clinical conditions in which this seems to be no essential pre-requisite for the occurrence of angina pectoris at all: *"Some patients who develop pain when walking slowly or in connection with emotions, are able to carry out relatively strenuous muscular work, such as sawing wood, lifting heavy objects and the like, without difficulty, despite a presumably greater increase of cardiac output during these latter activities".* [49]

So, Raab referred to those conditions which were precisely at variance with the conditions related to typical angina of effort. In his opinion the term "sympathetic stimulation" should be understood "with due regard to its **biochemical implications**" because the heart did not work harder, but wasted its oxygen. Elsewhere he stated: *"The balance between adrenergic and cholinergic chemical influences upon myocardial oxygen economy can be assumed to be of decisive significance for the **metabolic and structural state** of the myocardium in conjunction with the* *behaviour of the coronary blood supply*". [50] This biochemical and pathological activity deviated from the notion of the work done by the heart which was derived from hemodynamics. Indeed, this hemodynamic concept redefined ischemic heart disease. Either it was angina pectoris or myocardial infarction. These two categories were drifting apart. But clinical practice continued to relax its definition of both categories because of patients in which the symptoms and signs were neither typical for myocardial infarction nor for angina pectoris. To this varied group of "atypical" patients terms like "acute atypical coronary insufficiency", "intermediate syndrome", "coronary failure", "Prinzmetal`s variant form of angina pectoris", "angina decubitus" and "status anginosus" were applied. By that time angina of effort had become the dominant form of angina pectoris.

Anglo-American medical views of angina pectoris during the 1970s.

During the 1960s coronary angiography had become a major diagnostic technique in cardiology and cardiac surgery. The technique enabled clinicians to visualize occlusions of one, two or three major branches or smaller vessels of the coronary system. Concepts such as "one-vessel-disease", "two-vessel-disease" and "three-vessel-disease", though already known, now entered the clinic to characterize the various subsets of occlusive coronary artery disease. Coronary angiography supported the view that there existed a **direct** relationship between fixed coronary stenosis and the clinical manifestations of the disease.[51] The division of labour between cardiologists and cardiac surgeons entered a new era and became the subject of controversy.[52]

In his 1972' article, published under the apt title "Some Comments and Reflections on Changing Interests and New Developments in Angina Pectoris", Friedberg commented that *"rather suddenly angina pectoris has become a glamour subject, intellectually and clinically exciting in almost every aspect - pathology, pathophysiology, diagnosis, treatment. Not long ago it was difficult to spark a bright glow of interest in angina pectoris, except possibly by reading Heberden's sharp delineation of the clinical picture (...). Any further discussion was regarded as dull and drab".* [53]

True, we should be careful with such comments. Whenever a branch of medicine comes into prosperity or becomes revolutionized it is common for the medical profession either to dissociate the innovating period from the preceding era or to reduce the break with the past to the view of new wine in old bottles.[54] Friedberg's article seems to fall into the latter category since he argued that *"the pathology of angina pectoris has provoked renewed interest, not because of new discoveries but because of the increased importance of familiarity with old observations, and because of the possibility of visualizing coronary pathology in vivo".* [55]

Yet, he hit on a relevant feature in arguing that if the host of drugs designed to promote coronary blood flow had been successful, there would not have been such a spectacular evolution of coronary surgical procedures.[56] While the concept of coronary vasodilation had been defeated in the pharmaceutical sector, it had been in gaining wind in surgical therapy of angina pectoris. When the spectacular rise of coronary bypass surgery heralded the revival of the concept of coronary vasodilation, it struck back like a boomerang on cardiology.In this sense the defeated concept revived the battle between cardiology and cardiac surgery. This battle was fought at the level of therapy, clinical symptomatology and pathogenetic mechanisms. Between these levels new links emerged with major consequences for clinical taxonomy.

At the **therapeutic** level conflicting views about the benefits and risks of medical versus surgical therapy emerged. The essence of managing angina pectoris became whether or not to do coronary bypass surgery and conflict arose about defining the therapeutic and prognostic indicators. The surgical technique revolutionized the management of angina pectoris but precise diagnosis became essential.[57] The question became, not how and why surgical therapy mattered but if it really did matter.

This controversial issue revolutionized the therapeutic perspective on angina pectoris. *"Prior to coronary arteriography"*, as Friedberg wrote, *"physicians treated most of their patients with angina pectoris without serious thought of surgery, reassured by the knowledge that the angina was of only moderate severity and frequency, was responsive to rest and nitroglycerin, and did not seriously interfere with the patient's work. Furthermore, the vast majority of such patients continued in this manner for many years"*. [58] Now this approach was turned upside down. Taking the pyramid as a metaphor for the management of angina pectoris, the significance of this change in perspective is readily explainable. The base of the pyramid rested firmly in general medical practice for a long time. With the advent of coronary angiography and cardiac surgery it became placed upon its apex, and in so doing new subsets of angina pectoris were distinguished.

With this latter point **clinical symptomatology** becomes an issue and the peaceful distinction between angina pectoris and myocardial infarction was disturbed. The feverish activity to reclassify the subsets of patients intermediate between angina pectoris and myocardial infarction illustrates this. This intermediate zone which during the 1960s was perceived as being very small, became subject to intensive research. As a result stress came to lie on the heterogeneity of angina pectoris.[59]

In counteracting the claims made by cardiac surgeons, cardiologists attempted to correlate the subsets of patients with occlusive coronary disease, visualized on arteriograms, with the differential courses of the disease in their patients observed at the bedside. The nosologic entity angina pectoris became subdivided. Some categories, for example 'pre-infarction angina', still reflected the search for indicators as harborer of infarction or sudden death. Other terms denoted more complex prognostic or therapeutic features. This is the case with "stable" versus "unstable" angina; and to a certain extent this holds also true for "angina at rest". However, other terms stressed that certain forms of angina clearly deviated from typical exertional angina, for example, "Prinzmetal's variant form of angina" and "vasospastic angina".

Pathogenetic mechanisms also deserve a closer look. The 1970s witnessed the reappearance of the concept of coronary vasospasm that had been relegated to the graveyard of worthless concepts in cardiology. The concept of coronary spasm representing the functional factors operating in angina by mechanisms not yet understood, underlies the clinical entity of 'Prinzmetal's variant form of angina pectoris. Accordingly, this syndrome was the focus of increasing attention for the role of functional mechanisms in angina pectoris. The syndrome had been delineated by Prinzmetal and his colleagues in 1959. Since the syndrome exhibited clinical and electrocardiographical features that deviated from classical angina, they coined the term "variant form of angina pectoris". Biochemical and physiological mechanisms were superimposed on this clinical entity. The authors hypothesized that the attacks were the consequence of coronary spasm. So, here was a syndrome in which myocardial ischemia appeared to be precipitated by a reduction in myocardial oxygen delivery secondary to coronary spasm rather than by an increase in myocardial oxygen demand in the face of a simple organic narrowing of the coronary vessels.

During the 1960s this form of angina pectoris had been relegated to the margins of cardiovascular research and medical practice. It now attracted attention again. Though no one exactly knew what was going on behind the scenes in the heart's microstructure and coronary vascular system, the deeply ingrained appeal to functional mechanisms evoked new enthusiasm. This pathogenetic mechanism was extended to other forms of angina pectoris. It even entered the classic and typical form of exertional angina from which it was excluded many years ago.[60] Accordingly, several tests were developed to visualize vasospastic angina at the bedside, notably the cold pressor test and the ergonovine test. Both provocation tests presume that vascular tone of the coronary vessels is increased by neural, humoral-hormonal and endothelial factors.[61] The cold pressor test, for example, leads to a marked stimulation of the sympathetic system with concomitant rise of the vasomotor tone. In this sense, "irritability" and "over-excitability" of the vegetative system, once old-fashioned terms, reappeared on the cardiological scene.

Angina pectoris appeared as a continuous spectrum between "fixed" and "variable" obstruction, between typical, exertional angina and atypical, non-exertional angina at the other end. Between these limits of the spectrum most of the patients are encountered in clinical practice as Maseri stated in 1985.[62]

Hillis and Braunwald summarized the state of the art in the field: *"It is now clear that in many - perhaps most - patients with symptomatic coronary artery disease, there is some combination of these two cases of myocardial ischemia. (..) It is important to determine the position of a given patient with coronary artery disease within this spectrum and to adjust therapy appropriately".* [63]

This shift in pathogenetic views probably reached its zenith in the concept of dynamic obstruction. This was defined as an obstruction, not fixed by stenosis but capable of changing in degree depending on the vasomotor tone in the remaining normal wall segment. Various observations demonstrated that not all coronary obstructions were fixed and concentric: "It was shown that half of these obstructions were, in fact, of an eccentric type and, therefore, usually still contained large sections of normal arterial wall with functioning smooth muscle cells which had the ability to contract and expand and thus to change the degree of obstruction".[64] In this concept functional and pathological views merged in a new symbiotic relationship.[65]

The road to this concept was beset with many obstacles. It is noteworthy that the conflicting views about the pathogenetic role of vasospasm was carried on within the technique of angiography itself. Coronary spasm had been observed many times during application of this technique but it was considered to be an artefact caused by the mechanical irritation of the vessel wall. Somewhat later, after the concept of spasm reappeared in cardiology, the same technique was used to provide unequivocal evidence for the theory of coronary spasm.[66] It is paradoxical that the same technique that supported the pathological view of fixed stenosis so strongly, at the same time enabled clinicians to propose such deviating pathogenetic mechanisms.

6.3. Disease profiles of angina pectoris in Anglo-American medicine: cognitive dimensions.

Figure 6.1 approximates clinical taxonomy of angina pectoris during the 1950s.[67]

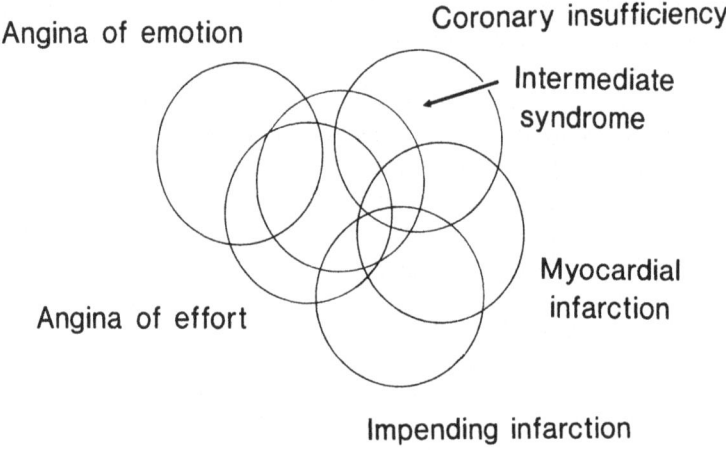

Figure 6.1
Profiles of angina pectoris in Anglo-American medicine, 1950-1960.

Angina of effort is a well-defined nosologic entity as is myocardial infarction. At the top left the profile of angina of emotion is depicted which intersects with that of angina of effort. The **intermediate** zone between angina of effort and myocardial infarction is represented by the categories coronary insufficiency, intermediate syndrome and impending infarction. This area was considered an ill-defined borderline state and it has been designated by various terms such as atypical or anomalous angina; severe angina; angina of rest; angina decubitus; coronary failure; slight coronary attacks; angina major; pre-infarction angina; false angina; forme fruste or spasmodic angina; and sub-endocardial infarction.[68] This sequence of terms raises the question if it is merely a matter of labels. However, this is not the case. These terms denoted different (sub)sets meaning that:
a. the disease characteristics as elements of the set differ; for example: the extent to which sets encompass (types of) electrocardiographical signs;
b. the values of disease characteristics differ; for example: the taking of nitroglycerin is very often used, yet its value differs (50 tablets daily or 300 tablets per week);
c. the priorities of disease characteristics vary; for example: the term intermediate syndrome

emphasizes prolonged chest pain of cardiac origin, intermediate in intensity, duration, and character between that of angina pectoris and acute myocardial infarction; in contrast, the term impending infarction stresses those characteristics that are warning signs of myocardial infarction.

A variety of profiles could have been shown but this intermediate zone has been oversimplified to the three illustrated. This choice is to some extent arbitrary but the three terms denote three different aspects central to the discussion amongst cardiologists. Coronary insufficiency stresses the pathogenetic aspect, i.e. the pathogenetic mechanism underlying the disease, and attempts to relate this to the symptoms and signs observed. The intermediate syndrome expresses the opinion that there is a distinct entity between the two major forms of coronary heart disease. Impending infarction emphasizes the attempt to find warning symptoms or signs as the precursor of myocardial infarction.

Since medical views about myocardial infarction were not taken into account, figure 6.1 oversimplifies the case. The very reason for depicting this clinical category is that clinicians, when discussing the various forms of angina pectoris, refer to potential overlapping with myocardial infarction.

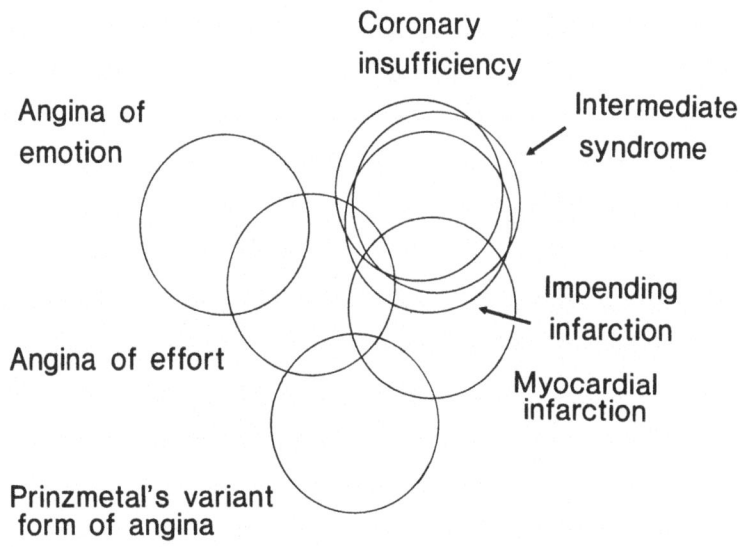

Figure 6.2
Profiles of angina pectoris in Anglo-Saxon medicine, 1960-1970.

Figure 6.2 designates the spectrum of disease profiles of angina pectoris in Anglo-Saxon medicine during the 1960s. It is similar to that depicted in figure 6.1. The major difference is the appearance of a previously undefined form of angina pectoris, i.e. "Prinzmetal's variant form of angina pectoris".

Table 6.1
Clinical and electrocardiographical differences
between classic and variant forms of angina pectoris.

Variant Form	Classic Form
Clinical Differences	
Exertion usually does not precipitate pain	Exertion usually precipitates pain
Emotional upset does not produce pain	Emotional upset frequently produces pain
Pain is frequently more severe and of longer duration than in classic angina	Pain usually is less severe and of shorter duration than in variant form
Attack often consists of series of pains, occurring in cyclic and remarkably regular pattern	Pain is not cyclic
If pain is not cyclic, period of increasing pain is equal to period of decreasing pain	Period of increasing pain is longer than period of decreasing pain
Pain often occurs at about same time each day	Pain does not occur regularly each day unless related to exercise or emotion
Arrhythmias, most often ventricular, occur in about 50% of cases in which severe pain is present,	Arrhythmias are not as common
It is theorized that attacks are precipitated by hypertonus of single narrowed large coronary artery; this syndrome occurs only when large coronary artery is involved	There is diffuse coronary artery disease*
Pain ceases immediately after myocardial infarction	Pain usually persists after myocardial infarction†
Electrocardiographic Differences	
S-T segments are elevated transiently during attack; reciprocal S-T depression occurs in standard leads	S-T segments generally show depression during pain; reciprocal S-T elevation is not observed in standard leads
S-T and T wave changes during an attack may seem to "improve" previously abnormal ECG	Spurious electrocardiographic "improvement" does not occur during an attack
Areas of myocardium which give rise to S-T elevation during attacks correspond to distribution of large coronary artery	Areas of myocardium which give rise to S-T depression are diffuse and do not correspond to distribution of any single large coronary artery*
Areas of heart giving rise to S-T elevation are sites of future myocardial infarction	Sites of future infarction are not predictable
R wave may become taller during severe attack	QRS complex usually is unaffected by attack
Exercise does not produce pain but in some instances may produce S-T depression	Exercise may produce pain and characteristic depression of S-T segment

Reproduced with permission from Prinzmetal et al. (1960).

The table as published by Prinzmetal and his colleagues shows the many differences between angina of effort and the variant form of angina pectoris.

Both profiles encompass fifteen characteristics, i.e. nine clinical and six electrocardiographical.[69] Presumably, the differences are listed according to the priorities of the characteristics. The most important difference concerns exertion. The authors introduced this variant type of angina pectoris as follows: "Nonexertional angina in itself has been long known to occur in heart disease. Heberden referred to it first in 1772 and again in 1802. Therefore, to identify this syndrome and to set it apart from other forms of nonexertional angina, the authors have chosen the term "a variant form of angina pectoris".[70]

While taking those forms of angina pectoris that deviated from classic angina and having no relationship to exertion, the authors created a new profile.

This leads to an examination of the profiles of angina during the period 1970 - 1980.

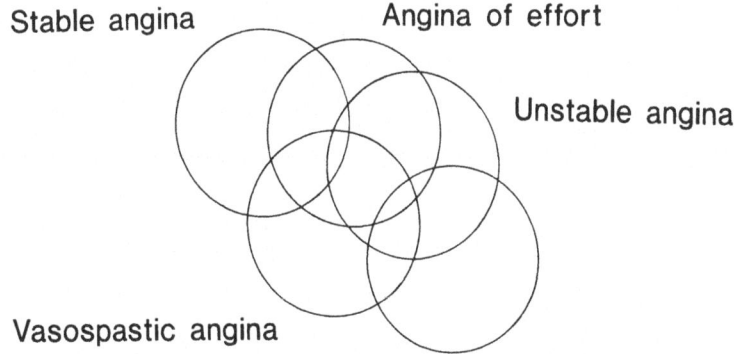

Figure 6.3
Profiles of angina pectoris in Anglo-American medicine, 1970-1980.

This picture that emerges is completely different from the preceding ones. Three categories, i.e. stable, unstable and vasospastic angina, appeared. To some extent this appears to be merely a matter of labeling. Unstable angina, for example, has also been called pre-infarctional angina.[71] In this sense, this category resembles other terms including: intermediate syndrome, coronary failure, pre-infarction angina and status anginosus. However, major differences are also seen. New characteristics were added to the category of unstable angina, for example, to predict the patient's prognosis on the basis of electrocardiographic findings. Other characteristics were removed while values and priorities of characteristics were changed. For example, while the term pre-infarctional angina stressed the fact that patients develop myocardial infarction, many authors noted that this was not the case, hence they preferred to use the term unstable angina.

Accordingly, other features became more important in recognizing the patients at risk but this does not mean that the risk of myocardial infarction was neglected. On the contrary, clinicians attempted to find other markers of this high-risk subgroup and there was some differentiation of the category of unstable angina to several subgroups. The incentive was the need to assess this risk, and it was strengthened when the therapy of saphenous vein graft bypass became available.

As Gazes and co-workers in their study on pre-infarctional (unstable) angina noted: *"The objective of this study was to determine the survival rate of this group and to discover whether it was possible to predict the patient's prognosis on the basis of electrocardiographic findings. Now that saphenous vein graft bypass techniques for direct myocardial revascularization have been developed, recording the natural history of pre-infarctional angina has become even more important. There are at present no specific criteria for selection of surgical candidates. The ubiquitous nature of angina makes it very difficult to pick out those patients with this symptom who would probably die without surgical intervention. It would be helpful if types of angina pectoris could be defined and distinguished by their natural history".* [72]

The foregoing notes on terminology express the fact that disease profiles are not static but dynamic entities, though, as noted earlier, myocardial infarction is treated as a static entity. The category of angina of effort is changed in two respects. Firstly, its position in the spectre of the various forms of angina has altered. Since other categories such as stable and unstable angina appeared, its relationships with other profiles (i.e. its intersections) are changed. Secondly, the category itself has changed, though not fundamentally.

The changes with respect to Prinzmetal's variant form of angina, however, are substantial. This category was differentiated by way of increasingly new techniques and procedures.[73] Thus, modern ECG-monitoring procedures revealed that the electrocardiographic feature of ST-segment elevation, attributed by Prinzmetal and colleagues to variant form of angina, was in fact commonly associated with many forms of anginal pain. As a result this feature was given a lower priority.

Another example is that Prinzmetal and his colleagues had postulated proximal severe lesions in one major coronary branch with "temporary increased tonus". By way of coronary arteriogram it was shown that proximal single-vessel lesions occurred in only some cases. Selzer et al. therefore attempted to differentiate the category of variant form of angina into two categories: *"The purpose of this report is to present findings in 29 patients with variant angina, to point out the differences between patients with and without coronary artery disease who have these clinical features, and to show that variant angina with a normal coronary arteriogram represents a distinctive clinical syndrome".* [74]

6.4. Disease profiles of angina pectoris in Anglo-American medicine: social dimensions.

Social maps of medical knowledge

This section tries to capture the social dimensions of clinical taxonomy of angina pectoris in Anglo-American medicine.[75] Figure 6.4 represents the situation in the 1950s.

Since angina of effort and myocardial infarction were well-defined and widely acknowledged nosologic entities, their profiles are depicted as two large squares. Angina of emotion is still a separate category, yet nearly completely incorporated into the picture of angina of effort. The intermediate zone represented by the categories coronary insufficiency, intermediate syndrome and impending infarction, was considered as consisting of a miscellaneous group of patients.

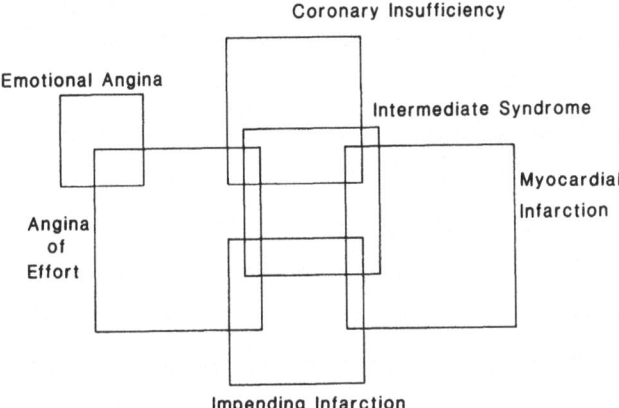

Figure 6.4
Profiles of angina pectoris in Anglo-American medicine, 1950-1960: social dimensions.

The various terms were not well accepted nor were they central to the diagnosis of angina pectoris. Therefore, the three squares are shown smaller than those of angina pectoris and myocardial infarction. As discussed earlier, the intermediate zone can be differentiated to cover all the proposed terms. Graphically this would have yielded two large squares and a lot of little squares with varying intersections. With due regard to graphical limitations the geography of the clinical world has been deliberately simplified.

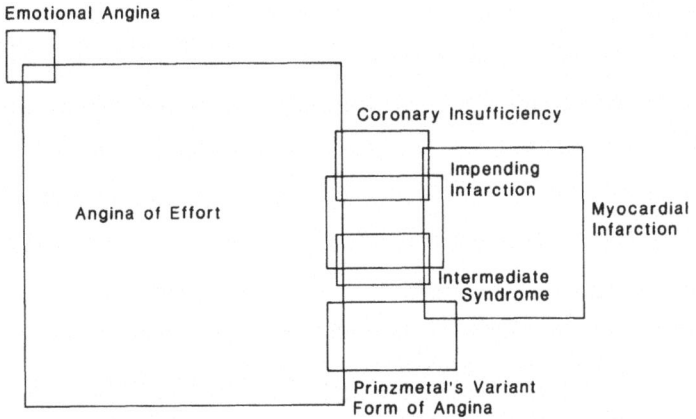

Figure 6.5
Profiles of angina pectoris in Anglo-American medicine, 1960-1970: social dimensions.

Figure 6.5 shows that angina of effort has become even more dominant and as a result, the intermediate zone is disintegrated into little spots. Particularly, the category of coronary insufficiency deserves further comment. It was still being referred to in Anglo-Saxon medicine in the 1960s. Friedberg, for example, discussed the term acute coronary insufficiency even in 1966, so this concept must have been in general use in medical practice until well into the 1960s.[76] It had, however, lost its influential position in clinical research, therapeutic evaluation and cardiology.

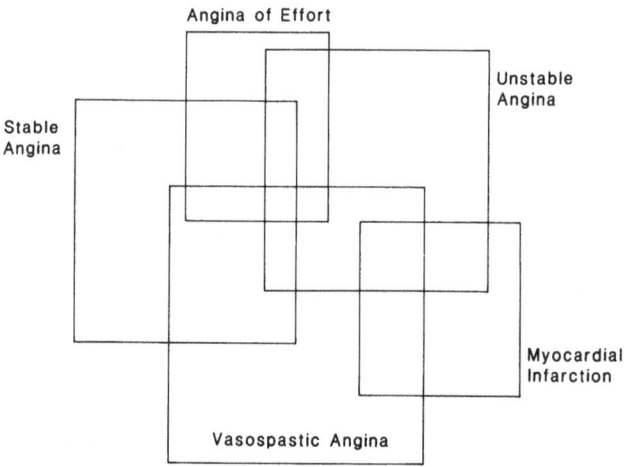

Figure 6.6
Profiles of angina pectoris in Anglo-American medicine, 1970-1980: social dimensions.

Figure 6.6 shows the increased attention to vasospastic and other forms of angina pectoris. It stresses that the bulwark of interest of angina of effort declined. Since the cognitive dimensions of the various types of angina pectoris have been discussed above, the scheme will speak for itself.

Regional variability

The question arises to what extent these maps cover Anglo-American medical views. The present research is based on textbooks, scientific and medical journals, and interviews with clinicians and fundamental cardiovascular research workers and general practitioners are not represented. To gain a better understanding of the medical views amongst general practitioners, particularly those in the United Kingdom, the journals **The Practitioner** and **The Journal of the College of General Practitioners** were screened using as key-words angina pectoris, (coronary) vasodilators, dipyridamole, ß-(adrenoceptor) blocking agents/blockade, nitrites/nitrates and propranolol.[77]
Seventeen articles were retrieved, a disappointing result. No review of the disease itself was provided but only therapeutic evaluations. Some of them were double-blind trials but did not define the enrolled patients except in one case where it was stated: "Angina was diagnosed

clinically on the basis of typical cardiac pain coming on with effort and being relieved by rest".[78] This is typical angina of effort. Obviously, this evidence is insufficient to delineate the views of angina pectoris held by general practitioners.

In restricting the analysis to clinical medicine, distinct classifications were used. In 1965 Gorlin, for example, classified angina pectoris as follows[79]:

a. angina of effort
b. angina with tachycardia
c. spontaneous angina
d. angina of emotion
e. angina of deglutition (angina with eating)
f. angina with cold wind
g. nocturnal angina
h. angina in aortic stenosis

At face value the forms of angina discussed by Gorlin, except angina of effort and of emotion, are at variance with the categories depicted in the cognitive (figure 6.2) and social map (figure 6.5) representing Anglo-American taxonomy during the 1960s. Closer examination, however, yields a more balanced view.

Categories c., d. and h. were characterized as states of hypersympathicotony, that is, states that reflect increased sympathetic drive of the heart and express the excess of cardiac work to be done while there is inadequate overall coronary reserve. These states are characterized by increase in pressure, acceleration of heart rate, increased vigour of contraction and elevation of cardiac work which are very much similar to those of angina of effort. Nocturnal angina occurs while the patient sleeps. A possible mechanism was an increase in sympathetic discharge in reaction to a dream. As in angina of emotion, nocturnal angina mimicked angina of effort because the stressful situation during a dream was relieved on awaking and the pain subsided. The same applies to category b., e.g., angina with tachycardia.

So, Gorlin classified these patterns of anginal pain by using the precipitating events which were interpreted in terms of the concept of the disturbed balance of oxygen supply and demand. In this respect, Gorlin's classification comes close to the one discussed with respect to figure 6.2.[80]

In contrast, Gorlin discussed aspects that deviate from the medical views during the 1960s. For instance, he argued that nocturnal angina may be caused by other mechanisms amongst which early heart failure was a possible candidate. Gorlin believed that many patients with coronary heart disease have **subliminal** heart failure. However, the major discrepancy with the already dominant view is that Gorlin stresses the dual origin of the categories c., d., f. and g. This is best illustrated with spontaneous angina (or angina at rest). The patients suffering from this condition according to Gorlin were usually tense, nervous, or fearful, hence they suffered from a tendency to generalized sympathetic discharge. One origin was that this state of hypersympathicotony led to a discernable hemodynamic change which *"would not seem to be enough of a mechanical load to precipitate angina through demand-energy imbalance alone"*. [81] The other origin was a severe vasoconstrictor episode which occurred frequently with sympathetic nervous discharge.[82]

Thus, almost invariably angina pectoris occurs in the presence of obstructive coronary artery disease and is precipitated by a set of circumstances which disturbs the balance between oxygen supply and oxygen demand, often through a rise in mechanical load, i.e. in oxygen demand. Yet, in some people superimposed constriction impairs coronary flow. Consequently, Gorlin attributed to both the long-acting and short-acting nitrites the important role of preventing or mitigating such constrictor episodes. With his contribution to the theory of coronary spasm Gorlin evidently deviated from the dominant view in the English speaking medical world.

Throughout the historical period described many differences in explaining various forms of angina are seen. I have discussed one with respect to coronary insufficiency; another is the further development of the concept of coronary spasm. During the first half of the 1970s conflicting opinions were put forward and some clinicians clearly opposed this concept. MacAlpin stated: *"Current teaching about classic, exertional angina pectoris therefore states that it is the result of increases in myocardial oxygen demand in the face of a limited coronary blood flow. No allowance for arterial spasm is needed in this framework"*. [83] In a typical clinical fashion Scherf and Cohen had a similar comment: *"The fact that individual cases and small series continue to be reported (...) lends credence to the role of variant angina as a medical curiosity"*. [84]

This issue of regional variability underlines the attempt of this chapter to provide cognitive and social maps of medical views and their changes using profiles as the principal pigeon-holes of medical knowledge. The cognitive and social maps drawn can be detailed to cover the wide range of medical views. For example, Gorlin's scheme can be easily translated into a cognitive map. This map depicts circles - denoting categories c., d., f. and g. - which variably intersect the circle representing angina of effort on the one hand and the circle representing Prinzmetal's variant form of angina on the other. In a social map the circles would be enlarged or reduced according to the impact of Gorlin's scheme. This impact can be measured by a qualitative or quantitative standard. [85]

The aim of this study was to perform a broad contextual analysis and not to account for differences in British and American medicine. [86] Furthermore, the maps depicted above are snapshots of the geography of the clinician's world, and together they reveal a **dynamic** pattern. The number of snapshots may be increased depending from the purpose of the study and the degree of precision strived for.

In principle it is possible to use quantitative methods and though the nature of this study is essentially qualitative, it may be worthwhile to provide some additional quantitative data. The increased attention to atypical and vasospastic forms of angina pectoris is illustrated by figure 6.7 taken from the article of Kübler and Tillmans. [87]

The increase in number of publications under the headings unstable angina and Prinzmetal's variant angina shows that both types of angina form a rapidly expanding field.

A citation analysis of Prinzmetal's articles on the variant form of angina yields the following picture (figure 6.8).

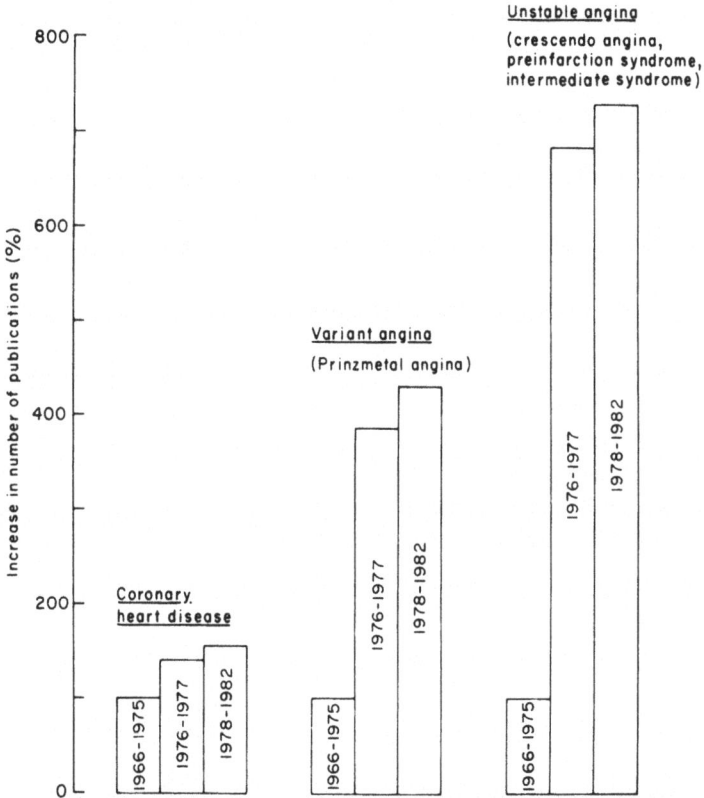

Figure 6.7 Increase in number of publications under different headings. The mean number of publications per year over the period 1976-1977 and 1978-1982 are expressed in (%) of the average number of publications per year over the period 1966-1975, corresponding to 100%.
Reproduced with permission from Kübler and Tillmans (1985).

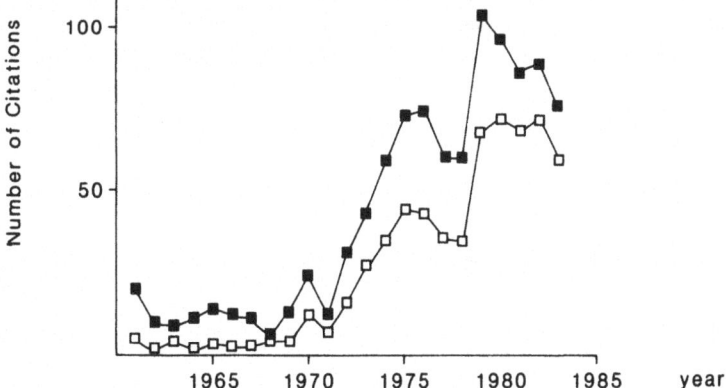

Figure 6.8
Number of citations, from the SCI, to Prinzmetal (1959) (□); and Prinzmetal ("set") (■).

One curve represents the citations per year with regard to the total set of articles that were published by Prinzmetal et al. during 1959 - 1961 on variant angina (namely 5 articles).[88] The other represents the most frequently cited article. Both curves show a similar pattern that to some extent differs from that suggested by the previous figure. During the period 1970 - 1975 there is a rapidly growing interest concerning the syndrome, while this increase is less significant in the scheme of Kübler and Tillmans. A difference in methodology could account for this. The authors counted the **mean number** of publications per year over the period 1966 - 1975, while in this study the citations of Prinzmetal's articles **per year** were counted.

6.5. Anti-anginal drugs in the light of changing views of angina pectoris.

The concepts of drug and disease profiles may now be applied to the historical material presented; the information about the drugs is derived from the preceding chapter and Venn-diagrams will be used to visualize some major developments. Panels a) to f) in figure 6.8 represent the state of affairs in 1960, 1964, 1968 and so forth, up to and including 1980. The symbols denote the sets representing the drugs or forms of angina. For simplicity only the names of the drugs or types of angina concerned will be used.

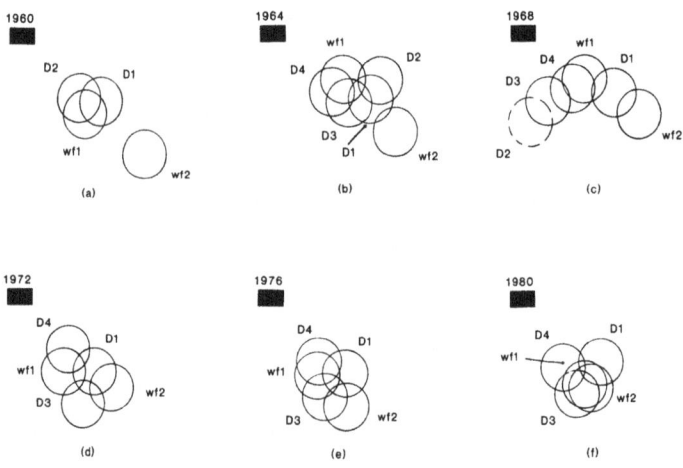

D1 = of(nitrates)
D2 = of(dipyridamole)
D3 = of(verapamil)
D4 = of(propranolol)

wf1 = wf(angina of effort)
wf2 = (Prinzmetal's variant form of angina

Figure 6.9
Development of operational functional drug profiles
of anti-anginal drugs in view of the changing
wished for functional profiles.

The first panel (figure 6.9(a)) represents the nitrites and dipyridamole with respect to angina of effort. The nitrites were recognized as a well-established therapy, and dipyridamole evoked enthusiasm. The circle representing Prinzmetal's variant form of angina is depicted with dotted lines. It was published but not well-known at the time.

The second panel (figure 6.9(b)) represents a complex situation because verapamil and propranolol entered the scene. Verapamil intersects both propranolol and nitrites, being discussed as a coronary vasodilator and beta blocker. Prinzmetal's variant form of angina is acknowledged as a distinct entity, though it was still considered as a medical curiosity. The nitrites were recognized as an useful therapy of this syndrome, at least in some cases, hence the intersection between the two profiles. Dipyridamole was already relegated to the margins of anti-anginal treatment. The drug is still considered as a coronary vasodilator but with disappointing clinical results.

The third panel (figure 6.9(c)) shows a clearly changed situation. Dipyridamole is pushed to the margins of the field, and hence is depicted as a dotted circle, though the drug was intensively used in clinical research to define the mechanism of action of the nitrites.[89] In due course, the effects of dipyridamole on platelet aggregation were revealed which might be beneficial in reducing thromboembolic complications following cardiac valve replacement.[90] Similarly but not so dramatically, verapamil was pushed aside. Its unstable position in the field is represented by the small intersections with propranolol and angina of effort. Its relationship with the nitrites changed dramatically because the mechanism of action of the nitrites was explained differently. The category of coronary vasodilators was divided into two classes, i.e. the nitrites and the "classic" coronary vasodilators.

The fourth panel (figure 6.9(d)) shows another pattern. Dipyridamole has been left out because it had played its part. Though the relationships between nitrites and propranolol regarding angina of effort remain stable, there is a marked change with respect to verapamil. The drug is now classified as a calcium antagonist and intersects both types of angina. As described in the preceding chapter, it is more suitable to let D3 represent nifedipine. In any case, the drug is dissociated from the class of beta blocking agents.

The fifth (figure 6.9(e)) and sixth (figure 6.9(f)) panels are similar in visualizing two major trends in the field. One trend is the increasing absorption of angina of effort by Prinzmetal's variant form of angina which actually represents the range of vasospastic forms of angina. The other trend is that, as a result, verapamil encroaches on anti-anginal therapy in the same way. Consequently, the beta blockers were discarded, even though they were the first choice drugs in angina of effort next to the nitrites.[91] The profile of angina of effort diverged into the new subsets of angina. In other words "pure" angina of effort was in danger of becoming a medical curiosity.

Finally some additional comments with respect to the diagram above. Each snapshot represents profiles present at that particular moment. Hence, the six snapshots characterize the body of knowledge at $t_1, t_2, ..., t_6$, where t denotes the moment of recording ("t" could range from a fraction of a second to a period of years). It is therefore more correct to use separate symbols to denote the profiles of the drugs and diseases in the snapshots, i.e. by using of(x^t) and wf(P^t). Clearly, the dynamics of profiles involve (a) absence\presence of characteristics; (b) values and (c) priorities of characteristics. Venn-diagrams are not suited for visualizing this dynamic process. In fact, Venn-diagrams are also not suited for representing the (logical) relationships between sets when dealing with more than three or four sets. However, logical relationships between the sets is not an issue here. The purpose is merely to visualize some major developments. Similarly, the cognitive maps representing the snapshots can be translated into social maps.

6.6. Conclusions

The title of this chapter "Metamorphosis of a Disease" focuses on the fundamental changes that took place in medical views about angina pectoris in the English speaking world. A fundamental tenet of Anglo-American cardiology became that ischemia (lack of blood) to the heart muscle is the cause of angina pectoris. This is the essence of what might be conveniently called the coronary, or ischemic, theory.[92]

Basically, the idea is of a fixed obstruction caused by anatomical lesions in the coronary system. During the 1940s and 1950s this structural aspect of the disease was connected to the variety of circumstances under which angina pectoris as a symptom complex arose in the patient's daily life. Hence, the syndrome angina of effort was recognized which encompasses, in addition to the structural lesion, a functional aspect which is the critical balance between oxygen supply and demand of the heart.

In this respect, the sympathetic system as the mediator between the outside world and the internal milieu of human organism attracted attention. Though various and sometimes conflicting interpretations were given to the role of the sympathetic system, the dominant view emerged that it mediated the stress. This stress, somehow initiated outside or inside the human organism, imposed an increased mechanical load upon the heart.

Proponents of the basic views about the role of the sympathetic system were encouraged to evaluate the clinical symptoms and signs in terms of these views. In contrast, opponents like Raab, for example, in trying to make a good case out of his biochemical view of the oxygen-wasting effects of the catecholamines, put emphasis on clinical phenomena such as the walk-through phenomenon, which fell outside the view of exertional angina that was coming to dominate cardiology.

This attests to the fact that views about the etiology or pathogenesis of the disease affect the way syndromes as complexes of symptoms and signs, are constructed. Yet, the reverse is also true. The symptoms and signs that attract attention of clinicians determine the framework for proposing theories of etiology and pathogenesis. One major consequence was that the syndrome of acute coronary insufficiency which actually emphasized the structural aspect, was pushed aside, not instantaneously, but gradually, being replaced by the physiological, i.e. hemodynamic, concept of oxygen supply and demand. Another consequence was that the concept of coronary vasospasm was gradually removed from cardiology.

In this changing world, the syndrome angina of effort became the dominant category in the clinical taxonomy of angina pectoris. Most striking is that these changes occurred in a web of concepts which, each by itself, signified the various aspects of angina pectoris. Thus, the various theories of pain which evolved through history, influenced the way patterns of pain were registered in the consulting-room. But the same might be said with respect to other symptoms and signs, be they biochemical, hemodynamic, electrocardiographical or otherwise. Furthermore, taking chest pain as one example, this symptom might be observed in many other clinical conditions. Yet, each condition finds itself in another web of theoretical and medical concepts. In fact, the history of gall-bladder disease, lung disease, inflammation of the pancreas, stomach or intestine which may cause similar patterns of pain, have not been accounted for.

This betrays the dual character of differential diagnosis in medicine. To differentiate angina pectoris from other diseases is a two-way process. Changing views about angina pectoris have major consequences with respect to the diagnosis of other diseases, and vice versa. This is another reason why taxonomy is so important in medicine. Heterogeneous pieces of knowledge have to be integrated in order to investigate and to treat disease.

Taking profiles as the pigeon-holes in which clinicians store their knowledge - in a taxonomic manner - the changes in profiles of angina pectoris have been described. Cognitive and social maps of these profiles have been constructed to illustrate the usefulness of the concept of profile as well as to mark the shifts in medical opinion about angina pectoris at several crucial moments.

Having indicated the late 1950s and early 1960s as one critical time period in which the syndrome of angina of effort became increasingly important, it is interesting to see that right then a new variant form of angina pectoris was created. This attests to the curious conflict between old and new, common and deviant knowledge or whatever terms are available to designate this conflict. For it is evident that to mark a **variant** form of a disease another picture, the **common** type, must be established and well-known. Simultaneously, this is evidence that this variant form has been neglected for quite some time.

Pivotal to the history of angina pectoris is how the bulwark of angina of effort, so dominant during the 1960s, and largely reinforced by the success of the beta blockers, decayed during the first part of the 1970s. What started as an underground activity, reached its full-blown expression in the course of the 1970s when the role of vasospasm attracted much attention, so much so that the syndrome of exertional angina threatened to become a medical curiosity itself.

This study has attempted to describe the crucial developments in Anglo-American, especially British, cardiology: the introduction of techniques in cardiology, the striving for objectivity in therapeutic evaluation and the battle between various therapies. Noteworthy is that the conflict between cardiac surgery and cardiology has particularly been a struggle between medical (pharmacotherapeutic) and surgical therapy. Hence, we should realize that drug discovery is part of a broader process of innovation in medical therapy.

In particular, this study attempts to give flesh and blood to what is here called the "physiological" or "hemodynamic", approach that ruled Anglo-American cardiology during the 1950s and 1960s. When screening the various medical and cardiological journal to investigate this approach, an editorial of the American Journal of Cardiology was found as a typical example of what Robinson termed the "engineering approach" (much in line with the mood of the time). The editorial was published under the title "The Hemodynamic Concept of Atherosclerosis", and one passage goes as follows:

"The hemodynamic concept of atherosclerosis was developed by correlating atherosclerotic lesions found at autopsy with their localization as determined by hydraulic principles. It was then demonstrated with

the aid of model hydraulic systems built to the precise specifications of blood vessels obtained at autopsy. Flow in these models, as well as in the arterial tree generally, is streamline or laminar rather than turbulent. The forces and principles involved are directly comparable to those which prevail in all hydraulic systems. The flow of rivers and streams in their boundaries, the flight of the airplane, the insect and the bird, the movement of a ship in the water or a fish in the depths and the circulation of the blood in our arteries and veins are in major degree varied expressions of the laws of fluid mechanics. Everywhere in this domain, the laws of fluid mechanics must control". [93]

This engineering, or more precisely, hemodynamic approach, greatly reinforced by the techniques of cardiac catheterization and exercise tests, stimulated the development of the beta blockers. This class of drugs provided the tools to unravel the mechanisms pertinent to this hemodynamic approach, and simultaneously elicited bodily responses which could be measured with these techniques. This is important in a discipline like cardiology which has grown up amongst a surplus of techniques.

An attempt has been made to account for this approach in cardiology, particularly in British cardiology. British cardiology largely seemed to be anti-research, anti-clinical-science, anti-industry, and last but not least, anti-therapy. Still, various other events occurred which stimulated the development of the hemodynamic approach and the beta blockers: the rise of clinical pharmacology in the bosom of cardiology, acquaintance with controlling cardiovascular disease through interfering with the sympathetic drive, the great influence of Paul Wood and the involvement of a young generation of clinical research workers like Dollery, Prichard, Taylor and many others who educated a whole generation of British clinicians and introduced the principles of beta blockade.

However, a lacuna in the empirical material remains which makes it difficult to mark more precisely the balance of forces between the opposing streams in British cardiology which have evolved through generations of British physicians. In this sense, Wood's textbook in which he attempts to come to terms with these traditions, by attempting *"to maintain a proper balance between man and instruments, between experienced opinion and statistics, between traditional views and the heterodox, between bed-side medicine and special tests, between the practical and the academic, and so to link the past with present"*, partly fills this lacuna. It illustrates the decades of struggle in clinical medicine, and it attempts to satisfy the romantic retrospection towards a particular period in the history of medicine. In that period, a clinician could boast of his being a "genuine" clinician who listened to the voice of nature, not to technical results. As Silk commented on this long-lasting struggle in British cardiology:

"Cardiology seems to be too technical, too many technical methods and if you like..we have lost something. We are seeking our lost youth, a lost youth based on clinical practice. And people feel that nowadays, looking back to the days when you had the stethoscope that then you were a good clinician". [94]

Chapter 7.   Targeting in drug research and the medical scene

The beta blocker project at Boehringer against the background of different views in German and Anglo-American medicine

7.1 Introduction

At Boehringer Ingelheim several beta blocking compounds were developed early on in the race. Boehringer's scientists possessed the compound Lg 32 that turned out to become the most successful beta blocker, e.g. propranolol, even before the ICI scientists discovered the compound. Although there was so much potential, Boehringer was eventually left empty handed with only memories of a period that could have brought so much success to the company. This suggests that Boehringer had the compounds but not the right ideas. However, such a view about failure, or success, in pharmaceutical research neglects the medical side of the story of industrial development. The crucial point is what the "right" ideas were and why they were picked up at one place and not at the other. If the Boehringer project is considered against the background of medical perceptions of cardiovascular disease and therapy, the failure at Boehringer is seen in quite a different light. For, neither success nor failure are without cause.

The story begins at a time when no scientist or clinician had ever heard of a "beta blocker". Part 1 of this chapter, sections 7.2.1. - 7.2.3., provide the medical background in Germany against which the beta blocker project at Boehringer Ingelheim must be considered. Three medical areas of the utmost importance to the development of the Boehringer project are described. Firstly, the development of the coronary vasodilator concept in German versus Anglo-American medicine will be discussed (7.2.1). This has been touched upon several times but now the differential course of this concept in both medical settings will be more precisely delineated. Secondly, the German medical views on heart failure will be described (7.2.2). In highlighting German and Anglo-American intellectual frameworks to investigate heart failure three typical German disease profiles of heart failure will be discussed: "heart failure of effort", "old age heart" and "heart failure in angina pectoris". Thirdly, the German medical views about angina pectoris will be analysed (7.2.3). From this it becomes abundantly clear that the German concepts markedly differed from those of their Anglo-Saxon colleagues as described in Chapter 6.

The second part of this chapter (7.3.) concerns the development of the beta blocker project at Boehringer while in the third part the theory of drug and disease profile will be used to mark some critical points in the development of this project (7.4.).

Part 1. The medical scene- Different views in German and Anglo-American medicine

---

7.2.1 The coronary vasodilator concept

7.2.1.1. Introduction

Beta blockers introduced a view of how anti-anginal drugs could produce beneficial effect in angina patients. This view clashed with the coronary vasodilator concept that was imprinted on the minds of many physicians for such a long time. After the introduction of amyl nitrite, independently by Richardson and Brunton, a whole array of nitrites and nitrates were introduced in medical practice. However nitroglycerine, first used in 1879 by Murrell, became the reference drug.[1]

The term "nitrites" applies therefore to a heterogeneous group of compounds, but their basic action was believed to be the relaxation of smooth muscle, the most prominent and important of which was the dilation of blood vessels. The nitrites were, and still are employed both in the treatment of acute attacks of pain, and the prevention of anginal episodes. The prophylactic use of nitrites led to the development of long-acting nitrites that were beset with many problems. This unsatisfactory state of prophylaxis in angina pectoris set the scene for the decline of the coronary vasodilator concept and the introduction of the beta blockers in the 1960s.

This will be discussed in further detail in this section. First the concepts about nitrites and angina pectoris as they became dominant during the 1950s will be reviewed briefly (7.3.2.). Next the evolution of the coronary vasodilator concept in Anglo-American (7.3.3) and German (7.3.4) medicine will be discussed. Contextual differences are illustrated with the help of a bibliometrical analysis of medical perceptions of the clinical results with some anti-anginal drugs (7.3.5).

7.2.1.2 The early history of the coronary vasodilator concept

After Brunton's successful introduction of amyl nitrite, his textbook of pharmacology in 1885 became the international leader and went through several editions.[2] In the 1897 edition Brunton described his first experiences with amyl nitrite in the treatment of angina as follows:

"Many years ago, when I was a resident physician, I had a case of angina pectoris under my care. I used to go at all hours of the day and night and take tracings of the man's pulse. I found that during the attack of angina pectoris the pulse became very hard indeed, and the oscillations became very small. He had a certain amount of aortic regurgitation, and his normal pulse wave was very large. As the man's pain came on, the pulse became smaller and quicker, and when the pain was excessive the pulse became very rapid, but hardly perceptible. Now, it is almost impossible to explain such a change in

the pulse as we have here without assuming that the peripheral arterioles had become enormously contracted. It therefore occurred to me that if one were able to dilate the arterioles the man's pain ought to subside. I knew that nitrite of amyl had the effect of dilating the vessels and I tried it, with the result that no sooner had the flushing of the face occurred, and the vessels begun to dilate, than the pain disappeared. Since that time nitrite of amyl has become recognized as regular remedy for the paroxysms of angina pectoris". [3]

Brunton believed that anginal pain was relieved by amyl nitrite through the relaxation of peripheral arteries. His belief fitted the commonly held view at that time that angina was caused by paroxysmal spasms of (otherwise normal) peripheral arteries. According to this view vasomotor spasm increased blood pressure, hence hampered the heart's ability to pump out blood, leading to cardiac distension and cardiac pain. [4]

Brunton's detailed description has been quoted to illustrate that therapeutics is in constant change. In 1941 and 1955 the first two editions of Goodman & Gilman's influential textbook **The Pharmacological Basis of Therapeutics** quoted Brunton's textbook to dismiss his ideas and to illustrate that *"the clinical efficacy of a particular therapy is no proof of the theory underlying that therapy".* [5] Later editions again referred to Brunton's ideas but then to establish that Brunton was more nearly correct than had been suspected. [6] The therapeutic interpretation of the action of amyl nitrate shifted depending on the pathological theory about angina pectoris that was held at the time.

Brunton's view belonged to a variety of theories put forward in the 19th century to explain anginal pain. According to Lie these theories can be grouped together into three prominent schools of thought: coronary theories, nervous theories (the most popular during the 19th century) and aortic theories. [7] The coronary theory proposed atherosclerotic narrowing of the coronary arteries as the cause; nervous theories laid the origin of angina pectoris in a diseased nervous system; aortic theories in a diseased aorta leading to hypersensitive pain fibers in the beginning of the aorta.

The flaw of the coronary theory - a continuous thread in medical thinking about angina pectoris throughout the centuries - was the lack of consistent correlation between the clinical picture and pathological findings. Autopsy evidence in some patients with angina showed no organic lesions in the coronary arteries; while other patients with organic lesions did not suffer from angina pectoris. Various schools of thought put forward theories to explain this. Most protagonists of the coronary theory during the first two decades of this century postulated in addition to atherosclerosis coronary spasm as a cause of angina. This postulate of a coronary spasm was in fact a combination of the coronary theory with the nervous theory. [8] Controversy over these theories reigned until in the late 1920s and early 1930s the coronary theory emerged victorious. Thereafter the aortic and nervous theories, and the theory of coronary spasm were abandoned. [9] In the meantime myocardial infarction had been recognized as a disease entity distinct from angina pectoris. [10]

Fixed coronary artery stenosis was thought to be the cause of myocardial ischemia. [11] Emphasis shifted to the coronary circulation per se, and the new pathophysiological concept of "coronary insufficiency", emerged. [12] The original view of Parry (1799) that the narrowed coronary arteries provided sufficient blood to nourish the heart at rest, but not when the needs of the heart were augmented during exertion, was restored. [13] This concept had been translated into the straightforward therapeutic objective: "Dilate the coronary blood vessels to increase the blood and oxygen supply to the heart and to restore the critical imbalance!". The nitrites were thought to dilate coronary vessels, hence were termed "coronary vasodilators", and were taken as the model for a highly desirable complex of pharmacological properties. Pharmacologists were constantly on the alert for drugs that exerted a specific dilating action on the coronary vessels. A whole array of coronary vasodilators, mainly derivatives of khellin, xanthine, papaverine - known to be potent smooth muscle relaxant agents -, were introduced in medical practice.

7.2.1.3. The rise and decline of the coronary vasodilator concept in Anglo-American medicine.

The coronary theory and the theory of coronary vasospasm enforced the use of coronary vasodilators in the treatment of angina pectoris.[14] Emphasizing "spasm" as the cause of angina the basic action of the nitrites was conceived of as an "anti-spasmodic" effect. Focussing on the "ischemia" of the heart during exertion the "vasodilating" effect was stressed. The "spasm" theory moved the nitrites into pathological conditions like pylorospasm, bronchial spasm, urethral colic, migraine, Raynaud's disease and biliary colic in which spasm was considered the underlying mechanism of disease. The "ischemia" theory led clinicians to try the nitrites in various pathological conditions in which blood flow was impaired due to sclerosis such as claudicatio intermittens and cerebral vascular disorders.[15] Though it was eventually defeated, the theory of coronary spasm remained influential in Anglo-American cardiology during the 1930s and 1940s. Evidence of this is found in the repeated publications to expel the theory from medicine.[16] MacAlpin refers to Kattus who remembers that even in the early 1940s coronary spasm was still an influential explanation for anginal attacks.[17] In contrast, MacAlpin notes: *"On the contrary, during my own medical school days of the late 1950s, I was taught that coronary spasm probably did not exist. I well remember that at national cardiology meetings during the 1960s there was great reluctance even to use the term coronary arterial spasm".* [18] Dispersed through his historical review he refers to British and American spokesman vehemently arguing against coronary spasm as the cause of angina pectoris.[19]

With the turn of medical thinking towards the hemodynamic view as described in chapter 6, the theory of coronary spasm was finally defeated. Within the framework of the laws of hydrodynamics and pump mechanics that reflected the classic idea of Harvey - the heart as a pump and the circulation as a pipe-line system - it is impossible imagine pumps and pipe-lines falling into spasm. By the 1950s the 'spasm' theory had declined and the concept of coronary vasodilation relied solely upon the theory of coronary insufficiency.[20]

During the 1950s scepticism about the coronary vasodilators began to grow in the Anglo-American world. Clinicians had set the task of evaluating the classic and newly developed coronary vasodilators, yet their methods of assessing the benefits of therapy profoundly changed.

Firstly, electrocardiographical techniques and standardized exercise tests were accepted as the standard for the evaluation of anti-anginal drugs.[21] Secondly, the controlled clinical trial was introduced to evaluate cardiovascular drugs. Silber and Katz commented in 1953 on the state of affairs with respect to the coronary vasodilators: *"It is apparent, from even a casual survey of the literature dealing with the medical treatment of angina, that confusion and conflicting reports surround the use of each of the coronary drugs currently in favour. Such discrepancy in results has as its basis the poorly designed clinical experiment"*. [22]

The repeated inability to show beneficial effects in controlled clinical trials evoked much frustration as expressed by Traks et al.: *"It is a distressing fact that many substances which pharmacologically appear to be promising later fail to fulfill this promise in the course of direct clinical trial"*. [23] Clinical medicine urged experimental research to explain why nitroglycerine was the only effective coronary vasodilator.

Initially, physiologists refined the coronary vasodilator concept. In the early 1950s Gregg and Sabiston had proposed a new classification differentiating between benign and malign vasodilation.[24] Malign vasodilators increased coronary blood flow but did so by increasing the metabolic requirements of the heart. Benign vasodilators in contrast increased coronary blood flow without increasing cardiac oxygen consumption, and this is as Gregg and Sabiston pointed out, *"obviously an excellent situation for the heart, in that it obtains its blood flow cheaply"*. [25] This classification gave a new meaning to the saying of Sir William Osler (1897) that *"the patient with angina should learn to live within the income of his circulation"*. [26] This classification defined the criteria to be met by new **benign** coronary vasodilators. Yet after initial enthusiastic endorsement, most of these new agents fell into disrepute or lost popularity and the nitrites remained an important form of anti-anginal treatment. A new approach to the mechanism of action of the nitrates evolved (see chapter 5).

7.2.1.4. The coronary vasodilator concept - a firmly rooted principle in German medicine.

In German-speaking countries, i.e. West-Germany, Switzerland and Austria, the situation was quite different in the 1950s and 1960s. New benign coronary vasodilators were coming off the production line of German pharmaceutical companies (table 7.1).

The Belgian-French region was also committed to the coronary vasodilator concept, but West-Germany formed the focus.[27] Though the pharmacologists of these companies were acquainted with the scepticism in Anglo-American medicine, their research was intricately connected with the German medical world which firmly believed that coronary vasodilation was beneficial in the angina-patient.

Table 7.1
Coronary vasodilators developed by pharmaceutical industries in German speaking
countries and Belgium-France.

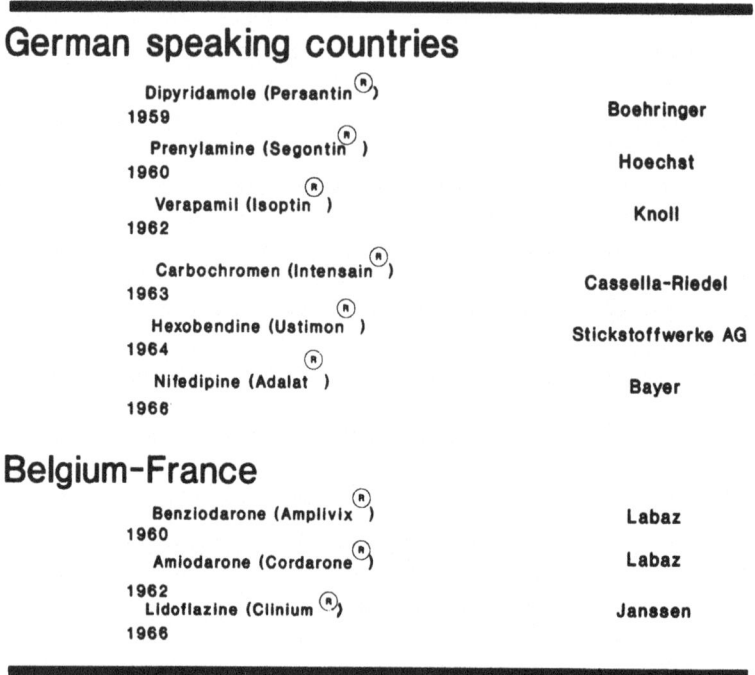

German speaking countries

Dipyridamole (Persantin®) 1959	Boehringer
Prenylamine (Segontin®) 1960	Hoechst
Verapamil (Isoptin®) 1962	Knoll
Carbochromen (Intensain®) 1963	Cassella-Riedel
Hexobendine (Ustimon®) 1964	Stickstoffwerke AG
Nifedipine (Adalat®) 1966	Bayer

Belgium-France

Benziodarone (Amplivix®) 1960	Labaz
Amiodarone (Cordarone®) 1962	Labaz
Lidoflazine (Clinium®) 1966	Janssen

At a symposium about coronary vasodilators in 1969 the German cardiologist Kreutzer commented as follows: *"There is certainly no therapeutic principle, despite the numerous experimental results, of which the clinical assessment is so varying as of the medicative coronary vasodilation. The data concerning the clinical effectiveness in the case of angina pectoris range from 0 to 90%. Particularly in the German language literature there are many research papers that report exceptionally small doses in an exceptionally short time. (...) In contrast there are negative evaluations, not least from the Anglo-Saxon literature, that at times even go so far as to totally reject this substance. Hence Fisch writes in a general review that none of these medications (he refers to Persantin, Segontin and Amplivix) can be recommended for the treatment of angina pectoris".* [28] The German cardiologist Lichtlen noticed the same phenomenon when discussing the state of affairs of anti-anginal treatment in 1972. In his review about prenylamine (Segontin), he commented: *"Accordingly, the clinical results - usually based on double blind tests - with regard to the anti-anginal effect are contradictory too. Whereas most Anglo-Saxon authors - with one exception - report on the negative clinical results with angina pectoris, the German and French authors present numerous positive results".* [29]

During the interviews for this study many examples were given of the peculiar attitudes of German clinicians regarding beta blockade and coronary vasodilation and many interesting tales were heard. The following anecdote told by Kaltenbach perfectly illustrates the strong influence of the coronary vasodilator concept in German medicine: *"And I can still remember when I had this discussion with some colleagues in Freiburg and how I then raised my objections. They said: 'Yes, but Kaltenbach, listen. If your mother now suffered from coronary complaints, would you deny her the coronary dilators? Surely, you cannot do that'".* [30]

When confronted with this era in German medicine around the 1950s, German clinicians seem to be rather reluctant to recall this period. They have a sense of shame about the state of "immaturity" as Kaltenbach called it.[31] Bender pointed to the enormous gap between clinical institutes and experimental medicine: *"(..) one must say that in Germany, different from in the USA, there is a strong division in general - not here in Münster - between experimental research and the hospital, so that one doesn't know what the other does, and they have developed in separate ways"*; and in fact, he argues that this gap has continued to widen ever since.[32] Kaltenbach pointed out: *"Perhaps the physicians who used to be in charge at that time simply were not doctors to whom scientific thought was very dear, who had been educated in a medical science which was organised in a very different way".* [33]

More particularly, two methodological issues were relevant.

First, the use of exercise tests did not influence German medicine to the same extent as it did in the British and American speaking world, although exercise testing was essentially developed by pioneers like Knipping and Reindell: *"Exercise tests were a stepchild in many hospitals. For example, in Düsseldorf they had started early with cardiac surgery but diagnostically, they were concentrating totally on cardiac catheterization. This could be expected since for the most part patients with vitia and teratism were treated, not coronary patients".* [34]

This had consequences for the selection of patients for cardiovascular research and therapeutic evaluation of anti-anginal treatment: *"And especially in relation with the testing of such medicines, we were presented again and again with studies with classic coronary dilators such as Persantin. And then I had to ask again and again: What exactly do you define as angina pectoris? If all chest troubles are regarded as angina pectoris, even Luminal can be miraculous medicine; but that hasn't got anything to do with the effect on the coronary insufficiency".* [35]

Indeed, German journals contained many therapeutic evaluations of anti-anginal treatment that defined their object, i.e. the angina pectoris patient, very differently in comparison to Anglo-Saxon studies.[36] The German classification of angina pectoris will be discussed in more detail in section 7.2.3.

Secondly, the double-blind controlled clinical trial was not as influential in German medicine as in the Anglo-American context. Several German clinicians pointed out that this fact is related to the social structure of medicine and health care in West-Germany. Pfennigsdorf stated: *"Realization of a placebo-controlled double-blind crossover study of angina pectoris usually means that the patient must participate in the study for at least 10-12 weeks. Since most German hospitals do not have their own number of ambulant cases at their disposal, as a rule the patients can be recruited for e.g. examination of the effectiveness of coronary medicines with permission of the attending general practitioner only. Problems may arise on these occasions, since it is not seldom that the general practitioner in attendance is afraid to "lose" his patients".* [37]

Against this background the differential course that the coronary vasodilator concept took in Germany, must be considered. Still, this is not to say that German medical views about coronary vasodilation were simple or irrational. The concept of coronary insufficiency was accepted as was the classification of benign and malign vasodilation. Moreover, the new views on the mechanism of action of the nitrites were accepted as well. However, these new theoretical insights were included within the German framework of the coronary vasodilator concept. This framework had two points of support.

The **first** point of support was that pathology and biochemistry formed the frame of reference for discussing the benefits of coronary vasodilating treatment, not physiology. On the one hand this implied that the hemodynamic way of thinking was not as influential as in Anglo-American medicine, and on the other hand the coronary vasodilator concept was developed in two directions.

Firstly, it was hypothesized that coronary vasodilator agents improved the collateral circulation. It had been shown that prolonged administration of dipyridamole, for example, appeared to promote the development or enlargement of arterial anastomoses. So, it was not the **direct** dilation of coronary vessels that improved coronary blood flow but the **indirect** development of new meshes in the network of coronary vessels. In this sense the plasticity of the coronary circuit was of primary concern, a concept that was very akin to morphological and pathological thinking in German medicine.

This way of thinking seemed to enable German clinicians to stand on firm ground in the swamp of uncertainty that ruled the debate about the coronary vasodilators. In 1969 Kreutzer expressed this general feeling as follows: *"Therefore it is understandable that there are great uncertainties concerning the administration of coronary dilators in the hospital. Opinions range from total rejection to large-scale medication even in the case of functional complaints (..) Notwithstanding the frequently disappointing clinical effectiveness of coronary dilators and notwithstanding the difficulties in objectifying their effects, for the moment it does not seem justified to generally denounce their administration. Experimental results concerning the collateral development are so impressive that it is advisable to administer coronary dilators for at least as long as it has not been established beyond doubt that they do not favour collateral development in the human heart. However, up to now this evidence has not been produced".* [38]

Secondly, interference with the metabolism of the heart by coronary vasodilators was hypothesized. In this respect the theory of the potentiating effect on the action of adenosine attracted considerable attention. Adenosine represented one of the end products of the high-energy phosphates in the metabolism of the heart. It played a role as a regulator of the coronary circulation because it was a very potent vaso-active substance and it was believed to enhance the availability of substrates for heart metabolism.[39] Another aspect of this biochemical approach is that whenever beta blockade was discussed for its beneficial effects, the terms sympathetic stimulation and sympathetic inhibition should be understood with due regard to their biochemical implications, not merely their hemodynamic consequences concerning cardiac work. In this respect, Raab's hypothesis had considerable influence in German medicine.[40]

The **second** point of support was the nervous-vasomotor paradigm which formed the basis of the spasm theory. This not only influenced medical theory of angina pectoris, it also underlied the medical views about heart failure, low blood pressure, and other disturbances of the circulation. While the spasm theory was eliminated from Anglo-Saxon medical theory, it remained influential in Germany, though in a specific way. It went "underground", and occasionally explicit references to this theory appear in German medical textbooks and literature. Sometimes one finds obvious disagreement with the turn Anglo-Saxon medicine took. So the German physician Mainzer wrote in 1958: *"A classic observation by Gruber and Lanz proved, in addition to other facts, that coronary spasms can also occur with arteries that are intact. As a consequence of an epileptic fit with tightness of the chest, they were able to find myocardial necroses with perfect coronary arteries. Their observation has not been changed, not even as a result of the furious attacks undertaken by the English clinician Pickering, who referred to their notions as "a grotesque myth of idiots".* [41]

The spasm theory was concealed in concepts that did not betray their origin, but were used to signify the influence of the autonomic nervous system on the cardiovascular system. Thus, this theory keeps on playing a central role, though camouflaged, in pathology, biochemistry and physiology of heart and blood vessels. The following two sections about medical views of heart failure and angina pectoris illustrate this point.

It is remarkable that the nervous-vasomotor paradigm maintained its position in German medicine for such a long time, certainly when it had already been pushed aside in Anglo-American medicine during the 1930s and 1940s. Though a variety of factors such as the relative isolation of German medicine before and after the Second World War and its hierarchical organization, explains this continuity, it also springs from cultural traditions that stretch far back in German history. Payer stresses the deep-lying and lasting influence of the intellectual and cultural movement of "Romanticism" in German medicine. An important aspect of this influence is according to Payer "the notion of the synthesis or interplay of opposing forces" that underlies typical German disease entities such as vaso-vegetative dystonia, circulatory collapse and low blood pressure. [42] However, there are other cultural and social factors including therapeutic pluralism in German medicine associated with a close relation between regular and alternative medicine. The influence of pathological-biochemical and nervous theories on German medical views of heart failure and angina pectoris will become clear in the following sections.

7.2.1.5 Bibliometrical analysis

To illustrate the differential course and timing of the coronary vasodilator concept in Anglo-Saxon and German medicine a bibliometric analysis was performed. For this purpose I took Charlier's textbook **Antianginal Drugs** of 1971 reviewing about 2600 articles and papers in the field. [43]

Charlier reviewed 274 articles published during 1959 - 1969 about five coronary vasodilators relating to angina pectoris; another 165 articles about propranolol were reviewed. (table 7.2). This sample was taken as a database to perform a bibliometric analysis (see Appendix III for the methodology).

Although Charlier was a proponent of the coronary vasodilator concept and worked at the firm Labaz that developed a coronary vasodilator, he changed his ideas in favour of the Anglo-American views about angina and nitrites. [44] In his first book in 1961, entitled

Table 7.2
Number of articles relating to coronary vasodilators, and
propranolol published from 1959 to 1969
(reviewed by Charlier (1971)).

	Number of articles included in sample
Coronary vasodilators	
Prenylamine	48
Benziodarone	48
Dipyridamole	96
Carbochromen	46
Hexobendine	36
	- - -
	274
Beta blockers	
Propranolol	165

Coronary Vasodilators he defended the coronary vasodilator concept, in his second of 1971 he dismissed it.[45] Since Charlier took a position between that of the German and English speaking world, articles from both viewpoints were covered which is rather unique in medical literature of the 1960s.[46] Through his eyes perceptions in the two medical settings have been analyzed.

The citation results obtained yield clear-cut differences between the Anglo-Saxon and German medical context as shown by figures 7.1, 7.2 and 7.3.

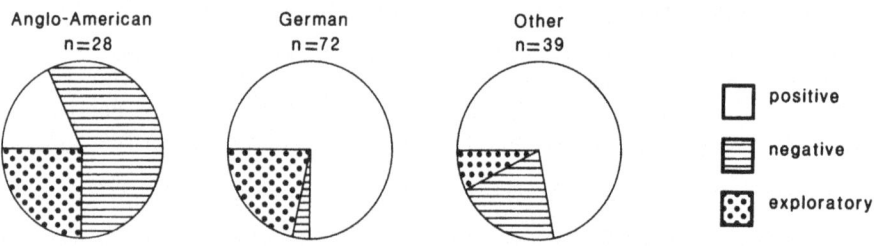

Figure 7.1
Distribution of type of clinical judgment about coronary vasodilators classified as positive, negative and exploratory in Anglo-American, German and "other" medicine.

Almost 60% of the clinical articles in Anglo-American journals about the coronary vasodilators were negative. In contrast, 75% of the clinical articles in Germanic journals were clearly positive. The journals of the "Other"-type take a position closer to the Germanic category, mainly because Belgian and French journals contained many positive clinical articles.

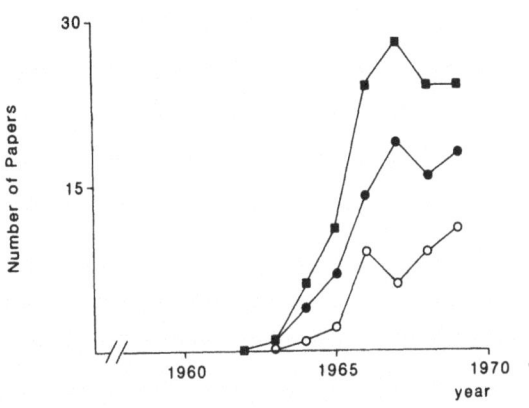

Figure 7.2
Number of articles on beta blockers published in Anglo-American medical literature:
(■) total number of articles
(●) number of clinical articles
(O) clinical articles with positive evaluation

The Anglo-Saxon world turned away from the coronary vasodilators and rapidly moved to the field of the beta blockers as shown in figure 7.2.[47] The steep curve for all three categories of articles indicates the rapid acceptance of the beta blockers.[48] Almost 90% of all the articles reviewed by Charlier appeared in Anglo-American journals. A similar figure representing the German situation is therefore impossible and irrelevant.

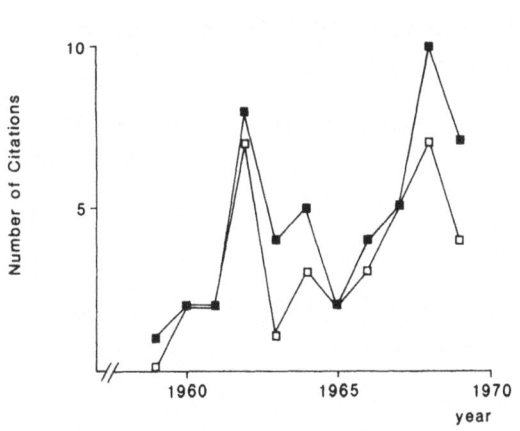

Figure 7.3
Number of articles on five coronary vasodilators (including dipyridamole) (■) in comparison with the number of articles on dipyridamole only in Anglo-American journals (□).

Almost all of the experimental and clinical articles about the coronary vasodilators published in Anglo-American journals concerned dipyridamole (figure 7.3). In the German context dipyridamole accounts for about 30% of all articles meaning that the compound is just one of the many coronary vasodilators used in clinical practice, though it was a highly appreciated drug. British and American doctors used dipyridamole as a tool to trace the mechanism of action of the nitrites, to mark the desired profile of new anti-anginal drugs and to differentiate between various mechanisms in experimental and clinical research. In short, dipyridamole was used as a technique to crack the mystique about the coronary vasodilator concept. In the German setting the same technique "fixed" the concept.

7.2.1.6 Conclusions

The coronary vasodilator concept maintained its established position in German medicine for a considerable time. Moreover, it was not a static view but was carried through to the frontiers of biochemical and pharmacological research in the German speaking countries. Conservatism in German medical practice formed a major impulse to German industries to develop new coronary vasodilators and to basic sciences to develop new concepts. In contrast, Anglo-American medicine had relegated the coronary vasodilators to the backseat of anti-anginal treatment at a much earlier stage.

7.2.2. Medical views about heart failure

7.2.2.1. Introduction

The definition, etiology and mechanism of heart failure have been debated for over a century, and are still a source of controversy. The survey of the achievements and trends in this particular field of medicine cannot be historical in the same sense as were the earlier sections concerning angina pectoris. This section about heart failure will therefore deal with the most prominent differences in the **frames of reference** between Anglo-Saxon and German definitions of heart failure. The hemodynamic framework in which Anglo-American physicians discussed heart failure will be covered (7.2.2.2.). In contrast, German physicians discussed the issue within a pathological-biochemical and ergometric framework (7.2.2.3.). Subsequently, three German disease profiles regarding heart failure will be described in more detail (7.2.2.4.).

7.2.2.2 Anglo-American medical views about congestive heart failure: Starling's Law of the Heart.

Since William Harvey the heart has been a major pre-occupation of the physiologist and the clinician. So essential is the pump function of the heart that, if the left ventricle expels one drop of blood less per beat than the right ventricle, within three to four hours about one litre additional blood would accumulate in the lungs which causes shortness of breath (dyspnea), cough and sputum secretion. If the reverse should occur, an equal amount of blood would accumulate on the venous or right side of the circulation with the result of venous distention, enlarged liver and peripheral edema.[49] Congestion (fluid retention) is so much a central feature of heart failure that Anglo-Saxon physicians called it **congestive** heart failure whereas German physicians coined the equivalent term "Stauung" ("Herzinsuffizienz mit Stauung").

Two diametrically opposed schools of medical thought concerning the mechanism of heart failure have governed medicine for decades. The theory of backward failure, which goes back as far as James Hope (1852), contended that heart failure causes a rise in pressure "backward", that is to say upstream from the failing heart. This theory was based on the clinical picture of left-sided heart failure that leads to an increase in pressure in the lung circulation and therefore to congestion of the lungs. Subsequently, right heart failure develops because of the increasing work load made upon the right heart with the result of congestion in the systemic vessels, liver and edema. The theory of backward failure explained the sequence of clinical manifestations of left heart failure that is still recognized as the most common form of congestive heart failure in medical practice.

After holding sway for nearly a century, this theory was replaced by the theory of forward heart failure, particularly expounded by the distinguished British clinician Sir James MacKenzie (1913). MacKenzie maintained that the clinical manifestations resulted directly from the inadequate discharge of blood into the arterial system.[50] For MacKenzie, the functional state of the heart was the key feature of heart failure; organic change of cardiac tissue was of no importance.[51] MacKenzie's views were broadly accepted by his contemporaries in the British medical world.[52]

In the following years, the ideas of cardiac failure were fundamentally revised, particularly Starling's concept (1918) and its translation into the clinician's view of heart failure.

In order to make this point clear it is necessary to trace some of the compensatory events of the normal and the failing heart as implied by Starling's concept. When the heart has to expel blood while there is an increased resistance to outflow, for example in the case of hypertension, it ejects less blood than it received. Consequently, the pressure in the heart rises, the heart becomes slightly dilated and this dilation makes the pressure return to normal and improves the contraction. The heart's output becomes larger until it ejects as much blood as it receives. In this way the equilibrium is restored.

The same mechanism operates when for some reason venous flow to the heart increases. In both cases the heart is able to adapt itself to changes over a wide range. However, when the heart fails, it no longer pumps as much blood as it receives and consequently, there is a rise in pressure as well as a dilation. In a sense, the heart acts like a bow. As the string is pulled out more strongly, the arrow darts off with more power and higher speed into the air. Similarly, the lengthening of the muscle fibers due to the dilation results in an increased force of contraction and propulsion of blood. This fundamental type of adjustment was coined with the term "Law of the heart" by Starling and his colleagues.

It took some time before clinicians started to translate Starling's concept in terms of the symptoms and signs seen at the bedside, but during the 1930s and 1940s it became to be known as **the Law of the Heart**.[53] Medical views about heart failure have been shaped largely by the work of Cournand in the USA and McMichael and Sharpey-Schaefer in England.[54] A theory of congestive heart failure in the centre of which stood the Law of the Heart. On the basis of hemodynamic monitoring in patients with cardiac failure made possible by cardiac catheterization it was demonstrated that elevation of the venous pressure was the primary mechanism in congestive heart failure. Though increased intra-cardiac pressure operated for some time as a compensatory mechanism for increasing cardiac output, sooner or later this would fail and overloading would occur.[55] British and American textbooks and medical literature continuously stress the applicability of Starling's law to man. Wood stated in his textbook that *"McMichael and Sharpey-Schaefer have developed a theory of congestive failure which is in accordance with Starling's Law of the heart"*. [56] Pickering declared in his 1958' paper delivered before the Washington State Heart Association that *"Starling's concept of the nature of heart failure was closely in accord with what actually happens in man"*. [57] Subsequent editions of the textbooks of Harrison, Hurst and Friedberg also testify to the applicability of Starling's law to man.[58] This is not to say that there was no opposition.[59] A large number of clinicians spoke and wrote about the discrepancies between the law and the observations in man.[60] Yet, heart failure was defined within the same intellectual and technical framework.The advent of cardiac catheterization techniques enabled clinicians to measure intra-cardiac pressures and cardiac outflow. Accordingly, congestive heart failure was defined within this hemodynamic framework. Despite the controversy, the general feeling was that Starling's law was applicable in man.[61]

By the end of the 1950s, however, awareness grew that myocardial contractility might be governed by other mechanisms than Starling's law alone. This realization came from two sources.

One source was the basic sciences trying to provide Starling's law with an ultrastructural basis. New insights were collected regarding the structural mechanisms underlying the contractile process of the heart's muscle. In this sense the characteristics of the bow's string itself formed more and more the centre of scientific interest. In as much as Braunwald's work on heart failure can be taken as reference for the way this concept entered cardiology, one has to conclude that the basic sciences provided "an ultrastructural basis of Starling's Law".[62] This basis consisted of two general properties of the heart's muscle, i.e.*"a change in initial muscle length which is the basis of the Starling mechanism and a change in the contractile state of the heart as brought about by an inotropic intervention"*. [63] Precisely this latter is in direct opposition with Starling's law of the heart as it had governed medical views for many years. The other reason to question Starling's law came from clinical practice. The autonomic nervous system attracted much attention from clinicians during the 1960s. The importance of the sympathetic drive in patients with heart failure was shown by the dramatic effects of beta blockade in these patients. Clinical experience with guanethidine   forecasted this event. Awareness grew that neurogenic reflex and humoral compensating mechanisms might be more important in circulatory adaptation than the operation of Frank-Starling's Law of the Heart.[64]

7.2.2.3. German medical views about heart failure: The master of the circulation?

How markedly different were German conceptions of heart failure! During the 1940s and 1950s when Anglo-American medicine was elaborating on Starling's law of the heart, German literature is filled with accounts of the inapplicability of Starling's views in man. Central to the German view seems to be the acknowledgement of the heart as a "part" of a "functional" system in which nervous and humoral mechanisms were crucial.

It is interesting to note that as early as in 1942, the Austrian clinician Wenckebach criticized the perception of the heart as the master of the circulation. In so doing he was backed by his colleague Rudolf Kaufmann who denounced the important role of the vegetative system to which the heart and the circulation were subordinated. In his address to the Society of Physicians at Vienna in 1926 Kaufmann criticized the view that the heart is the sovereign master of the organism: *"Actually, I think the matter is as follows: if we, following old opinions that were recently improved by W.R. Hess, divide the corporal functions into two categories, viz. on the one hand the animal functions, to which belong the functions of the senses, the functions of the nerves that attend to the muscles and the senses, and particularly the functions of the muscular system, and on the other hand the vegetative functions, to which belong digestion, excretion, and particularly respiration, the relation of the heart to these functions can then perhaps be expressed appropriately when we say: 'The heart is servant to the animal functions and slave to the vegetative functions of the organism'"*. [65]

These remarks were used by Wenckebach when discussing under the heading "ceteris non paribus" all the mechanisms that modify or transform the laws of hydrodynamics - which are treated under the heading "ceteris paribus" -to criticize the views of Harvey who compared the heart with King Charles I and ranked both with the sun, the centre of the universe on which everything turns. Subsequently, hereby referring to Kaufmann, he continued in writing: *"What would Harvey have said, had he lived to hear that statement? As an old, wise man he would have been comforted: He had already had to experience his king's head falling on the scaffold! For us it is an advance to have realised that the heart too must serve, not master, the well-being of the community"*. [66] It is interesting to note that in the early 1960s, i.e. when attention for extra-cardiac mechanisms rapidly grew, Anglo-American scientists, notably Louis N. Katz, held the view that the heart was *"as much the servant of the circulation as its master"*. [67]

Indeed, the glamour of the master role in the organism, if there is any, may have been attributed to the heart in Anglo-American medicine, German medicine assigned this honour to the vegetative system. The attention to a nervous and humoral mechanism was referred to by the German clinician Hans-Joachim Florian (1953) in terms of "a new way of thinking".[68] Noteworthy of this term "new" as Florian wrote *"seems to me the continuous dissociation from mechanistic to functional thinking as well as the realization that the heart is not merely a part of a circulatory system but organ in an organism"*. [69]

The healthy heart was able to adjust its pump function to the varying demands by means of nervous control mechanisms. The heart was capable of increasing its force of contraction, not on the basis of the Law of the Heart (or not alone), but due to "inotropic" mechanisms (as well), e.g. qualitative changes going on in the heart that increase its power. The simple analogy of the bow helps us to understand this remarkable change. Not the stretching of the bow's string, but the use of another string, stronger and more elastic, would increase the power with which the arrow darts off. The failing heart was not able to respond in this way. The functional state of the circulation influenced its structure and vice versa.

The description of some relevant pathogenetic concepts may illustrate this reciprocal relationship between structure and function.

Pathological strains imposed upon the heart were divided in two categories: pressure-load and volume-load.

A pathological pressure load in hypertension, hypertonic dysfunction or valvular stenosis is initially compensated by nervous and humoral control mechanisms that increase cardiac contractility. In addition hypertrophy of the heart, a structural compensation, develops in the course of weeks or months. This hypertrophy is essentially a normal and efficient mechanism of adaptation that merely arises under pathological conditions. There is no increase of cardiac inflow or intra-cardiac pressure. The size of the heart remains normal or even small instead of enlarged as in manifest cardiac failure.

A pathological volume load occurs in valvular insufficiency, cardiovascular shunts or malformation, arterio-venous aneurysm and in cases of increased cardiac output (anaemia, "high output hypertension", etc.). A regulative enlargement of the heart develops. This enlargement was not the result of a passive dilation ("stretching" and thus "lengthening" of the cardiac muscle fibers) caused by an increased filling pressure on the basis of the Starling mechanism but instead by some regulatory mechanism. The concept of "regulative enlargement" ("Regulative Herzvergrösserung") was developed in the context of sport medicine.[70] Presumably, enlargement of heart in sportsmen originated from a loss of muscle tonus induced by the parasympathetic part of the autonomic nervous system. This regulative dilation was considered as a precursor as well as a stimulus of subsequent hypertrophy.

The basic question arose whether or to what extent hypertrophy was compatible with normal activity of the heart. An important concept in German medical literature to answer this question was the "critical weight" of the hypertrophous heart. Beyond that critical point the supply of energy and oxygen was insufficient and the heart was unable to maintain its contractile function. Consequently, "contractile" or "muscular insufficiency" arose.[71] Beyond the point of "critical weight" compensatory mechanisms attempted to overcome this disturbance and are essentially the same as presupposed in Starling's law of the heart.[72] On the basis of the Starling' mechanism the heart dilated in order to restore its contractile function which was called "myogenic dilation" ("Myogene Dilatation").[73] Simultaneously, other mechanisms like morphological changes in the heart muscle, might add to this dilation. This adaptive dilation would succeed only partially. In general it was considered that when no improvement of the underlying disease occurred, oxygen and energy conditions were so poor that a vicious circle emerged and further structural damage occurred with the result of irreversible states of cardiac dilation.

Obviously, "hypertrophy" and "dilation" are essentially concepts from morphology, anatomy or histology. However, the changes in the heart were surmised from clinical and clinico-roentgenological studies as well. The view, that governed Anglo-American medicine, that dilation and hypertrophy are both compensatory mechanisms in response to the same stimuli, did not apply to German medicine.[74] At the bedside German clinicians attempted to delineate different forms and stages and distinct relationships between dilation and hypertrophy. A typical form of cardiac dilation as clinically encountered may illustrate this point.

In various patients with heart failure German clinicians observed an enlarged heart was present at rest but without an increase in pressure whereas during exercise the pressure rapidly increased.[75] This paradoxical state was perceived as contradictory to Starling's law of the heart because this implicated that dilation, e.g. enlargement, was not due to an increased pressure. The dilation was instead explained on the basis of **structural** changes in the hypertrophied heart. This change implied that a normal or only a slightly raised pressure was able to cause a marked dilation of the heart.

At this point the concepts of the German pathologist Linzbach during the 1940s and 1950s were very influential.[76] According to Linzbach this dilation originated from a re-structuring of cardiac muscle. This implicated a "slippage" or detrimental re-arrangement of muscle fibers in particular areas of the heart. This re-arrangement was due to morphological changes induced by necrosis, scarring and interstitial inflammatory changes in cardiac tissue. Thus, the heart was able to "flow out" under normal filling pressure as is the case in rest. This regional "overstretch" was coined with the term "plastic dilation" ("Plastische Gefügedilatation").[77]

It is interesting to note that German clinicians urged pathologists to throw up new concepts of dilation. For it was observed that severe states of dilation were capable of a rapid return to normal.[78] Subsequently, biochemical hypotheses were put forward that dilation resulted from a "loss of tonus" due to energetic disturbances. The German clinicians aware of their position contrasting with the Anglo-American views distinguished "energetic insufficiency" from "dynamic insufficiency". The latter denoted the hemodynamic characteristics exhibited by congestive heart failure, the former cardiac insufficiency in which energetic disturbances were central. To explain this difference Hegglin, a well known clinician in Zürich, drew upon the analogy with the petrol motor. A motor fails when the demands made upon it are too high, e.g. too heavy chassis, leaking valves, impassable roads, etc. ("hemodynamic insufficiency") but also when the fuel is inferior![79] Accordingly, Hegglin classified several forms of "energetic" heart failure during the 1940s and 1950s.[80] Though clinically acknowledged as a minority case, these energetic forms of heart failure were considered as well-defined nosologic entities and formed the target of frontier research in biochemistry. This is yet another aspect of the typical German intellectual framework. It explains why the pathological tradition in German medicine was occupied with biochemistry at a very early stage. The connection between biochemistry and pathology in German cardiovascular research formed a fertile soil for the experimental work of Fleckenstein who took up this issue of active tonicity of the heart muscle.[81]

In what follows three clinical profiles will be described that are the primary consequence of the German intellectual framework.

7.2.2.4. Three clinical profiles of heart failure

1. "Failure on effort"

German clinicians distinguished between heart failure in rest and during exercise ("Ruhe-insuffizienz" - "Bewegungsinsuffizienz").[82] Heart failure in rest ("Ruhe-insuffizienz") was defined as the state in which clinical manifestations, with or without congestion, were present at rest. Heart failure on effort ("Bewegungsinsuffizienz") denoted the state that cardiac performance is in accordance with the physical strain at rest, but not during exertion. Other terms for this category "Bewegungsinsuffizienz" were "Frühinsuffizienz" ("early failure"), "Latente Insuffizienz" ("latent failure") or "Präinsuffizienz" ("pre-failure"). Thus, heart failure was considered as a gradual phenomenon between two extremes: latent and manifest heart failure. The most extreme and severe form was the full-blown picture of congestive heart failure.

Diagnosis of the various stages of heart failure was performed by ergonomics using exercise as the standard of circulatory function. This ergometric approach was very popular in Scandinavian and German speaking countries.[83] Though various tests have been developed and tested in United States of America and Great Britain, Anglo-American physicians never accepted ergonomics as widely as Swedish or German medical doctors because of the variable results and the purported overlapping between normal subjects and cardiac patients.[84]

These problems were acknowledged by German physicians as well, but apparently their evaluation differed.[85] Various clinical centres in West-Germany developed new techniques and parameters to account for the overlap between normal and pathological circulatory function. Particularly the schools of Brauer and Knipping ("Brauer-Knippingschen Methode"), Reindell, Klepzig and Roskamm developed ergometric tests that were very influential in Germany. Furthermore, the Scandinavian schools of Nylin, Wallstedt, and Sjohstrom played a major role.[86] *"At that time, in the fifties, the Swedish school had an extremely good reputation. Indeed, I think they used to be really good",* as Kaltenbach stated.[87]

The method developed by Reindell and his group (H.W. Kirchhoff, K. König, K. Musshoff and H. Roskamm) is illustrative for the intricate relationship of "structure" and "function" in defining heart failure. Reindell and his colleagues worked at the Institute of Occupational and Sport Medicine at the Medical University Clinic of Freiburg and were very influential in German medicine. During the 1950s they published more than thirty articles, and during the period 1960 - 1965 about 35 articles concerning this method appeared in German medical journals.[88] Reindell together with Klepzig wrote the chapters on Diseases of Heart and Vessels in subsequent editions of the influential textbook of internal medicine edited by Heilmeyer, a well-respected and very influential German internist.[89]

The method was developed during the 1950s and early 1960s and was widely accepted in Germany. The basic idea of this test was to combine ergonomics as a function of the circulatory state and roentgenologic measures of the size of the heart as the standard for the pathological state of the heart. During an extensive series of studies the crucial parameters to measure function were standardized by reference to different aspects of the normal heart and the normal organism. Subsequently, these standardized parameters were correlated with the size of the heart, i.e. the structure. The values obtained were used to differentiate between respiratory and circulatory failure, between the normal and the pathological state of the heart, and in the latter case between organic and vegetative disturbances of the heart. Different forms of regulatory dysfunction ("normotonic", "hypertonic", "hypotonic") as well as their sites and consequences were established as were the various forms of and stages in heart failure.[90] Its significance laid in the diagnosis of the early and latent forms of heart failure amongst which "failure on effort" was a very prominent syndrome encountered in German medical practice.

2. "Old age heart"

Yet another clinical picture, e.g. the "old age heart" ("Das Altersherz") is illustrative, and it includes two major forms. Firstly, the "old age heart" in the clinico-pathological sense of the word, e.g. a heart that becomes "flabby" due to atrophy and other structural changes in the hypertrophied heart; the heart is like a limp bellows without elasticity and contractile power. This view is connected with a spectre of clinical signs that might be diagnosed particularly in people of over 60 years.

Secondly, the "old age heart" in a more physiological sense of the word. Due to the changes of the human organism with increasing age, physiological and biochemical processes are performed less efficiently. The various parameters representing the normal function of various organs and tissues are inclined to shift to the abnormal. Thus, a picture emerges in which old-age is conceived of as a stage in human life in which changes due to aging interfere with normal activity. Obviously this picture is germane to a broad range between normal and abnormal. In the German setting it concerns particularly people in the age class of 50 -60 years and precedes the group of elderly people of 60 years and older that have a flabby heart. Both forms have been recognized since the German clinician Wezler formulated the concept late in 1930s and early 1940s. On the one hand Wezler constructed the concept on the basis of pathological observations showing that the weight of the heart increased during life time but decreased in the elderly. These observations suggested that the heart lost its "functional mass" due to involutional changes. On the other hand he supported the concept of the old age heart in terms of "approaching limits of cardiac insufficiency" ("Näherrücken der Insuffizienzgrenze").

According to Wezler hypertrophy developed on the basis of a progressive increase in mechanical stress on the heart.[91] Beyond a critical point, somewhere occurring at the age of 55 years, a disproportion between the mass of the hypertrophied heart and the demands made upon it would arise. Thus, a divergence between the curves of heart weight and of exercise performance formed the physiological basis of the concept. In this sense Wezler's concept preludes the two basic terms of structure and function with which German physicians came to define heart failure. During the late 1950s and 1960s, the concept of old age heart was connected with and translated into those of failure on effort, early insufficiency or latent insufficiency.[92] However, it retained its status as a separate nosologic entity.

Thus, the concept of old age heart has a long tradition in German medicine, and it is still influential in contemporary practice.

3. Angina pectoris and heart failure.

The intensive evaluation of the active role of coronary insufficiency in the development of heart failure reflects in yet another way the intricate relationship between structure and function in German medicine. Whereas Anglo-American medicine disregarded any intimate relationship between coronary insufficiency (angina pectoris) and heart failure[93], German medical literature is full of pejorative references to this interrelationship. The various views that make up the typical German account can be summarized as follows. Angina pectoris was considered to be the disease associated with the development of structural changes of the heart in the long term. "Muscular insufficiency", that critical stage in heart failure, was believed to be the result of inadequate supply of oxygen and nutrients to the heart. Moreover, the risk of damage as well as the regenerative capacity of the heart's muscle was dependant on the adequacy of the coronary circulation. Angina pectoris was either a primary or a secondary cause in heart failure. The morphological characteristics describing angina pectoris and heart failure were the same. Hence, concepts like "necrosis", "rudimentary infarction", "dilation", "scarring" and "plastic dilation" were pertinent to both clinical pictures. In this sense the term structure figured most prominently in the description of both disease complexes, and there has been a considerable overlapping between angina pectoris and heart failure.

7.2.2.5 Disease profiles of heart failure in Anglo-American and German medicine

In summary, figure 7.4 approximates clinical taxonomy of heart failure in both medical settings.

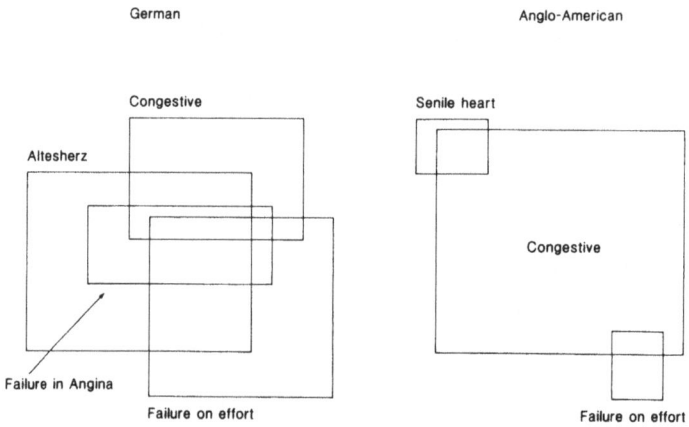

Figure 7.4
Disease profiles of heart failure in Anglo-American and German medicine, 1960-1970: the social impact.

Congestive heart failure is the dominant category in Anglo-American medicine, while in the German setting the situation is quite different. Here the three profiles as described above are substantial parts of the classification and are characterized by major overlap. The opposite category to failure on effort, namely failure at rest, is synonymous with congestive heart failure. At least it overlaps with congestive heart failure to a considerable extent and therefore it has been omitted from the graphical representation. Angina of effort is rather similar to the Anglo-American terms of grade 1 and grade 2 heart failure as proposed by the New York Heart Association during the 1920s. Though the category was familiar to physicians, it was not a dominant category. Therefore, the square denoting this category is relatively small in comparison with the squares representing the Anglo-American category congestive heart failure and the German nosologic entity failure on effort.

The senile heart was a well-defined category in the English speaking medical world but represented a very specific form of destruction of cardiac muscle. It differs quite markedly from the German old-age heart and it was not a very important concept.

To underline the marked differences between the views about heart failure in both medical worlds it is interesting to discuss some therapeutic aspects. Therapeutic strategies with regard to heart failure seem to have followed rather different courses. Dornhorst stated: *"There has always been a considerable difference in the attitudes to cardiac failure between French and German physicians on the one hand and the British on the other. (...) Somehow the continentals were always more interventionist".* [94]

Even in 1978 German physicians prescribed six times the amount of cardiac glycosides, the standard therapy of heart failure, as their British colleagues did. Moreover they are "winners" when comparing prescribing practices of cardiac glycosides in eight European countries (table 7.3).[95]

Table 7.3
Utilization of cardiac glycosides in eight European countries.
(The data derived from Friebel (1982)).

	DDD/1.000 Inhabitants daily
Federal Rep. Germany	64.29
France	8.81
Sweden	32.34
Finland	42.38
United Kingdom	10.16
Norway	18.76
Italy	16.65
Spain	7.29

These quantitative characteristics of German prescribing practice may be related to the typical patient profiles as described in foregoing sections. The profiles of old age heart and failure on effort are still very influential in German medicine and are responsible for the high prescription of cardiac glycosides.

It might be argued that the large amounts of cardiac glycosides prescribed are dependent upon social and economic factors and that there need not to be a direct relationship between patient profiles and prescribing practice. Yet, the clinicians when asked declared that cardiac glycosides were heavily used in the case of old age heart and failure on effort. Moreover qualitative data about the reasons why German physicians prescribe cardiac glycosides, notably arguments spelled out during the period 1940 - 1970, point in the same direction. Terms like "early digitalization" ("Frühdigitalisierung"), "Once digitalis, for ever digitalis" ("Einmal digitalis, immer Digitalis") or "Digitalis, milk for the elderly" ("Digitalis, Milch des Alters") betray the development of digitalis treatment within the confinement of typical German views of heart failure. Moreover, the development of cardiac glycosides as a treatment of **angina pectoris** took place in German medicine during the 1930s and 1940s and underlines the interdependency of heart failure and angina pectoris.

Thus, cardiac glycosides intersect with the German patient profiles of heart failure to a considerable extent. Behind the formal boundaries of scientific argument, German physicians were in conflict with their foreign colleagues, notably British and American clinicians, during informal meetings about the approach to cardiac failure. The next anecdote told to me by Chamberlain is evidence of this. Chamberlain recalled a clash with four German cardiologists around 1970 when he expressed his views about the minimal risks of beta blockers in heart failure and when he even dared to declare that the value of digitalis therapy might be less than generally presupposed: *"Their notion was that weakening the heart beat could impossibly be good for the heart; what you should be doing was toning it up (..)"*. [96] Indeed, digitalis was and still is perceived by German physicians as the "tonic" of the heart par excellence.

7.2.2.6. Conclusions

From the very outset medical views of heart failure have been mechanistic, and the laws of pump and fluid mechanics were considered to apply to the normal and failing pump and transport function of the circulatory system. In accordance with this mechanistic approach two diametrically opposed schools of thought have governed Anglo-American medical views about heart failure. The technique of cardiac catheterization enabled clinicians to apply the sophisticated and increasingly ingenious laws of pump and fluid mechanics to congestive heart failure.

The Law of the Heart was drawn into the clinical battle between forward and backward failure theories which in fact had been put forward to explain the clinical manifestations of heart failure, the key feature being congestion. This promptly raised the question of whether Starling's law was applicable or not.

However, a controversy about this law never arose. Rather this law was taken up in a more general scheme of circulatory adaptation. Starling's law of the heart became one of the first and major lines of defense called upon in circulatory adaptation to maintain the pump function.[97] Altogether, the terminology developed in the 1960s prepared the era of a more dynamic perspective on heart failure in which nervous and humoral mechanisms of adaptation, interacted with the mechanics of the heart and the circulation.[98]

German medicine took another direction. Structure and function were the leading terms with which German physicians defined heart failure. The strong emphasis on structure reflected the pathological tradition in German medicine which was certainly at variance with Anglo-American medical views. Similarly for the term function because this was not defined as the performance of the heart itself but as the functional capacity of the human organism. In this latter respect the performance of the heart was not defined in hemodynamic terms as was the case in Anglo-Saxon medicine but in terms of exercise capacity of the human being, i.e. an ergometric definition. The applicability of Starling's law was not so much denied but rather could not be settled in pathological-biochemical and ergometric terms.

What has been said is in no sense meant to be a definitive account of the Law of the Heart nor of the richness of Starling's experimental work.[99] The apparent discrepancies between German and Anglo-American medical **perceptions** of the (in)applicability of Starling's Law have been used to help sort out the differences between the intellectual frameworks within which heart failure was discussed. Using this example the analysis of the German medical views were confined to the three patient profiles which were encountered most frequently, which differed markedly from Anglo-American concepts and yet which could be considered the result of the typical German intellectual framework described above.

7.2.3. Angina pectoris and coronary insufficiency in German medicine

7.2.3.1. Introduction

In this section the German medical views about angina pectoris will be described. In contrast with the reconstruction of Anglo-American clinical taxonomy (chapter 6), it is not intended to provide a history of developments, rather emphasis lies on medical views as they emerged during the 1950s. These views marked the definition of angina pectoris at a time when the beta blockers were about to appear, and markedly influenced clinical thinking during the 1960s.

7.2.3.2. Coronary insufficiency

To characterize German views on angina pectoris a start can be made with the pathological concepts of Franz Büchner, a very influential pathologist in German speaking countries who worked at the Pathological Institute in Freiburg. During the 1930s and 1940s Büchner described various forms of coronary heart disease causing sudden death in patients who were found to have coronary atherosclerosis without coronary thrombosis or occlusion.

Nevertheless, their hearts were damaged ranging from small to severe pathological lesions. This damage was attributed to a state of acute coronary insufficiency ("Akute Koronarinsuffizienz"), i.e. an inadequate coronary blood supply. Coronary insufficiency denoted a clinical entity. It was built on selected cases who suffered from sudden death but not myocardial infarction in which "through-and-through" infarction of the heart was caused by thrombosis or occlusion of the coronary vessels.

Under the heading of coronary insufficiency ("Koronarinsuffizienz") the range of coronary disease was classified. This spectre represented a continuum from the mild, transient forms of angina pectoris to severe anginal states with prolonged pain accompanied by objective laboratory and electrocardiographic signs of infarction (but not through-and-through). In contrast to Büchner's intention, myocardial infarction became classified within the category coronary insufficiency as the most extreme form.

Obviously sudden death denoted a state of acute coronary insufficiency as did myocardial infarction. Chronic coronary insufficiency was considered as the repetitious occurrence of attacks of acute coronary insufficiency. This category denoted the collective noun of all forms of angina pectoris.

Three subcategories were distinguished: angina pectoris simplex, angina pectoris gravis and status anginosus. The first concerned attacks of anginal pain that lasted maximally ten to fifteen minutes and generally responded fairly well to nitroglycerin. The second referred to attacks that lasted more than fifteen minutes associated with electrocardiographical signs of myocardial ischemia. Finally, status anginosus included those patients with severe pain lasting from half an hour up to several days, commonly originating from rest; ECG changes were very similar to those developing in infarction. The latter category will be dismissed from this reconstruction because it is rather similar to the Anglo-American category "status anginosus".

At first sight the first category mimics angina of effort because the terms "angina simplex" and "angina ambulatoria" are sometimes used interchangeably. However, the duration of attacks (up to 10 - 15 minutes) is considerably longer than in the case of the Anglo-American category typical angina of effort in which the duration of the attack is two to three minutes. Therefore the category angina simplex included patients who would be classified by Anglo-Saxon physicians as angina at rest, angina decubitus and so forth. German physicians also considered angina simplex as a broader category than angina pectoris ambulatoria.

Figure 7.5 is taken from the German Medical Journal. The figure was presented by the German clinician Klaus Holzmann in his 1954[']article entitled "Possibilities of differentiation in angina pectoris".

It is interesting for three reasons. Firstly, it illustrates the three categories described above and their interrelationships. Secondly, it gives an impression about the quantitative relationship between the three entities.[100] The numbers (expressed in percentages) are based on 400 patients who visited the Department of Internal Medicine of the Zürich' Hospital (Switzerland) and who were diagnosed by Hofmann as suffering from angina pectoris. The sum of the percentages exceeds 100% because in 26% of the cases two or three forms of angina pectoris were encountered in the same patient.[101] The percentages are impressive. On the one hand the categories angina pectoris gravis and particularly status anginosus exceed the numbers encountered in Anglo-Saxon literature, based on a subjective

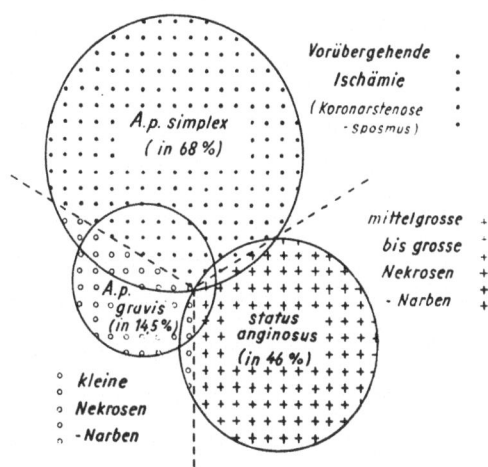

Figure 7.5
Classification of three forms of angina pectoris according to Holzmann: the relationships between the
clinical patterns and the influences on the heart ("kleine Nekrosen-Narben": little necroses-scars;
"Vorübergehende Ischämie (Koronarstenose-Spasmus)": transient ischemia (coronary stenosis-spasm;
"mittelgrosse bis grosse Nekrosen-Narben: moderate to large necroses-scars).
Reproduced with permission from Holzmann (1954).

impression. On the other hand, the simultaneous appearance of several forms of angina
pectoris, in Holzmann's sample in about 26% of the cases, reveals the emphasis on the
multiplicity and a-typicality of angina pectoris in German medicine. As Holzmann wrote:
*"All clinicians experienced in the field of angina pectoris have stressed ever since the multiplicity of
its symptomatology and its course"*. [102]
Thirdly, and most important, the division of three sectors that is depicted simultaneously
with the three forms of angina pectoris in this scheme is quite characteristic. The upper
sector denotes transient ischaemia whereas the left and right sectors below represent small
and severe spots of necrosis and scars respectively. This sectional division refers to the
pathological defect that is present in angina pectoris.
Whereas in Anglo-American medicine coronary insufficiency increasingly denoted a
physiological disturbance, German medicine laid emphasis on pathology. In this respect
angina pectoris was considered as a serious disorder because in the long term the heart would
become repeatedly damaged.[103] Even mild and transient forms of anginal attacks
purportedly evoked little spots of necrosis and structural damage in the heart.[104] This
pathological way of thinking affected anginal treatment as well.[105] Coronary vasodilators
and other therapeutic measures were not merely stopping or preventing anginal attacks, but
also preventing structural damage.[106] Coronary insufficiency was considered as an iterate
process of physiological disturbances associated with an impaired **function** that caused
pathological lesions, i.e. changes of **structure**. This vocabulary of function and structure,
e.g. of "organic" and "functional", inspired German medical perceptions about the role of
organic and functional factors in coronary insufficiency.

7.2.3.3. Organic and functional factors in German clinical taxonomy

When Büchner formulated his concept of coronary insufficiency, he explicitly rejected the theory of coronary spasm. However, this theory never completely disappeared from German medicine, but remained disguised as one of the functional factors in angina pectoris.

German usage of the term functional should be contrasted with Anglo-Saxon terminology. Comparative analysis is complicated by differences in epistemological frameworks in which medical knowledge about disease is organized. The conceptual scheme of etiology, pathogenesis, precipitating, contributory and predisposing causes, prognosis and treatment that pervaded the English speaking medical literature, is not used by German clinicians to the same extent. The comparative analysis of the term functional factors will be confined to etiology, precipitating factors and pathogenesis.

Etiology

Anglo-American medicine increasingly eliminated functional factors from etiology. This is not to deny their significance in heart disease. Functional factors were involved in disease entities such as functional heart disease, cardiac neurosis, nervous heart, soldier's heart and neurocirculatory asthenia. However, these clinical categories were considered as ill-defined syndromes of psychogenic or neurogenic origin and were disregarded as nosologic entities. Functional heart disease confronted the clinician with diagnostic difficulties. Its clinical significance lies in the sphere of differential diagnosis. As Levine stated in case of neurocirculatory asthenia: *"The importance of this condition is that it must be recognized and not confused with organic disease".* [107]

In contrast, German clinical taxonomy included functional factors as etiological causes in angina pectoris. This fitted in with the general attitude of German physicians of stressing the reciprocal relationship between organic and functional. Both were conceived of as two sides of the same process, originating from one or the other and leading from "transitory" to more or less "fixed" states of mal-adaptation. Accordingly, a sharp distinction between functional and organic factors was difficult or impossible. Textbooks continuously refer to clinical conditions in which the response of coronary insufficiency is evoked but apparently without organic lesions. In these conditions functional factors were predominant.[108] This is illustrated even more by clinical and experimental observations that functional factors were able to **cause** organic damage.[109]

Precipitating causes

Functional conditions as emotional states, psychic pain or neurosis, sexual intercourse and excitement were considered by British and American doctors as precipitating causes. Such causes included all clinical conditions which, because of their close and sequential relationship appeared to be concerned with the onset of the symptoms of a disease, in this case angina. These causes were considered typical when they revealed the same pattern as in exercise. The onset of pain is accompanied by the onset of the stimulus. When the latter disappears, pain rapidly vanishes. British and American clinicians considered physical exercise as the most frequent and most significant precipitating cause of angina pectoris[110], and whenever they stress typical angina pectoris, the relationship with physical exertion is described.[111]

In contrast, during this study three variants were found in German medicine. The first comes close to "angina of effort" and is called "angina pectoris ambulatoria". Yet, it formed a minority case in German clinical taxonomy.[112] The second variant treated exercise and all "functional" factors equally in the sense that they precipitate angina pectoris, whether this is typical or atypical. The third variant does the same except that **typical** angina is associated particularly with exertion, whereas other functional factors precipitate **atypical** angina. The latter two variants seem to be more prominent in German medicine.

Thus, Anglo-American usage of functional factors as precipitating causes applies to German medicine too but apparently two differences prevailed. First, German physicians left much more room for emotion, climate, psychic trauma in the complex of precipitating causes of angina pectoris. Second, they stressed the fluid transition between typical and atypical angina.

Pathogenesis

Anglo-American physicians considered the imbalance of supply and demand as the predominant pathogenetic mechanism in angina pectoris. Functional factors such as exercise, emotion, digestion or cold are superimposed on the structural defects of the coronary vessels such that the heart is unable to comply with the demands evoked by these precipitating causes. The anginal attack, therefore, is conceived of as a response by physiological mechanisms of adaptation that are in themselves **normal**. The term that denotes the normal status of these mechanisms is "mediation". The most significant mechanism by far that mediated between the human and its environment, be it internal or external, was considered to be the sympathetic system which formed the transit-house between the human being and his environment.

In German medicine, however, the **pathological** state of the autonomic system itself was very prominent. Amongst a variety of terms like "imbalance", "irritability", "hyperactivity", "hypo-activity", "dysfunction", "sensibility" and "lability", the term "dysregulation" ("Fehlsteuerung") was the most popular term to denote the **pathological** state of the autonomic system, i.e. a failure of adaptation evoked by whatever mechanism which results in an inadequate steering of cardiovascular reflex and control mechanisms.

This concept of dysregulation affected clinical taxonomy of cardiovascular disease in general as well as of coronary insufficiency in particular. In the former case the various cardiovascular circuits, e.g. coronary vessels, bio-electrical system, cardiac musculature and the peripheral vessels, were considered as triggers of dysregulation. Consequently, prototypes of both acute and chronic regulatory disturbances of the cardiovascular system were identified. A quite common classification, for example, was to divide the chronic regulatory disturbances in four major groups:

a. "hypertonic" disturbances of the general cardiovascular system;
b. "hypotonic" disturbances of the general cardiovascular system;
c. "regulatory disturbances of the heart" (dynamics, blood circulation, metabolism, sensibility);
d. "local regulatory disturbances".

Under these headings various clinical patterns were classified. Hypertension, for example fitted the pattern of "hypertonic" disturbances; hypotension that of hypotonic dysregulation while coronary insufficiency was related to regulatory disturbances of the heart. The objective of clinical diagnosis was to disentangle these basic regulatory patterns. The medical doctor was to watch carefully for the symptoms and signs that indicated the regulatory state of the cardiovascular system. Physicians asked for "nervous" symptoms to mark vaso-vegetative lability. They looked for sweaty hands and feet, redness or paleness and irregular breathing. Vasomotor reactions were tested with the patient in different postures: lying, recumbent, sitting and standing while watching various critical parameters. These "vegetative stigmata" marked the basic patterns of vegetative dystonia.

From the therapeutic point of view a variety of measures were available to the physicians to restore this undesirable state. In this sense drugs for lowering or increasing blood pressure were considered not simply as antihypertensive or antihypotensive agents. Drugs like Sympatol and Effortil which are alpha-adrenergic drugs were considered "stabilizers" of the vegetative system as well. The most prominent term that figured in German medical treatment, i.e. "Vegetative Umstimmung" which denotes the "tuning up" of the vegetative system, illustrates the typical German attitude to the vegetative system and its substantial role in cardiovascular disease.

Vegetative dysregulation was also an important component of coronary insufficiency in particular . Firstly, it might affect the coronary circulation. Normally the sufficient circulation of the heart was considered to be guaranteed with healthy coronary vessels and a vegetative regulation in good order. Accordingly, *"the clinical picture of coronary insufficiency can be evoked through a multiple co-operation of functional and organic changes in the coronary vessels"*. [113] Secondly, vegetative dysregulation might affect disturbances in the metabolic and energetic processes in the heart. Thirdly, vegetative dysregulation induced changes in sensibility of pain. In complex ways, therefore, the vegetative system might be involved in the syndrome of coronary insufficiency. This reflected the attention that the vegetative system attracted in German medicine. As we will see this becomes apparent in the multiplicity of forms of angina pectoris. Let us now consider the clinical patterns of angina pectoris in more detail.

The geography of angina pectoris in German medicine

In addition to the clinical patterns described above German physicians distinguished between "Angina Pectoris Vera" and "Pseudostenokardie". The former denoted all clinical patterns that are "true" angina pectoris, the latter those clinical conditions associated with angina-like complaints but without organic lesions. This terminology is confusing. For, "Angina pectoris vera" and "Pseudoangina" are quite opposite terms as are "Stenokardie" and "Pseudostenokardie". The former distinction, i.e. "Angina pectoris vera" and "Pseudoangina", refers to clinical symptomatology, the latter distinction to pathology; literally "Stenokardie" means "stenosis of the heart". In practice, however, these distinctions lost their significance. Hence, "Angina Pectoris Vera" was contrasted with "Pseudostenokardie".

Another clinical syndrome that is distinct from but closely related to "Angina Pectoris Vera" and "Pseudostenokardie" concerns vasomotor angina ("Angina pectoris vasomotorica"). This syndrome appears in patients on the basis of vegetative dystonia. Very often these patients are marked by "vegetative stigmata" and the nature and character of anginal pain is different from "real" angina. The syndrome most commonly affects subjects of thirty or forty years and very often females in critical stages of their lives, i.e. menstruation and menopause, psychic trauma, conflict and anxiety. Considering the type of patients as well as the circumstances related to the appearance of angina pectoris vasomotorica, the syndrome had much in common with "Pseudostenokardie".

On the other hand the anginal attacks could be very much like those of real angina pectoris. Under the surface of this similarity the major difference was that the coronary vessels in angina pectoris vasomotorica were structurally sound. Vegetative disturbances either affected the coronary vessels or changed the sensibility or nervous pathways of anginal pain. It is no wonder that considerable overlapping between angina pectoris vera and vasomotorica existed. The rather fluid boundaries between the syndromes were stressed and mixed forms were acknowledged.[114] Elderly people, for example, were susceptible to vasomotor lability but undoubtedly were beset with structurally defective coronary vessels as well. The idea of vasomotor changes on the basis of vegetative dystonia prominently figured in German medical practice.

Finally, we have one last form of angina pectoris to discuss: "Verkettungsangina". The term "Verkettungsangina" is difficult to translate but it essentially denoted the entanglement of a particular disorder with angina pectoris. This entanglement consisted of two possibilities. The first was that the underlying mechanism of some disorder elicited angina pectoris - with or without organic lesions of the coronary vessels. The second implied that a variety of disorders induced reflex changes in the nervous pathways thus modifying the symptoms and signs of angina pectoris. This concept of entanglement was introduced by the French physicians Froment, Gonin and Bruel who called this syndrome "Angor intrique". (1956, 1952) These authors described patients in which angina pectoris and another clinical disorder coexisted in such a complex way that atypical angina pectoris became manifest. Syndromes like radicular syndrome, peptic gastric or duodenal ulcer, gallbladder disease, diaphragmatic or para-esophageal hernia and vegetative dystonia were capable of transforming typical angina pectoris into atypical forms. So much emphasis was given to atypical angina that Froment formulated the thesis: "Whenever in angina pectoris precipitating factors, time course, radiation or reaction of the pain on administration of nitrites differ from the typical pattern, this is sufficient to search for the modifying factors that originate from simultaneously present disorders".[115] Atypical forms of angina pectoris formed a major concern to the physician.

The concept of "Angor intrique" was picked up readily and rapidly by German clinicians. Mainzer (1958) coined the term "Verkettungsangina"; Delius (1959) the term "implikative Kardialgie". However, German medical literature of the 1950s was already filled with observations that were similar to those of Froment and concerned the overlapping between angina pectoris and other chest pain syndromes.[116] It was particularly the renowned clinician Delius who developed and elaborated the concept of "Angor intrique", and following Froment two major forms were discerned by Keller, a co-worker of Delius (figure 7.6).

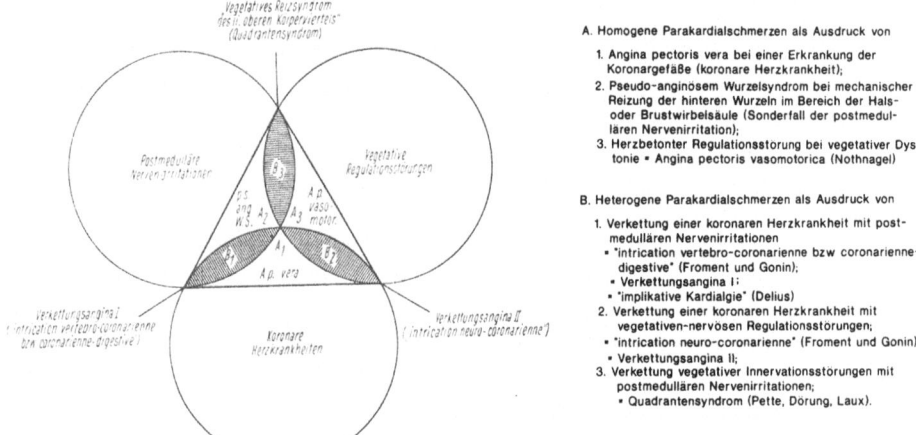

A. Homogene Parakardialschmerzen als Ausdruck von

1. Angina pectoris vera bei einer Erkrankung der Koronargefäße (koronare Herzkrankheit);
2. Pseudo-anginösem Wurzelsyndrom bei mechanischer Reizung der hinteren Wurzeln im Bereich der Hals- oder Brustwirbelsäule (Sonderfall der postmedullären Nervenirritation);
3. Herzbetonter Regulationsstörung bei vegetativer Dystonie • Angina pectoris vasomotorica (Nothnagel)

B. Heterogene Parakardialschmerzen als Ausdruck von

1. Verkettung einer koronaren Herzkrankheit mit postmedullären Nervenirritationen
   • "intrication vertebro-coronarienne bzw coronarienne-digestive" (Froment und Gonin);
   • Verkettungsangina I;
   • "implikative Kardialgie" (Delius)
2. Verkettung einer koronaren Herzkrankheit mit vegetativen-nervösen Regulationsstörungen;
   • "intrication neuro-coronarienne" (Froment und Gonin);
   • Verkettungsangina II;
3. Verkettung vegetativer Innervationsstörungen mit postmedullären Nervenirritationen;
   • Quadrantensyndrom (Pette, Dörung, Laux).

Figure 7.6
Classification of two forms of "Verkettungsangina" in German medicine.
Reproduced with permission from Keller (1960).

The first form concerned the entanglement of angina pectoris with vegetative dystonia ("intrication neuro-coronarienne" (Froment)), the second with vertebral or digestive pain syndromes ("intrication vertebro-coronarienne" or "intrication coronarienne-digestive" (Froment)). The third type of 'entanglement' is not of interest here. Both types of entanglement were conceived of as a type of two-way traffic one syndrome expressing the other that was yet clinically latent. In both cases atypical angina pectoris would arise though especially in the case of vertebral pain syndromes typical angina might appear as well.

The category "Verkettungsangina" did not represent the mere coexistence of two syndromes.

As Delius' colleague Keller wrote: *"If there is, for example, a second disease additional to but independent of a coronary disease, located outside the heart, then, as a rule its occurrence by no means results in mere co-existence. It much sooner leads to highly complicated linkage or entanglement, and new patho-genetic conditions come into existence that typically modify the usual clinical pattern of "stenocardiac" attack. That attacks of angina pectoris can be explained in this light, and that they take*

on a new, yet again typical shape under the influence of linkage, are facts that have not been known to clinical medicine for a long time and could only be proved during the last few years". [117]
This classification of "Verkettungsangina" as a separate category in clinical taxonomy makes the task of differential diagnosis of angina pectoris more difficult. This contrasts with the English speaking medical world. Clinical history, laboratory measurements or other investigations able to substantiate an alternative diagnosis, e.g. radicular syndrome, were sufficient to reject the possibility of angina pectoris. Anglo-Saxon textbooks repeatedly refer to the variety of conditions to which cardiac pain has too often erroneously been attributed.

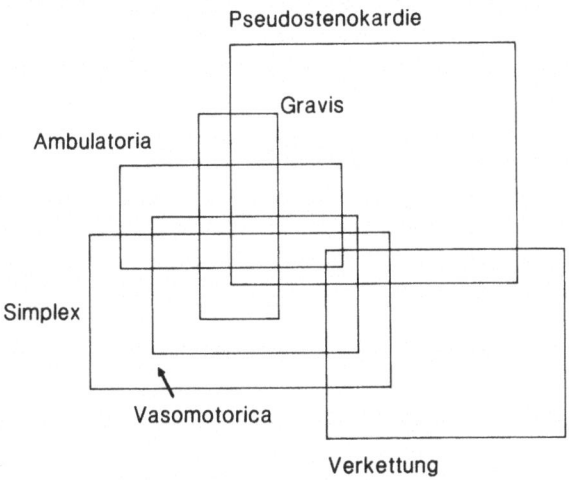

Figure 7.7
Profiles of angina pectoris in German medicine, 1960-1970: the social impact.

In summary figure 7.7 represents German taxonomy of angina pectoris around 1960. All the profiles represented have been explained in the text. It becomes clear that German physicians defined the "angina patient" quite differently to their Anglo-American colleagues.

Part 2. The influence of medical perceptions on targeting in drug research.

7.3. The beta blocker project at Boehringer Ingelheim.

Founded in 1885 by Albert Boehringer in Ingelheim on the Rhine, the chemical factory C.H. Boehringer Sohn has developed into an international pharmaceutical enterprise. The firm operates on a world-wide scale and consists of many companies active not only in pharmaceuticals but also in veterinary medicine, laboratory diagnosis, chemicals, bakery products and plant pesticides. Since the firm's advance into the territory of synthetic drugs in the second decade of this century, heart and lung diseases have been major targets of scientific research.

After some initial successes Sympatol, a preparation to stabilize the circulation, was developed in 1931. With this drug which is still available today, research into sympathomimetic compounds took a fresh start resulting in a variety of drugs. One of the most successful drugs was Aleudrin (isoprenaline), a medicine for the treatment of asthma that was introduced in 1942. Successors to this drug were orciprenaline (Alupent) and fenoterol (Berotec) introduced and developed during the 1960s. Boehringer was also successful in the field of heart medicine. In 1949 Vasculat, a medicine for the treatment of peripheral vascular disorders, and 1955 Effortil, also a preparation to stabilize the circulation, were introduced. Both products became important elements of cardiovascular treatment, particularly in the German speaking countries and are still available.

After the Second World War Boehringer established, in addition to its research department at Ingelheim a second research centre, i.e. the firm of Dr. Karl Thomae GmbH in Biberach, in the South of West-Germany. One of the early and major achievements of this research centre was the development and introduction in 1959 of dipyridamole (Persantin), a coronary vasodilating agent for the treatment of coronary heart disease which is still commercially the leading drug of the company. The research centres together developed more than fifty medicines amongst which are many therapeutically significant drugs.

Research into the sympathomimetic drugs unexpectedly branched into the realm of the beta blockers. Late in the 1950s the Boehringer scientists became aware of the publications about DCI: *"Then, towards the end of the fifties, we heard that a dichlorine derivative of Aludrin had been synthesized at Eli Lilly, one that hadn't been produced here up to then; and that was somewhat like an electric blow: 'Why didn't we make that?' 'Is that so difficult?' And so on. So... and of course with the remarkable feature that this compound also had blocking qualities. So actually it was DCI that put us on this matter, this discovery of DCI".* [118]

DCI and some derivatives of adrenaline and noradrenaline were synthesized. Dr. A. Engelhardt, the pharmacologist who had set up the experimental systems, performed the tests. Simultaneously, chemists at Boehringer expanded into a wide range of sympathomimetic drugs some of which after chlorine substitution were compared with DCI. About 1958 Dr. H.G. Köppe, chemist at Boehringer, was asked to search for new anorectic drugs, devoid of the central nervous side effects of Boehringer's drug, phenmetrazin (Preludrin), that had been on the market since 1950. The objective was to eliminate the unwanted effects while retaining the anorectic activity.[119] Since phenmetrazine can be considered as a cyclized form of phenethanolamine (fig. 7.8), it was decided to look for new variations in this class of compounds which after all had been the subject of extensive research within Boehringer for many years.[120] As a result of this, the class of 1-alkylamino-3-phenoxy-2-propanols unexpectedly yielded highly active and pure beta blocking compounds.

These compounds possessed no central stimulating activity though unfortunately also without anorectic activity. Some compounds were substituted with chlorine as was the case with dichloroisoprenaline.

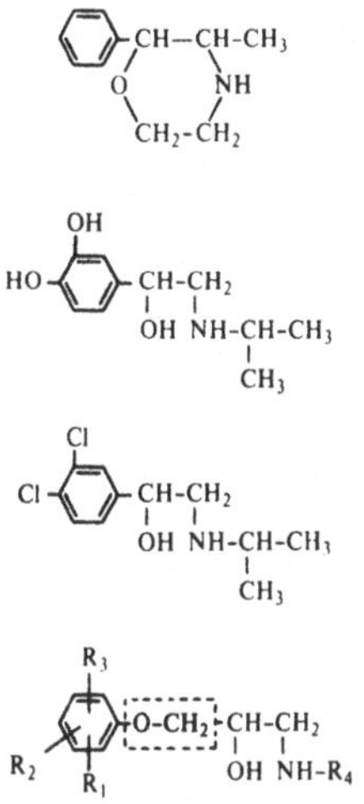

Phenmetrazine
Boehringer Ingelheim (1950)

Isoproterenol
Isoprenaline
Boehringer Ingelheim (1939)

Dichloroisoproterenol
Dichloroisoprenaline
(DCI) Lilly (1958)

1-Alkylamino-3-phenoxy-2-propanols
Kö 446: R_1, R_2, R_3 = 2,4,5-Cl_3;
$R_4 = C_2H_5$
Boehringer Ingelheim (1960)

Figure 7.8
Structural relationships between anorectic, anti-asthmatic and beta adrenoceptor blocking drugs. Reproduced with permission from Köppe (1983).

In May 1961 Engelhardt reported on this first compound, Kö 446 (figure 7.8):

"Kö 446 is a highly active β–adrenolytic. Its efficacy is between that of dichloroisoprenaline and dichloroadrenaline, but it differs from both these substances in that there is no intrinsic sympathomimetic activity. In a therapeutic trial with this substance, it would be possible to block a part of the sympathetic nervous system (the β–adrenoceptors) which it has so far not been possible to influence in terms of inhibition. Thus, further pharmacological investigation and possibly clinical testing appear to be called for". [121]

With Kö 446 the Boehringer scientists possessed a tool that superseded DCI. No clear-cut therapeutic objectives were associated with this novel type of drug: *"That was in itself purely for pharmacological reasons, because it was a new phenomenon that the sympathetic heart muscle could be blocked (...) And then I said to myself (...) that is in the first place a very interesting and new pharmacological finding, but I didn't have a concept yet for, let's say, a therapeutic use, but I just said to myself there should be a therapeutic use for it, in whatever way... theoretical considerations could be made about that. These implied at that time particularly the influence on the frequency of the heart, which has been demonstrated thereafter as the most important principle of the beta blockers. But I had no idea at the time what the implications would be for certain diseases and indications".* [122]
Though the bradycardial effect of Kö 446 was of interest, this was certainly not considered from the viewpoint of diminishing the heart's work; angina pectoris was not then being considered. Initially, the therapeutic considerations originated from the experiences with Aleudrin. This drug was beset with various difficulties amongst which the acceleration of the

heart was a disturbing effect. In this context some theoretical possibilities were discussed. First, one could try to find a compound that would stimulate beta receptors in the lungs, hence dilate the bronchi, yet at the same time with negligible effect on the beta receptors in the heart. This option fitted in with decision making at Boehringer but had already materialized in the compound orciprenaline. Amongst other advantages this drug had presumably fewer cardiovascular side-effects than isoprenaline. Another hypothesis was to find a beta blocking drug that slowed heart pace but had no effect in the lungs. Such a drug could be given to asthma patients in combination with Aleudrin to relieve the cardiovascular side-effects of the latter drug.

Had these hypotheses evoked concrete results, perhaps the development might have taken a different course. As Engelhardt stated: *"Of course. So if we had found something, it would have become a project at once. That's obvious! For such a finding would, of course, have been very similar to Boehringer's whole concept with Aludrin, wouldn't it? At the same time we were about to develop a successor to Aludrin, too. (..) That was orciprenaline, indeed"*. [123]

Yet, the hypotheses were competitive with the orciprenaline project. This drug was the direct result of the first option (and this was better than the second). In fact, right from the beginning there was not much credit for research on beta blocking agents. Graubner, head of the Medical Department - responsible for the therapeutic targeting at Boehringer, and in charge of the physicians at Boehringer and Thomae but also supervising the pharmacologists - requested Engelhardt to refrain from their research into sympatholytic drugs. [124]

However Engelhardt and Köppe continued to work on what might be called their "private project". The private character of their work may be illustrated in another way. Several derivatives were synthesized between June 13 and July 14 (1960); Kö 446 was synthesized July 14th 1960. [125] September 12, 1960 Dr. Köppe asked for pharmacological testing whereas Engelhardt presented the first results on May 19, 1961. Thus, there was a considerable time lag due to the fact that both had to perform experiments with established priority, e.g. the search for anorectic drugs for example. Moreover, the application forms during 1960 - 1961 in which Köppe requested pharmacological testing, were submitted with the heading "to test for anorectic activity". [126] Pharmacological results, however, referred to isoprenaline-antagonism; the form was signed only by Engelhardt, not by Graubner. This procedure was common practice, in later years also, and it enabled Engelhardt and Köppe to continue their research on the side-lines, simultaneously with well established projects at Boehringer. There was considerable freedom for exploring new ideas at the laboratory bench.

The above is not to deny the importance of the hypothetical ideas on asthma therapy within Boehringer. These ideas gave support to Engelhardt and Köppe's private research goals to investigate the beta blocking drugs. When results failed to materialize the legitimate basis for their experiments was unstable. Anti-arrhythmic therapy formed the sole basis of their research but this therapeutic target was of no interest to Boehringer.

Despite these reservations, a firm basis was found for further modification with the compound Kö 446 as the reference compound: "Well, at the beginning we have of course, together with Dr. Köppe, optimised respectively examined the molecules, and that took some time. Now what was decisive for this effect? Was it the chlorine substitution at the ring which we assumed at first? We soon noticed that this wasn't the case. And then we were to find a preparation or a substance that worked in the best possible way and that was only a little toxic".[127]

Further chemical manipulation yielded several compounds. Amongst the chlorine substituted derivatives, Kö 581 raised much interest as did the otherwise modified compounds, Kö 592 and Lg 32 (figure 7.9).

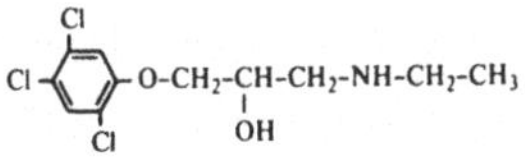

Kö 446

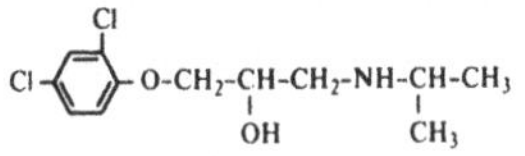

Kö 581

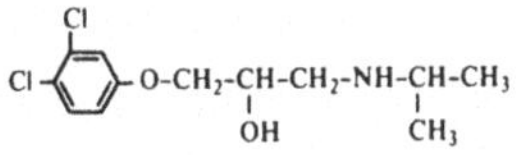

Kö 673

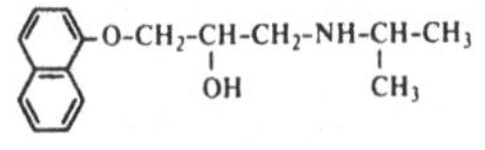

Lg 32

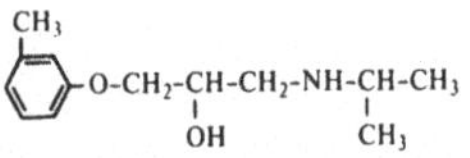

Kö 592

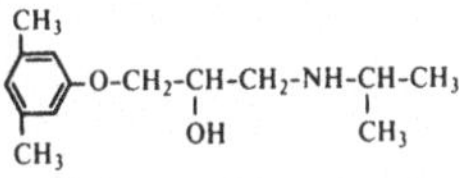

Kö 707

Figure 7.9
Synthesis and detection of beta adrenolytic effective 1-alkylamino-3-phenoxy-2-propanols (1960-1962, Boehringer Ingelheim).
Reproduced with permission from Köppe (1983).

The compounds referred to as Kö were both synthesized in the period from July to September 1961 and underwent pharmacological screening from September 1961 till the middle of 1962.[128] Lg 32, which became later known as propranolol,was descended from a series of compounds synthesized by Ludwig, a young chemist, who was appointed in the middle of 1960 to assist Dr. Köppe; hence, the abbreviation "Lg". The compound was purposefully synthesized on the basis of chemical precursors designed by Köppe - limited capacity delayed further development - and in 1961 this compound entered pharmacological screening for anorectic activity and was tested for beta blocking activity late in 1962.[129]

Pharmacological testing focussed on three actions: bradycardia, negative inotropic activity and isoprenaline antagonism.[130] Furthermore, acute toxicity tests were performed.[131] The first action was important for assessing the anti-arrhythmic potential. Negative inotropic activity was considered an unwanted property, in danger of producing cardio-depression. Isoprenaline antagonism was the reference for determining beta blockade.

Kö 592 exhibited a most interesting bradycardial action. June 1962, Engelhardt reported: *"Kö 592 is as yet the strongest bradycardiac substance among the related compounds, which may possibly indicate its applicability as an anti-arrhythmic medicine, but that must of course be tested emphatically"*. [132] This therapeutic target set the stage for further research and the reference drugs were DCI and quinidine. An optimal anti-arrhythmic action had to be found. Several critical parameters with respect to the electrical function of the heart were assessed - e.g. the effects on spontaneous beating, threshold and refractory period. In the early phase these "toxic" effects on rhythmic function were screened for with the help of the LD_{50} toxicity test.[133]

The negative action on heart muscle contraction was assessed by the effects on the amplitude of the force of contraction of the heart taking the cardio-depressive action of quinidine as the reference. From the very outset cardio-depression was part of the Boehringer project. However, we need to separate the meaning of the term "cardio-depression" from the specific meaning it received during the controversy about propranolol some years later. It was a general, yet strict parameter for any cardiovascular drug to be developed. In this sense, the research department had adapted this parameter as the norm for screening and further exploration. Dr. Lichterfeld, working at the Medical Department from 1962 onwards, stated that cardio-depression was spelled out at a very early stage and that it governed the discussions about the pros and cons of the various compounds.[134]

A new phase started when ICI revealed pronethalol in August 1962. Now the therapeutic domain was extended to the realm of anti-anginal treatment. Engelhardt commented on this apparently surprising event:

"No. It wasn't a surprise in itself. It was just that they had taken their thought a little further than we had ourselves, that is to say, aiming at a special disease. So, at angina pectoris, at the coronary disease and that seemed almost a paradox at that time, since the coronary therapeutic agents were based on coronary dilation. And now with these beta blockers that wasn't the case at all. They didn't have a coronary dilator effect, under certain conditions they even had the opposite effect. And nevertheless, they were applicable for a coronary disease. That was amazing". [135]

The ambiguity in this quotation is quite clear. It was no surprise when considering beta blockade in the light of its potential of sparing the heart or as the Germans say "Schonung des Herzens". But it was surprising from the viewpoint of the coronary vasodilator concept. Many questions had to be answered as Köppe stated: *"At the time (1961/1962) we did not know at all what considerations one could have about its applications, simply therapeutically. If one keeps the heart steady, what happens? Is that favorable? Is it possible to let the heart beat more economically? Does it help? Today it is easy to say, it helps an angina pectoris patient, isn`t it?"*. [136] These questions introduced conflict to the coronary vasodilator concept.

Still, ICI's entrance on the market and the novel therapeutic target provided new arguments in decision making within Boehringer. Attempts were made to bring beta blocker research into a further stage of development. In a letter, dated October 31, 1962 and directed to Dr. Graubner, Prof. K. Zeile, research director, Dr. Thomae, chemist at Boehringer working on anti-asthmatic drugs, and Dr. Köppe, Engelhardt reported the results of four compounds as summarized in table 7.4.

Table 7.4
Profiles of beta blocking agents at Boehringer.

	In vivo (guinea pig) bradycardial activity	Isoprenaline antagonism	Toxicity mice, LD 50 mg/kg s.c.
DCI	1	1	235
Kö 592	23	5	630
Kö 581	12	11	500
Th 293	-	5	860

Th 293 refers to a compound synthesized by
Dr. Thomae at Boehringer; reproduced with
permission from Engelhardt, Letter October 31, 1962.

The letter continues as follows: *"In the table the most important features of these compounds and the reference substance DCI are set against each other. All substances are considerably less toxic than DCI and they check the effect on the heart of Aludrin in a way which is 5-11 times stronger. They vary with respect to their own bradycardiac effect, which is absent in Th 293, but which in contrast, exceeds the effectiveness of DCI in Kö 592 and 582 by 12 and 23 times respectively. Their own bradycardiac effect might indicate an additional anti-arrhythmic effect on the heart".* [137]
This quotation is interesting for several reasons. Firstly, it signifies the process of profiling drugs at a very early stage in the discovery process. Secondly, it shows that selection of candidate compounds is influenced by the therapeutic target. The distinction between "own bradycardiac effect" ("bradykardische Eigenwirkung") and "isoprenaline antagonism" ("Aludringantagonismus") suggests that the bradycardial action overruled the beta blocking effect **per se**. [138] In any case, the potent bradycardial activity of Kö 592 was positively valued and Engelhardt added that, since the compound exhibited a somewhat better toxicity profile (LD_{50} test), this favoured Kö 592. [139]
Thirdly, the reference compound was DCI, since the comparative analysis with pronethalol was yet to be performed.

Larger amounts of the compounds were requested in order to perform more extensive pharmacological research. Engelhardt carefully described these investigations as serving the objective of elaborating and developing new methods and of comparing the compounds. Explicitly it was noticed that the investigations should not be labeled as "profound pharmocological testing" which within Boehringer denoted a pharmaceutical project in itself. In this respect, the therapeutic target had to be approved by the Medical Department and that would have rejected such a proposal.[140] Though the request was backed up by Prof. Zeile, Graubner's permission was decisive in moving from the research department into further stages of development.

Scepticism about this new direction in anti-anginal treatment prevailed due to prominence of the concept of coronary vasodilation: *"So surely the concept of coronary dilation in practical medicine had become very firmly established here, hadn't it. (...) And now there were these beta blockers, coronary therapeutic agents without a coronary dilator effect and that was difficult to understand"*. [141] Lichterfeld pointed into the same direction: *"Also at Boehringer thinking towards the therapeutic principle of coronary dilation had been influenced by Persantin. There was only a slow reorientation, which was instigated by the lack of clinical success of pure coronary dilation"*. [142] In fact, there was speculation within Boehringer to develop beta-stimulating drugs to support "coronary training" therapy.[143] This speculation is evidence of the strong research tradition on sympathomimetic drugs as well: *"The research of the company was up to then directed at the agonists of the adrenergic alpha and beta receptors. New and a turn of 180 degrees was the development of inhibitors of the sympathetic innervation and the way of thinking that was related to it"*. [144]

By that time, dipyridamole (Persantin) was introduced to the market and the compound attracted much clinical interest, particularly in the German medical world. Numerous clinical articles, many of them presenting positive results in anti-anginal treatment, were published in German medical journals.[145] For example, more than 30 clinical articles about dipyridamole appeared during 1959 till 1961.[146] However, the initiative was lacking as commented by Engelhardt: *"Here at Boehringer we actually lacked the impetus or the consensus to lead the way with the substances"*. [147] The project remained an affair for the Research Department as Köppe stated resignedly: *"Even from the beginning people were cautious when they saw this new therapeutic potential, it was purely a matter for research. We continued with it but there was no follow-up in subsequent departments"*. [148] According to Lichterfeld it was decided in 1964, on the basis of the necessary pre-clinical studies, to test Kö 592 clinically. Thereafter, the development of the drug, in fact of any drug at this stage, was the full responsibility of the Medical Department.[149] The possibility that management preferred to stimulate dipyridamole at the cost of the beta blocker project seems to be unlikely. According to Lichterfeld projects at Boehringer Ingelheim and Dr. Karl Thomae were considered to be competitive; they were not managed jointly.

So, for some time research on beta blocking agents was carried out in a reserved atmosphere. In the context of this waiting game further chemical modification and pharmacological screening went on. In a narrowed-down selection the compound Kö 592 was favored.[150] It showed potent negative chronotropic activity while having the least cardio-depressive action and the most advantageous toxicity profile. Lg 32 was not regarded as optimal because of its strong cardio-depressive activity.[151] The compound remained a reference compound to mark the properties of Kö 592: *"Lg 32 is half to twice as effective as quinidine and consequently has a stronger cardio-depressive effect on the isolated atrium than Kö 592"*. [152] April 1963 Engelhardt reported: *"Combined the tests have shown so far that Kö 592 is a specific beta-adrenolytic agent and offers these kind of advantages, as opposed to the substances that we have hitherto known. We recommend extensive pharmacological testing and we suggest that a patent application be made and that the separation of isomers is started"*. [153]

Subsequently, the compound was profiled with respect to pronethalol. Kö 592 was considered more potent than pronethalol while having no intrinsic activity.[154] Yet, there were some problems too. The activity after oral administration was limited due to rapid metabolism in the liver. Furthermore, the compound did cause disturbing skin reactions at the place of injection in animals.

"The concept of early clinical testing of Kö 592", as Lichterfeld commented, *"was determined through clinical-pharmacological questions in the research in healthy volunteers, such as establishing dose-response and time-response for the isoprenaline-antagonistic effect and its intrinsic effects, i.e. the effects per se. The parameters hinted at adrenergically induced functions of the heart and the circulation, bronchi and metabolism, in order to get some clues about potential indications and contra-indications"*. [155]

The major problem, however, remained the cardio-depressive activity which was studied by several academic and clinical centres.[156] The critical action was the effect of Kö 592 on the period of isometric contraction of the heart ("Anspannungszeit"). The normal range was supposed to be between 0.07 - 0.09 second; in the case of Kö 592 the duration of this period came close to the values measured in athletes (0.15 sec.). The standard values of this period, determined under a variety of conditions, had originated from the studies of Reindell and his group during the 1950s. The prolongation of the period of isometric contraction indicated the transition of the normal cardiovascular function to the pathological state of heart failure. Thus, this parameter defined the boundaries of cardio-depression. The Reindell school considerably influenced medical opinion at Boehringer.[157] Several studies with Kö 592 were performed, directly[158] or indirectly[159], by Reindell and colleagues and other investigators also used the concepts developed by Reindell.[160] Similarly these different groups studied propranolol and other beta blocking compounds.[161]

Another important feature of these studies is the primary interest in functional hypersympathicotonic heart disorders. On the basis of functional-ergometric studies scientists drew upon the similarity between the state of the heart during physical therapy, i.e. training, and beta blockade. The similarity of action was attributed to an altered state of the sympathetic nervous system, an desirable effect in case of vegetative disorders; and in fact, physical exercise was an important therapy in this area. Accordingly patients with vasoregulatory asthenia, "vegetative Dystonie" and hyperkinetic heart syndrome, effort syndrome and soldier's heart became the first group of patients in clinical trials. This decision was based on the unlikelihood of heart failure in these patients and the above-mentioned disorders became the target of beta blocker research in German speaking countries. As early as in 1964, as Lichterfeld commented, these mostly hypersympathicotonic disorders were also chosen as a logical approach for a substance inhibiting sympathetic tone by blocking beta-receptors.[162] Lichterfeld added, German disease classifications markedly differed in comparison with those in Anglo-American medicine; one major difference being the dominance of vegetative disorders in German medicine.[163]

This is not to say that at that time angina pectoris was no longer in the picture. Indeed it was and labeling the new target as an expansion of the area of application would be a better way of expressing the developments. However, underneath this wave of expansion a fundamental change of course was occurring. The reason for the medical department to change its tack was the concern about the dramatic experiences with propranolol. The risk of cardiac insufficiency was spelled out in the German medical world, particularly during pharmacological and medical meetings.[164] The risk of heart failure was taken so seriously by the Boehringer physicians that it was decided to shift emphasis from cardiac diseases to functional heart disorders. In the former case the pathological state of the heart might be susceptible to failure, in the latter the normal heart was able to compensate the negative effects. The **normal** not the **pathological** heart would mark the steady course of the further development of Kö 592.

In the mean time, however, the further development of Kö 592 was affected by a dramatic event. In April 1963 a patent application for the class of 1-Aryloxy-2-hydroxy-3-isopropylamino-propane was asked for by Köppe.[165] A procedure that usually took no more that one or two weeks now lasted several months and the patent was applied for August 26, 1963.[166] The reasons for this delay are not very clear but obviously the lack of high priority of the project may have been important.[167] But the delay turned out to be disastrous for the project.

The publication of propranolol in May 1964 came as an unpleasant surprise, but there was still a feeling of confidence in having a competitive compound. However, this feeling of confidence was shattered, when in March 1965 Boehringer received a letter from ICI claiming the patent rights of Kö 592 and related compounds. The Patent Department of Boehringer concluded that without permission of ICI continuing research was difficult. Several proposals were made to come to an agreement but were repeatedly rejected by ICI.[168]

The critical decision whether to stop or to continue had to be taken. In the course of 1964 in depth pharmacology of Kö 592 had been performed as well as studies in human volunteers; and early in 1965 clinical studies had started. The Patent Department suggested that clinical testing be continued despite the seemingly hopelessness of Boehringer's position. This was supported by the fact that the chemists had their own method of chemical synthesis of Kö 592 which was not included in the ICI patent.[169] In the prevailing patent law of various countries this was sufficient to market the drug.

Yet, who took the decision and for what reasons is not clear but it was decided to stop the project. It has been suggested that the discussion about heart failure formed an important drawback to reaching a positive decision.[170] Contributing to this may have been the fact that German medical views were easily spelled out in managerial decision taking because several physicians filled important managerial functions.[171]

Obviously, the decision in itself must be considered in the context of ethical, legal, commercial and managerial considerations. There were other interesting projects going on with apparently more chance of success such as the fenoterol and the catapresan project. In any case, it was decided to stop clinical investigations and for some time Kö 592 would be used as a scientific tool in animal and human pharmacology.[172]

In 1967 the deadlock in which beta blocker research found itself, resolved. ICI changed its mind and allowed Boehringer to continue with Kö 592, though the market potential of this drug was severely restricted. Boehringer had permission to market in Mid- and East European countries, for example, but not in Anglo-Saxon and Scandinavian countries. Still, although Kö 592 could be developed after all, prospects remained gloomy. It was acknowledged that the differences between alprenolol and propranolol were probably greater than those between propranolol and Kö 592. Clinically higher doses of Kö 592 were needed in comparison with propranolol due to troublesome resorption. But since propranolol had become the reference drug there were still some possibilities, particularly with respect to the cardio-depressive action of propranolol. March 8th, 1967, Engelhardt noted for propranolol: *"Every measured parameter showed a dose dependent change towards a cardiac depression. The heart rate and the force of contraction of the right ventricle were affected in particular and more strongly so than after Kö 592"*: [173] And some weeks later: *"Compared to quinidinesulphate, propranolol was, with regard to the negative inotropic effect 5.9 (3.1 - 9.3) times stronger, with regard to the negative chronotropic effect 1.3 (0.9 - 1.5) times stronger, with regard to the negative bathmotropic effect 2.6 (1.8 - 3.7) times stronger, with regard to extension of the refractory period 2.1 (1.5 - 2.4) times stronger. Among the tested beta-adrenolytic agents propranolol showed the strongest cardio-depressive effect on the atria of isolated guinea pigs"*. [174] This shows that cardio-depression as induced by quinidine was taken as the reference point for determining the clinical risk of heart failure. However, from the clinical point of view this apparent advantage of a small cardio-depressive activity of Kö 592 was considered uncertain, particularly because the compound had caused fatal events in the clinic as well.

The profile of Kö 592 described above was made up during a meeting initiated by the Medical Department to prepare the introduction of the compound. It was concluded: *"It looks as if the warning of the German clinicians against the release of beta receptor blockers for outpatients is also justified in the case of Kö 592 and it also looks as if Kö 592 cannot be a preparation for general practice"*. [175] Moreover, it was concluded: *"Owing to the present level of knowledge it is not likely that beta receptor blockers will be found that can become therapeutic agents for extensive application in general practice"*. [176]

In the German medical context the term 'practice' had a particular meaning. For it denoted not only the general practitioner but also the clinician in private practice. The proportion of clinicians working in private practice - and not in a hospital - was apparently much larger in Germany than for example the United Kingdom or the United States of America.[177] Since German medical experts had advised using beta blockers only where reanimation facilities were available - and where careful pre- or co-medication with digitalis could be tried - the majority of physicians treating angina pectoris were not in the position to use beta blockers. The considerations quoted above illustrate that the risk of cardiac insufficiency played a prominent role in Boehringer's decision taking.[178] Lichterfeld commented that it was very difficult to persuade German physicians that the risk of beta blockade was only relative. It was the negative attitude of the German physician in general that was the stumbling block to therapeutic decision making at the Department. The therapeutic concepts were there but the readiness of the German physician was lacking, and hence brought about a feeling of resignation within the firm some time after introduction to the market: *"But I don't think the reason was that we had the wrong concepts. We had the concepts that were in the air, including angina pectoris and labile hypertension. But there was of course a restraining effect, since every representative knew 'somehow or other there is some danger in this stuff'. And then there wasn't an actual breakthrough and people became disheartened so that they didn't see the business through to the end but continued with their usual activities".* [179] Moreover, it was difficult to find opinion leaders in German cardiology who were prepared to throw their full weight into beta blockade.

There were, however, other reasons why it was hard to continue research. In contrast with other countries, clinical pharmacology developed slowly in German medicine. Both to the general public and the medical profession clinical experiments with patients were out of favour since the War. This negative attitude affected the development of clinical research, clinical trial methodology and therapeutic experiments in many ways: side-effects of new drugs were regarded suspiciously; general practitioners were reluctant to enroll patients into trials; and the practice of starting at low doses and carefully increasing the dose was not easily accepted whereas in other, notably Anglo-American countries high(er) doses were used from the outset. With respect to beta blockers in particular this was reflected in the practice of using digitalis as a pre- or co-medication with beta blockers. Proposals such as that of Prichard to go up to very high doses until a satisfactory effect was achieved was inconceivable in German practice. These particular aspects of common medical practice and the social structure of German medicine were suggested many times in the course of this study by various industrial and clinical scientists. [180]

When considering the Boehringer project in itself, the delay due to the suspension of clinical research for two years formed a major setback to the further development of Kö 592 because other firms had contacted the major clinical research centres in West-Germany. It took another three years before Kö 592 was introduced as Doberol.

It is interesting to see how the Medical Department of Boehringer envisaged the drug at the time of introduction. The major differences between Doberol and propranolol were summarized as follows:

"In a pharmacological and toxical way, Kö 592 has more therapeutic width. Beta-adrenolytic doses and negative inotropic doses have been moved further apart than in the case of propranolol.

Direct and indirect indications seem to hint at smaller cardio-depressive effects of Kö 592 in pharmacological experiments and in preliminary clinical findings". [181]

These conclusions were largely in accordance with those drawn around 1967. Yet, cardio-depression, negative inotropic action and heart failure were not synonymous terms anymore.

Therapeutically the major problem was the deleterious effect of the desired result, i.e. beta blockade. The physicians at Boehringer were so impressed by the dramatic responses of beta blockers in heart failure that any attempt to separate beta blocking and cardio-depressive action was considered of scientific not of therapeutic value.

Evidence of this is the comment of the Medical Department: *"These results may not lead to the faulty conclusion that Kö 592 can be used in the case of heart failure with less care than propranolol. The beta-adrenolytic action itself, i.e. the immanent main action, can lead to a worsening of the clinical picture in the case of heart failure, as a result of inhibition of the compensatory reinforced sympathetic drive. It follows that this "side-effect" is the therapeutic principle itself; in clinical-therapeutical dosage this cannot be ascribed to its cardio-depressive properties"*. [182] Less cardio-depression was no longer a feature that could be turned to advantage in the market. Despite its distinct experimental profile Kö 592 was just another beta blocker.

In 1970 Kö 592 was introduced as Doberol on the market with a broad scope of indications: functional heart disorders (palpitations, accelerated pulse, pseudo-anginal complaints), labile juvenile hypertension which was considered as a hypertonic regulatory disturbance, angina pectoris (prophylactic and intermittent treatment) and furthermore cardiovascular symptoms associated with hyperthyroidism and (post)menopausal syndrome, hyperkinetic heart syndrome and tachycardia. Specific instructions ("Besondere Hinweise") included pre-digitalization of patients with (latent forms of) cardiac insufficiency.

About the same time Boehringer introduced a combination preparation of Kö 592 and dipyridamole, e.g. Beta-Persantin. This combination preparation was claimed to be advantageous because the reduction of the coronary circulation due to beta blockade was nullified by Persantin dilating the coronary vessels. In the German context this argument still had impact. In this way the company attempted to merge the old and new therapeutic principle in the treatment of angina pectoris.

Part 3. Application of the theory of drug and disease profile

7.4 Theoretical analysis of the Boehringer project against the background of medical views about angina pectoris and heart failure

Introduction

In this section the theory of (drug and disease) profile will be applied to highlight three critical stages of the Boehringer project:
1. The period 1959 - 1961: the discovery of DCI and Kö 446;
2. The period 1962 - 1964: angina pectoris as a new therapeutic target;
3. The period 1961 - 1970: the problem of cardio-depression.

In general the epistemological language of drug and disease profiles will be used but at specific places the set-theoretical model will be applied. In either case disease profiles and functional - not structural - drug profiles are the subject of analysis.

In speaking about critical stages the same procedure as used in chapter 5 and 6 will be followed in that attention will be focussed only on snapshots of a dynamic process. The analogy to a film is appropriate since the shots represent stationary scenes of what should be in motion. Complexities and specifications of the scenery are neglected in order to let the leading figures be seen in their true colours.

1. The period 1959 - 1961: the discovery of DCI and Kö 446.

The first critical stage was marked by the discovery of DCI and Kö 446. Two wished for functional profiles were discussed with respect to Kö 446: a selective bronchodilator (wf_1) and an anti-arrhythmic drug (wf_2). These profiles were considered as perfect treatments of asthma (P_1) and (particular forms of) cardiac arrhythmia (P_2).

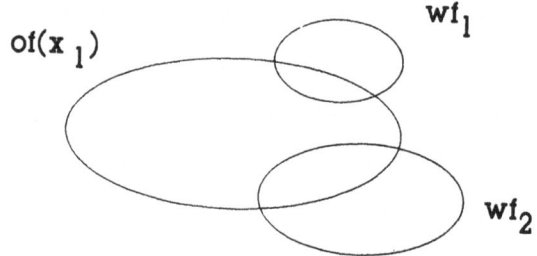

Figure 7.10
The representation of the functional profiles relating to the discovery of Kö 592.

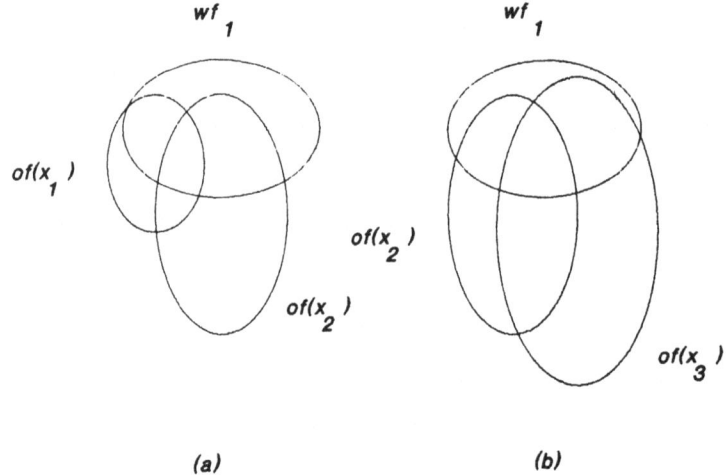

(a)   (b)

Figure 7.11
The compound Kö 446 in the context of bronchodilator research: Kö 446 (x_1); isoprenaline (x_2); and an improved candidate compound (x_3) which is either a new compound with "orciprenaline"-like activity or a combination preparation of isoprenaline and some other compound annulling the side-effects of the former component.

The intersection of $of(x_1)$ (= Kö 446) with both wf_1 and wf_2 was not empty, though it was evaluated differently (figure 7.10). To clarify this it is convenient to consider these cases separately.

Kö 446 (of(x_1) was unsuccessful in comparison with isoprenaline (of(x_2)) (figure 7.11(a)). One option was to transform Kö 446 in order to achieve a drug (of(x_3)) that would be better than isoprenaline: | of(x_3) Δ wf$_1$ | < | of(x_2) Δ wf$_1$ | (see figure 7.11(b)). This option conflicted with the state of affairs at Boehringer at the time. Orciprenaline-like compounds had been produced and superseded isoprenaline with respect to duration of action, route of administration and side-effects amongst which cardiac arrhythmias. Even if a compound x_3 had been found, it would have been estimated insufficient in comparison with orciprenaline, the latter having passed some critical toxicological and pharmacological tests.

The other option was to find a compound with anti-arrhythmic activity which did not block the beneficial effects of isoprenaline (Aleudrin).[183] This means an attempt to find a combination preparation that would fit wf$_1$.[184] Both options remained hypothetical but also unacceptable in the sense that orciprenaline made a better case than any foreseeable compound implicated by the options.

As a result the Boehringer scientists were urged to discuss Kö 446 with respect to anti-arrhythmic activity per se (wf$_2$) (figure 7.12(a)).

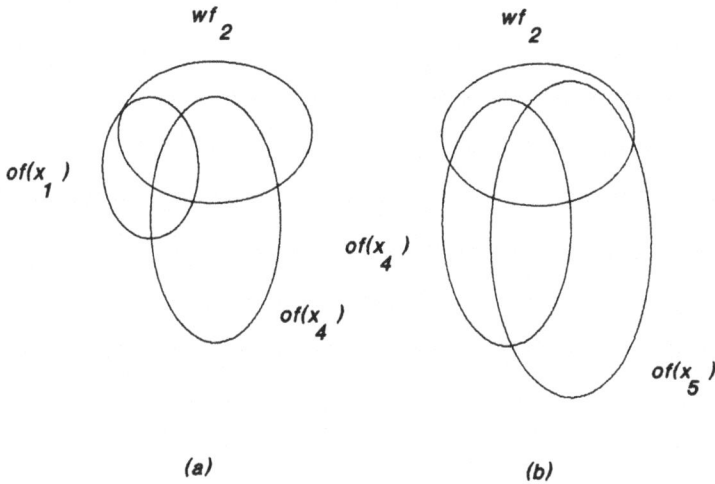

(a)   **(b)**

Figure 7.12
The compound Kö 446 in the context of anti-arrhythmic research.
Kö 446 = x_1; quinidine = x_4; and the compound searched for = x_5.

However, Kö 446 was not good enough for two reasons. First, cardiac arrhythmia was not accepted as a therapeutic target in itself. Second, even if this target had been accepted, Kö 446 would not have been good enough either. For, quinidine (of(x_4)) as the reference compound clearly superseded Kö 446: $|\text{of}(x_4) \vartriangle wf_2| < |\text{of}(x_1) \vartriangle wf_2|$ (fig. 7.12(a)). The objective was to find a compound x_5 such that in any case: $|\text{of}(x_5) \vartriangle wf_2| < |\text{of}(x_4) \vartriangle wf_2|$ (fig. 7.12(b)). Kö 592, another trial, came close to the desired compound but some uncertainties remained.

Up to now the (operational and wished for) functional drug profiles have been discussed in an unspecified manner. However, as described, in this early stage of the project three parameters were at stake, i.e. anti-arrhythmic action, beta blocking activity and toxicity (LD_{50} test). The Boehringer scientists operated with **"restricted"** profiles, that is, they selected certain elements as the targets for profiling their drugs. These restricted profiles also played a substantial role in the synthesis of a series of compound (Kö- and Lg-series) in order to find suitable compounds for further pharmacological research.

A pragmatic attitude regarding the wished for profile dominated. By using reference compounds that represented the therapeutically desired effects, notably quinidine and dichloroisoprenaline, patterns of biological action were dissected and evaluated. With respect to the selection of Kö 592 at the time it is sufficient to state that the criteria to "coarsen" value-ranges in order to differentiate between significant patterns of biological activity were developing in the course of the project.

2. The period 1962 - 1964: angina pectoris as a new therapeutic target.

The second stage started when pronethalol was launched by ICI. Angina pectoris (P_3) entered as a new disease target in the Boehringer project. Hence another wished for (functional) drug profile (wf_3) came to the fore, an event which is likely to occur in the course of any industrial project.

The (spectrum of) disease profiles of angina pectoris differed between the Anglo-American and German medical settings. Let P_a denote the profile of angina pectoris in the Anglo-American medical context; and P_g in the German (table 7.5).

Table 7.5
Disease profiles of angina pectoris in Anglo-American
and German medical context, 1960-1970.

Anglo-American	German
P_{a1} • Angina of effort	P_{g1} • Angina ambulatoria
P_{a2} • Angina of emotion	P_{g2} • Angina simplex
P_{a3} • Coronary insufficiency	P_{g3} • Angina gravis
P_{a4} • Intermediate syndrome	P_{g4} • Pseudostenokardie
P_{a5} • Pre-infarction syndrome	P_{g5} • Angina vasomotorica
P_{a6} • Variant angina	P_{g6} • Verkettungsangina

Semantic differences between the disease profiles in both contexts were important. Despite the similarities - for example, between P_{a1} and P_{g1} - the differences were significant. To some extent this was due to the nature of the parameters included in the profiles, and also to the values and priorities of these elements. Recall, for example, the discussion of the three variants of angina of effort in the German context, and the different values of criteria to classify angina of effort (P_{a1}) and angina simplex (P_{g2}) respectively. The major difference, however, consisted in the dominance of angina of effort in the one context, and the varying range of profiles in the other.

Similarly, therapeutic practices in Anglo-American and German medicine were remarkably distinct. In contrast to the unconditional rejection by Anglo-American physicians that the coronary vasodilators met with, it enjoyed enormous popularity in German medicine. In other words, the wished for drug profile of "coronary vasodilation" was a legitimate objective to strive for in one setting, and ignored in the other. However, reducing the coronary vasodilator concept to opposing attitudes fails to explain the situation fully. Firstly, a broader set of therapies with the objective of improving coronary blood flow existed in German medicine ranging from pharmaceutical compounds to alternative types of treatment, e.g. exercise therapy. To dismiss the coronary vasodilator concept in Germany was to eliminate a whole practice: $of(x) \cap wf(P_g) \neq \emptyset; x = x_1, ..., x_n (n \neq \infty)$. Secondly, this concept was embedded in a much broader view to improve blood flow in tissues poorly perfused by pathological blood vessels. Hence, there were cerebral, coronary, and peripheral vasodilators in German medical practice: $wf(ap) \subseteq wf(id)$, where ap denotes "angina pectoris" and id "ischemic disorders". Thirdly, the theory of coronary spasm was still present, and supported the objective of dilating coronary vessels. When s denotes "coronary spasm" and s' "antispasmodic action", then: $s \in P_g; s \notin P_a; s' \in wf(P_g)$; and $s' \notin wf(P_a)$.

These contextual differences with respect to disease and wished for functional drug profiles are complex and go beyond the power of the representation of Venn-diagrams. Yet, this is a graphical, not a principal problem. Basically, these differences mean that the target "angina of effort" and the strategy to hit the target therapeutically, i.e. the wished for functional drug profile, as set forth by the ICI team did not fit the intellectual climate of the Boehringer project.

The analogy of the heat-guided missile might help to clarify this point. Such a missile speeds through a universe in which many objects glide with varying "profiles of heat". This projectile finds and hits its target due to its capacity to differentiate between the heat of the target in contrast with other objects that may radiate heat as well. When searching for its target, it meets numerous objects hereby continuously matching the registered "profiles of heat" with its computer stored profiles until the perfect match is made. Accordingly, the maps of disease profiles in both medical settings may be transformed into maps with varying contrasts between white and black representing the spectrum between "hot" and "cold" spots comparable to our universe of heat.

If the drug to be developed is the missile, then it is clear that the target for the beta blockers, i.e. angina of effort, as defined within the Anglo-American context, had a different "heat profile" in the German universe. Consequently, the "profiles of heat" sorted out by Anglo-American scientists and clinicians in order to lead the drug to its target were not adequate for the German universe. The same applies to the wished for functional drug profiles. In terms of the analogy of the missile, the conceptions of how to hit the target - the angle for hitting, target point, hitting power, etc. - markedly differed. This implied a different conceptualization of the wished for profile.

Obviously we may elaborate on this analogy with decisions about the type of objects to hit, and the purpose of the hit. In military terms total destruction is the final goal, but in medicine the objectives are multiple - the acceptability of loss of life and the way to reach the target may affect the types of missiles to be developed.

When reducing the complexities of the situation, the following important point may be represented with the help of simple Venn-diagrams.

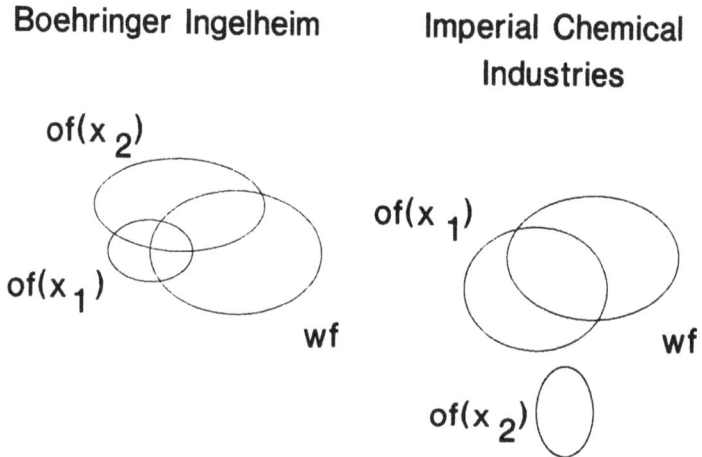

Figure 7.13
The different situation at Boehringer and ICI in the search for new anti-anginal drugs: beta blockers (x_1); coronary vasodilator (x_2); and wf = wished for functional drug profile with respect to angina pectoris.

Boehringer project:
$of(x_2) \cap wf \neq \emptyset$; $|of(x_2) \vartriangle wf| < |of(x_1) \vartriangle wf|$.
ICI project:
$of(x_1) \cap wf \neq \emptyset$; $of(x_2) \cap wf = \emptyset$.

While the ICI team operated in a therapeutic vacuum - no prophylactic therapy for angina pectoris existed - the area in which the Boehringer team operated was filled with a broad set of coronary vasodilating agents. Most prominent of all was Boehringer's own dipyridamole. Further, the coronary vasodilator concept had been interpreted in terms of the sympathetic nervous system. Thus, sympathomimetic drugs were considered as a therapeutic approach - oxyfedrine embodied this way of thinking. This immediately collided with the aim of developing sympatholytic drugs for the treatment of angina pectoris.

When 'm' denotes sympathomimetic action and 'l' "sympatholytic action, then: $m \in wf(P_g)$; and $l \in wf(P_g)$. This leads to a contradiction because $l = \neg m$.

3. The period 1962 - 1970: the problem of cardio-depression

The third stage revolves around the problem of cardio-depression. When feeling started to run high about heart failure precipitated or aggravated by propranolol, the discussion evolved around the question whether the technology, i.e. beta blockers, or the clinician was to blame for the problem. This question was approached in two ways. One was the attempt to develop a compound not as dangerous as propranolol; the other the attempt to assess the patients most at risk. In both respects the prevailing German medical views guided the Boehringer project. Just as with angina pectoris this influenced the development of Kö 592. Both lines of investigation repeatedly intersected, but the sequence of events will be described in a chronological order.

In the early phase of the Boehringer project cardio-depression was just an unwanted effect. Standard procedures, including comparison with quinidine, were used to assess this aspect of cardiovascular drugs. Cardio-depression represented a **variety** of more or less interrelated characteristics which can be divided into "electrical" and "mechanical" characteristics. The former (threshold, refractory period, etc.) entered the project at a later time.[185] Initially, the mechanical characteristic, i.e. the amplitude of the force of contraction, served as the standard. Negative effects on the mechanical function of the various compounds (the Kö- and Lg-series) were compared with those of quinidine. This matched common practice in pharmaceutical research, but cardio-depression in Germany was a highly unwanted effect. Evidence of this is the speed with which compound Lg 32 disappeared, particularly when compared with Kö 582 and Kö 592.

In due course, functional characteristics such as the relative ejection period, duration of systole, and, particularly, the period of isometric contraction became crucial standards to evaluate compounds. In other words, the priority of functional characteristics was the subject of discussion. In addition, there was discussion about the **values** of those characteristics: what was normal; and what was pathological? Standards derived from the German medical scene, particularly those elaborated by Reindell and his colleagues, were decisive in the Boehringer project.

Let 'c' represent "cardio-depressive action", and 'l' (= low), 'm' (= moderate) and 'h' (= high) the value of this functional characteristic. Furthermore, let 'd' denote "reduction of the demand of the heart", and 'l' (= low), 'm' (= moderate) and 'h' (= high) the value of this functional characteristic. Then, $c_{l \, v \, m} \in wf$, where wf denotes the wished for functional drug profile with respect to angina pectoris such that heart failure is not precipitated or aggravated, and

$$wf = \{d_h, c_{l \, v \, m}\}.$$

Since propranolol possessed a much stronger cardio-depressive activity than Kö 592:

(i) of(x_1) = {d_h, $c_{l \ v \ m}$} (x_1 = Kö 592);
(ii) of$(x_2$ = {d_h, c_h}   (x_2 = propranolol);

On the basis of (i) and (ii),

(iii) of(x_1) ∆ wf) ⊆ (of(x_2) ∆ wf)

Thus, Kö 592 was evaluated as a better drug than propranolol. Since (iii) is valid on the basis of (i) and (ii), the soundness of the procedure of "coarsening" of the values of c' was relevant. That is, whether the criteria for the subdivision of the range of values into low, moderate and high were valid. If so, then no doubt it follows that: $c_{l \ v \ m} \in$ of(x_1); and $c_h \in$ of(x_2). The fact that propranolol was two times more cardio-depressive than Kö 592 is not very impressive in this respect but sufficient to establish Kö 592 as an optimum within a series of compounds. In addition, propranolol was about six times more cardio-depressive than quinidine. Still, these findings did not resolve the issue where to draw the line to achieve clinically relevant values. In this respect the values with regard to the duration of the period of isometric contraction established by Reindell and his colleagues were much more convincing.

When the view persisted that beta blockers indeed caused heart failure, the typical clinical procedure of minimizing risks as much as possible by selecting patients at risk, became the subject of scientific interest. The assumption was that there were two categories of angina patients: those associated without and those with (subliminal) heart failure. If P_1 represents angina pectoris, P_2 heart failure and $P_{1,2} = P_1 \cup P_2$, then:
P_1 = angina patients without heart failure;
$P_{1,2}$ = angina patient with (subliminal) heart failure.
Since the spectrum of disease profiles of angina pectoris and heart failure differed in both medical contexts - that is: $P_{a1,2} \neq P_{g1,2}$ - the same remarks as in the preceding section about angina pectoris apply. The selection of patients at risk, i.e. the distinction between $P_{1,2}$ and P_1, meant something quite different to a German physician than to a Anglo-American physician. To the former the boundaries both between angina pectoris and heart failure, and frank and subliminal heart failure were fluid, while to the Anglo-American physician they were quite clear. The option of laying the burden of proof with the physician in prescribing beta blockers, was unrealistic in the German medical context. So much so that Boehringer's medical department choose to focus on cardiovascular disorders associated with an unimpaired cardiac function.

Due to the similarities between the effects of exercise therapy in functional heart disorders and the effects of beta blockers in the cardiovascular system, hypersympathotonic disorders became a new therapeutic target. In short, a new wished for (functional) drug profile (wf) was introduced. The sequence of events is depicted in figure (7.14).

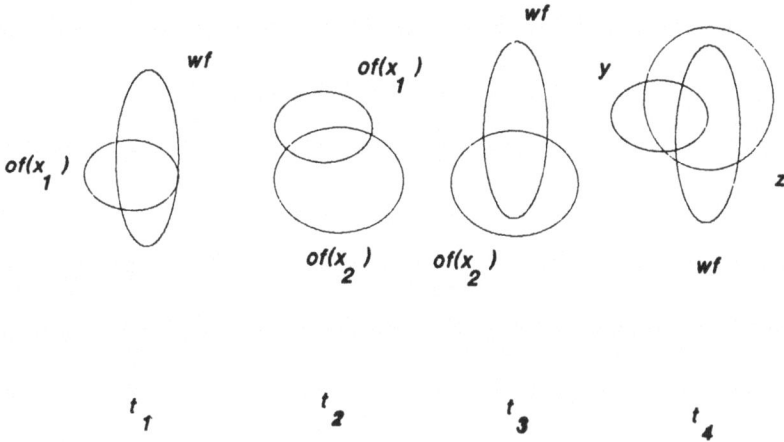

Figure 7.14
The sequence of events in recognizing the similarity of action between beta blocker and exercise therapy
in functional heart disorders.
Exercise therapy (x_1); beta blocker (x_2); wf is in this case the wished for functional drug profile with respect
to functional heart disorders - the change of wf from t_1 and t_4 not being depicted.
Question at t_4: $y = x_1$ and $z = x_2$; or $y = x_2$ and $z = x_1$?

At time t_1 the use of exercise therapy $(of(x_1))$ in the treatment of functional heart disorders
is depicted $(of(x_1) \cap wf \neq \emptyset)$.[186] It must be noted that 'P' represents a spectrum P_i $(i = 1, ...,$
$n; n \neq \infty)$ of disease profiles of functional heart disorders. Similarly, it must be noted that
'wf' represents a spectrum wf_i $(i = 1, ..., n; n \neq \infty)$ of wished for functional drug profiles with
respect to P. The joint action of these w's was supposed to be the change over of the
vegetative system ("Vegetative Umstimmung").
Subsequently, the similarity - being defined as a non-empty intersection between profiles
- between exercise therapy and beta blockade $(of(x_2))$ is recognized: $of(x_1) \cap of(x_2) \neq \emptyset$. On
the basis of the heuristic rule described in chapter 2, it was concluded: $(of(x_2) \cap wf \neq \emptyset)$.
Finally, the question became whether beta blockade was a better therapy than exercise
therapy: $| of(y) \Delta wf | < | of(z) \Delta wf |$ (figure (7.14))?

In the late 1960s a critical change of opinion occurred. Characteristics such as cardio-
depression, negative inotropic action and reduced cardiac output, once almost synonymous,
were separated.
The statement about Kö 592 that "negative inotropic or cardio-depressive doses" and "beta
blocking doses" lie further apart with respect to Kö 592 compared to those of propranolol,
lost significance. The blockade of the sympathetic drive of the heart by beta blockers became
the issue. This was explicitly discussed in the medical reports of Boehringer, and accordingly
considered in decision making. Moreover, the therapeutic situation had changed. New beta
blocking compounds, e.g. alprenolol and oxprenolol, with intrinsic activity emerged, and

made a better case for competing with propranolol. However, the clinical opinion began to conclude that patients with immanent or manifest heart failure should be excluded from treatment with beta blockers, with or without intrinsic activity. The burden came to lie on the shoulders of the physicians in selecting the right patients and the German physicians had set themselves a difficult task.

7.5. Conclusions

Several factors resulted in the dramatic events described above. The fact that a competitor possessed the patent rights, that the angina pectoris market was rather small at that time and that several other projects with seemingly more chance of prosperity were developing, were reasons for the lack of initiative at Boehringer. But these reasons also expressed current medical views.

Initially Aleudrin formed the context for discussing therapeutic objectives and were to some extent counterproductive. When angina pectoris came into the picture, this affected the dipyridamole project since dipyridamole was considered as the ideal coronary vasodilator. Considering the prosperous future forecasted by German clinicians it was no wonder that a new project trying to put forward a new direction in anti-anginal treatment was shrouded with a mist of caution and reservation.

Boehringer had the difficult task of deciding between two different principles in anti-anginal treatment. It was a stroke of co-incidence that the principles had materialized into two compounds, one being Kö 592 at Ingelheim, the other dipyridamole at Thomae. Presumably, it rarely happens that one and the same firm is the stage of such a paradigmatic clash with all its consequences. This contrasts with the situation at ICI. On the Anglo-American medical scene the coronary vasodilator concept had past its prime. In this respect a vacuum existed with respect to therapy for angina pectoris which could be rapidly filled by the new therapeutic principle.

Another prominent feature was the concern about heart failure which deeply affected the Boehringer project. German medical views, particularly the view of heart failure on effort developed by the Reindell school, influenced the standards for screening. Simultaneously, the great risk of heart failure influenced the change of course, i.e. to study the normal heart and thus minimize risk of damage and decompensation of the heart. In addition, the initiative for this was the similarity of the effects of beta blockade with those of physical therapy in coronary training, another typical German approach.

Heart failure remained a limiting factor in the further development and acceptance of beta blockade in German medicine. Once cardio-depression and beta blockade were disentangled, the Kö 592 project fell into a vacuum because there was no way to claim a privileged position with a compound that exerted a low degree of cardio-depressive action. The compound was finally marketed in 1970 but the market was very restricted. German physicians remained hostile to the drug, not to the compound in particular but to beta blockade in general.

Characteristic of this climate is the publication of an educational book in 1980 entitled **Keine Angst vorm Beta-Block (No Fear from Beta Blockade)** published by the German Physicians' publishing-firm with a foreword that opens as follows: *"In discussions with* *colleagues from general practice or the hospital, it all the time occurs that some physician or other expresses his fear for the use of beta blockers".* [187]

The sequence of events described above were disappointing to the Boehringer scientists who were left with memories and no success. Resignation pervades the following passage of an interview (RV) with Engelhardt (E) and Köppe (K):

E: *"We had to work hard on that physician - he no longer works for the company now - in other words, it was difficult to convince him"*
RV: *"But does that mean that actually the whole concept was questioned?"*
E: *"Right, right! That's how it was"*
(...) [188]
E: *"It was disappointing in the end and it all led to the situation that in priority we were behind ICI with our patent"*
K: *"Although we might have been in the lead by one or two years. There are situations in life that one cannot control by oneself from a certain position. Please also consider that we were at least 25 years younger so there were older persons in higher positions. And then, it isn't very simple to transform a new, surprising discovery into a marketable medicine. That is especially difficult if there is still a certain amount of risk, for instance that there was cardiac depression, and it was known, well, it was feared. You know that in Germany the beta blockers have become a really large field of medicine later, only much later, which had already been recognized in England and the Scandinavian countries years before that".* [189]

The history of the Boehringer project shows that the medical setting is pivotal to drug discovery. Therapeutic targeting at Boehringer involved distinct medical traditions, which is abundantly clear from the medical views that entered decision taking. However original or revolutionary we believe our ideas to be, they are inevitably part of a continuing tradition which owes its nature to previous experiences and which will continue even after they seemed to have been absorbed by the new views. The medical views about angina pectoris, heart failure and coronary vasodilation attest to this point. These concepts stretched back to previous periods in German medicine but casted a shadow over the future as well. They formed the soil of the beta blocker project at Boehringer and it turned out to be infertile. As Lichterfeld commented: *"But, looking back, it also became clear to me how completely we were embedded as a company in the German medical setting. (..) That it wasn't the failure of certain people, but a problem of the medical setting".* [190]

Chapter 8. Search processes, profiles and therapeutic practice in drug discovery

8.1. Introduction

In this chapter the proposal to use set theory to describe the process of matching drug and disease profiles as discussed in chapter 2 will be further developed by examining the search process in drug discovery (8.2), making some critical comments (8.3) and studying how medical practice functions as a source of new drugs (8.4).

8.2. The search process in drug discovery

Pathways of developing drugs can be long or short, with varying degrees of complexity and crossing of routes. These pathways can be projected onto the changing patterns of knowledge about drugs and diseases. The set-theoretical model enables us to specify and to trace the contributions from the various scientific disciplines. It also provides us with a set of terms or "grammar" from set theory, with which to describe the process of rapprochement between medicinal compounds and diseases (see appendix IV). Different developmental pathways familiar from the literature, such as indication-development, screening, drug design, molecular modification and chance discoveries can be re-interpreted and shown as special examples in this general model. They differ in the degree to which the searching process is limited by the use of more or less sophisticated techniques derived from drug design and structure-activity relationship studies.

In the following, screening is taken as an example for re-examination in terms of the set-theoretical model. The intention is to show that both screening and rational drug design can be reduced to three basic components which relate to the nature of the rules and the profiles in the search process. The screening is limited to the search for one drug for one disease, that is, with one particular profile in mind. The following six steps are possible:

Step 1: Look for a suitable drug x for disease E, and formulate a wished for profile, sub-divided into a structural (ws) and functional (wf) profile:
a) Regarding the wished for functional profile, one has in principle one or several (experimental or clinical) effects in mind which are therapeutically desirable (wf ≠ ø);
b) Regarding the wished for structural profile, one doesn't know the desired chemical structure for the drug to be found (ws = ø).

Step 2: A specific screening model is selected to detect a limited number of critical characteristics which will decide if a compound is of interest; this is a **restricted** (functional) profile[1]:

a) **Restriction** of the wished for functional profile:

$wf^r \subseteq wf$ (the superscript 'r' denotes "restricted");

b) **Restriction** of the operational functional profile:

$of^r(x) \subseteq of(x)$.

Heuristic rule: if compound x_1 is functionally more like the restricted wished for profile than x_2, then x_1 is more like the wished for profile than x_2:

$$|of^r(x_1) \, \Delta \, wf^r| < |of^r(x_2) \, \Delta \, wf^r| \quad \rightarrow \quad |of(x_1) \, \Delta \, wf| < |of(x_2) \, \Delta \, wf|$$

Step 3: A series of compounds is synthesized: x_n ($n = 1, 2, ..k$; $k \neq \infty$).

Step 4: Two potential compounds are found: $of(x_1) \cap wf \neq \emptyset$; $of(x_2) \cap wf \neq \emptyset$; for all $n \neq 1, 2$: $of(x_n) \cap wf = \emptyset$.

Step 5: The compounds of interest are tested in further test-systems:

a) **Extension** of the restricted wished for functional profile:

$wf^r \subseteq wf^{er} \subseteq wf$ (the superscript 'er' denotes "extended restricted");

b) **Extension** of the restricted operational functional profile:

$of^r(x) \subseteq of^{er}(x) \subseteq of(x)$.

Heuristic rule: if compound x_1 in the extended series of experimental systems is functionally more like the wished for profile than x_2, then x_1 is more like the wished for profile than x_2:

$$|of^{er}(x_1) \, \Delta \, wf^{er}| < |of^{er}(x_2) \, \Delta \, wf^{er}| \quad \rightarrow \quad |of(x_1) \, \Delta \, wf| < |of(x_2) \, \Delta \, wf|$$

Step 6: The search process is successfully completed, if a compound gives positive results, on one or more counts in the extended series of experiments.

Successful: $of(x) \cap wf \neq \emptyset$; $|of(x) \, \Delta \, wf^{er}| < |of(x) \, \Delta \, wf^r|$

The route of random screening is re-interpreted in terms of this model.

Without many problems the changes relating to drug and disease profiles can be described in terms of the set-theoretical model, at least in a broad sense.[2]

The above interpretation shows especially, however, the type of rules that play a role in the search process. Until now the description of (the type of) changes in the domain of drug and disease profiles was central. How those changes are induced has only been briefly indicated here. Theories, daring hypotheses, innovative technical principles, new experimental systems, clinical observations and chance discoveries can induce these changes and can be regarded as rules which are stored in a separate space.

There are two important points relating to the nature of the rules used in screening and they are that the search for the structural profile is done blind while the search for the functional profile is not.[3] An experimental system is chosen that allows for quantitative tests on the one hand and represents a key feature of the disease on the other. However, so little is known about this key feature that there is no way of judging the relevance of the system for the disease in question, and even less about the desired chemical structure of compounds that could cure the defect. These two points can be illustrated by the following three basic elements in terms of the model (fig. 8.1).

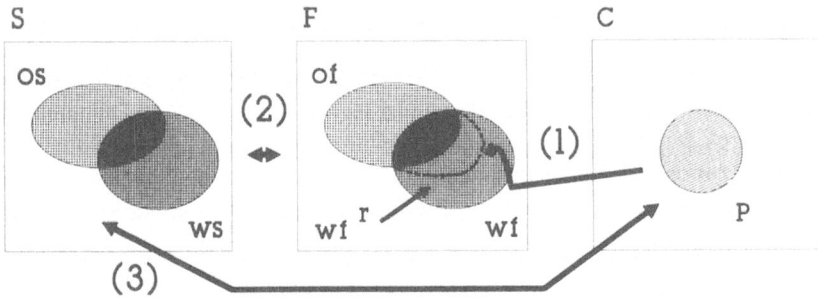

Figure 8.1
Three basic elements in the search process in drug discovery.

In figure 8.1 these elements are indicated by the arrows (1), (2), (3):

ad (1): The therapeutic relevance of the experimental model: the wished for functional profile is reduced to a number of relevant characteristics, i.e. $wf^c \subseteq wf$; and includes an exchange between domains F and C.

ad (2): The exchange between domains S and F, i.e. between wf and ws.

ad (3): The exchange between domains C and S: knowledge of the pathogenesis of disease produces insights concerning the (wished for) structural components of drugs; or reversely.

Not only screening, but also the other processes in drug discovery can be brought back to these three elements. The number of possible directions in which the search can take place can be restricted by making rational predictions about (1), (2) and (3). This can be illustrated by the choice of the test system which is first used in the drug search process. Any model used in the detection and characterization of a potential new drug, as Drews suggests, can be globally oriented towards a particular clinical utility and can be directed at a particular mechanistic or molecular parameter, with a large range of possibilities extending between these two extremes.[4]

Which of these possibilities have relevance for the therapeutic objective depends, Drews comments, *"on several factors: first, on the maturity of the scientific and/or therapeutic discipline in which we are working; secondly, on the amount of information already available with respect to a particular compound; thirdly, on the degree to which the therapeutic relevance of a particular experimental model has been demonstrated".* [5] Acknowledging the increasing levels of organization and complexity - sub-cellular, cellular and so forth till whole organisms - it does mean that at some particular level of the organism, models are used representing some key feature of the disease for which treatment is sought. At which level depends on the factors enumerated by Drews.

If we apply this to the stepwise method established for the screening procedure, then the three factors, although overlapping, determine in various ways the search process. We can begin with the third factor named by Drews. The therapeutic relevance guarantees the second and fifth step in the scheme outlined; the second factor gives the possibility for comparison with steps 3, 5 and 6 and provides clues for the chemist as to which chemical structures are important. In a sense the second factor determines the search process in a way that has not been described in the preceding series, that is, the process relating to the wished for and operational structural profile. The first factor, the maturity of the discipline, influences all six steps in the search process. As a general heuristic rule, Drews proposes that in mature scientific disciplines one can begin with very specific test systems; while in young research areas only general models can be used. Specifically, one is sure of the therapeutic relevance of the chosen system and that brings us back to the third factor.

Whichever way we look at it, we end up with the three basic elements as described above. If the therapeutic climate is ready, if there is good information about effective compounds and if there is reliable knowledge about the relevance of the experimental model, that is, the three factors stated by Drews, then the search can be more specific than in the case of screening. If the key feature of the disease, reflected in the experimental model, can be converted to molecular-mechanical parameters, then the whole battery of drug design and SAR techniques can be applied to the search process. As Davey stated: *"Compare what we are doing in the case of rheumatoid arthritis with what we did when we went in search of a beta-blocking drug. In terms of disease we were talking about the prevention of angina and heart attacks. In laboratory terms we were talking about blocking the action of catecholamines on particular receptors in the heart. This is the kind of situation that we must try to create for the great problem areas which remain. People might say that mental illness, rheumatoid arthritis, and many of the others will never be reduced to such simple terms. Who knows?".* [6]

Davey points out the ideal situation for every industrial researcher: the better the understanding of the disease at the molecular level, the more precisely one can compose the structural and functional profiles of the drugs. While clinicians were discussing the prevention of angina pectoris and heart attacks, scientists could debate the blockade of catecholamines on specific receptors. Knowledge of these compounds and receptors enabled scientists to create structural and functional profiles which were important for clinical practice. Thus, using the structure-activity relationship (SAR) techniques available to the chemist and the biologist, the large number of choices can be greatly restricted. In this way present day pharmaceutical research distinguishes itself from a few decades ago, when screening and trial and error were the chief tools available.

However, the present situation should not be overestimated, as illustrated by the following example, given by Austel and Kutter for searching for wished for structural profiles. Imagine that rational drug design strategy indicates that an indole-like compound would be a suitable lead-compound (ws = {i}; i = indole-like structure).

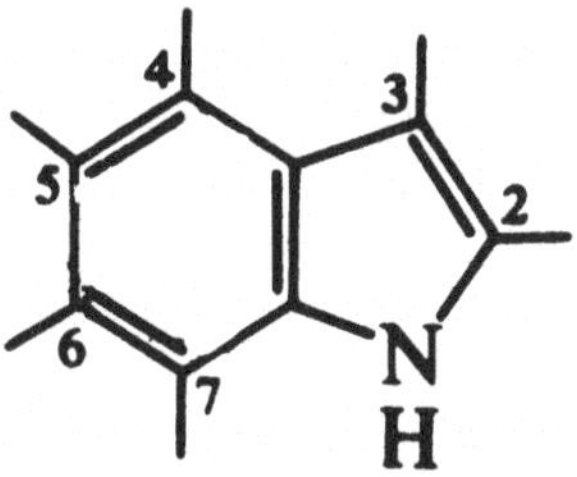

(72)

Figure 8.2
The basic structure of indole.
Reproduced with permission from Austel and Kutter (1980).

There are an infinite number of substitutes possible in the positions from 2 to 7 of this basic structure (figure 8.2). *"At this point"*, as Austel and Kutter comment, *"the creativity of the medicinal chemist, his ability to produce ideas, comes into operation. In this context, the term "idea" refers to chemical structures conceived by the medicinal chemist"*. [7]

The strategy that the chemist can follow is to choose a limited number of types of substituents that show sufficient spread in chemical potential, and to vary these types in a limited number of conditions. This creative stage, in Austel and Kutter's example, in which 31 substitution types were chosen (and which were varied on average 5 times each), for the seven positions, still results in a collection of 16.500 compounds. This enormous number of compounds would take an experienced chemist at least 150 years to synthesize, and that is not even including the testing stage.

In the second phase, the chemist again chooses a representative sample analogous to the random sample in sociological research. The chemist thus obtains a realistic number of compounds to be synthesized and which can be tested by the biologist. Even using a rational approach, the creativity of the scientist is indispensable.

The question is, whether this search process in drug discovery can be completely described in terms of the developed model. Let us assume that the process of innovation can be reconstructed in terms of profiles and rules. Then on the basis of an incompletely defined model - the partial definition of the concept of profile and the unspecified use of the rules - it is not possible to give a definite answer. Also, even if the intuition that the concept of profile can be made operational in terms of set theory is correct, the following opposing argument could be made. Since profiles consist of thousands of characteristics, or more, often of a composite nature, the model quickly comes up against technical and practical limits. An exact reconstruction of the discovery process is impossible.

This argument is valid in theory but not convincing from the practical viewpoint. Scientists regard profiles as finite sets and reduce large sets of parameters to smaller ones, which are manageable in their research. These operations can be reconstructed, just as the resulting profiles and the changes within. A more cautious position has to be adopted with respect to the rules applied by the scientists. Defining these rules, brings us to the territory of heuristics and statistics. These rules can be partially defined in the language of set theory and therefore in terms of the developed model.

Support for the model can be found in the work of Austel and Kutter, which, as far as is known to the author, is the only study in which set theory is used to discuss the process of drug discovery.[8] Their basic premises differ from the present model, in that they make no distinction between the three domains S, F and C, nor between wished for and operational profiles. They also do not distinguish between formal and heuristic rules and their analysis does not include the concept of profile.

However, as in the present model, the authors apply set theory principles to drug discovery, specifically to the development of the new cardiotonic drug AR-L 115 within their own company; and they also apply these principles to the basic strategies in drug research.[9] Their analysis has its starting point in medicinal chemistry which focuses on the molecular-structural and physical-chemical properties of the compounds. In terms of the present model, the **structural** properties of drugs - i.e. domain S and the interaction with domain F - are central, an aspect which has received little attention in this study. In addition, they are more specific about the rules of the search process, than in the current study, and they introduce the useful approach of regarding the search process as an interaction between creative and systematic, valuative phases.

If the principles of Austel and Kutter's study can be re-formulated in terms of the present model, then this model becomes all the more plausible. Indeed, the differences as well as the similarities can be re-stated in terms of the current model. The quite detailed description of the strategies of drug design and the development of AR-L 115 can therefore also be described in the terms of the present set-theoretical model

8.3. Evaluation of the theory of drug discovery

8.3.1. Introduction

The drug discovery process can be reconstructed with the help of the theory developed in this study. In this section two questions will be discussed: What is the role actually played by profiles in drug discovery (8.3.2.), and to what degree is the assumption that the discovery process can be reconstructed in terms of knowledge and rules, correct (8.3.3.)?

8.3.2. The epistemological status of the concept of profile

In this thesis, the concept of profile and the model derived from it, has been used as a set of binoculars to look at the (contextual) developments in the medical world from a great height. Some developments at lower levels, especially in industrial research projects have been examined at close range. But this instrument has not been used as a microscope to describe the creative processes at a micro-level in detail.

This binocular approach could suggest that the essential character of the process of innovation has not been included in the analysis. This suggestion arises from the belief that the essential character of the discovery process should be observed at the micro-level, i.e. the more one descends to the micro level in the scientific world, the closer one comes to the point where the innovative process unfolds. After all, the creative ideas are born at the laboratory bench.

The story of Prinzmetal's introduction of an alternative profile of angina pectoris to the medical world illustrates this point. The "newness" of this phenomenon had to be made visible in the consulting rooms and the researchers' laboratories. How Prinzmetal and colleagues created this profile and how they blended clinical experience, new techniques and theoretical insights to delineate this variant type of angina requires a reconstruction of the local situation in which they worked. But this reconstruction has not been performed in this study. However, Prinzmetal's publication was "new" in the medical world, and also at this level the "newness" had to be verified. We have seen in chapter 6 how this variant version of angina pectoris was pushed to one side, only to re-appear at the centre of scientific research in the 1970s. The discovery process therefore also takes place at the macro-level.

More important, is that the separation into levels in the discovery process brings other, more fundamental problems to the fore. The question is whether, by looking through the microscope, quite different structures than the profiles discussed in this study are made visible. Just as the epidemiologist uses the binoculars, for example, to study the migration pattern of micro-organisms in populations and thereby reduces his object to specific basic components, the microbiologist uses the microscope to study the micro-organisms themselves, and he sees quite different types of structures. Similarly profiles studied through the binoculars are in danger of loosing their structure at the micro-level.

In other words the epistemological status of the concept of profile is at stake here. What role is actually played by profiles at the laboratory bench and in the consulting room? When medicinal chemists design and synthesize new compounds, do profiles of (known) compounds play an important role? And when clinicians notice unsuspected complaints or signs in a patient, are they able to do this on the basis of a pattern of knowledge in the form of a profile? This author is of the impression that they play a role at the laboratory bench or in the consulting-room. In the interviews during the research for this thesis, participants used the concept of profile naturally: the chemists when drawing chemical structures on the blackboard and creatively imagining new ones; the biologists when discussing structure-activity patterns; and the clinicians in grasping the differences between the various subsets of patients, e.g. responders and non-responders on medical therapy, and the variant types of clinical patterns versus the general disease categories. However, further research is necessary to verify this impression.

In any case, whether or not profiles are important, still other knowledge structures play a role. Scientists experiment, develop equipment, and produce graphs, charts, vibrations and other phenomena. They are constantly busy separating signal from noise, stable effects from unstable, and relevant details from irrelevant. That cognitive structures other than profiles are involved is highly likely.[10]

However, the fact remains that the concept of profile has revealed an important means of representing medical knowledge. The structure of medical knowledge has been enjoying increasing interest in medical-philosophical circles in recent years. The main point of discussion is to what degree this knowledge deviates from scientific knowledge.[11] The starting point is the fact that few theories in the biological and medical sciences can approach the mathematical precision and the predictive power of thermodynamics, mechanics and quantum theory. Medicine lacks such a theoretical structure as a result of the individuality of the subject: the sick patient. The practical application of biomedical knowledge makes claims on the proposed theories and the arguments to be used. Schaffner resorts to the concept of "exemplar" as introduced by Kuhn; via "exemplars", i.e. specific but representative situations scientists learn how to apply the generalizations of the relevant scientific discipline. It is not a question of direct application of laws or theories but of adaptation and modification of the generalization through which the basic problem can be solved. In this way Newton's Second Law of Motion ($f = ma$) - an example used by Kuhn to explain the concept of exemplar - can take different forms depending on the basic problem. For example to describe free fall the law is transformed to $mg = m\ (d^2s/dt^2)$; and for the pendulum $mg.\sin\theta = -ml\ (d^2\theta/dt^2)$. The law $f = ma$ represents a group of symbolic generalizations with their related series of standard problems which together form the fine structure of the scientific discipline concerned.

According to Schaffner in the biomedical sciences, the familiarity with a series of exemplars ("prototypes") plays a more important role than in the physical sciences because medical theories have a more limited application and a less perfect agreement with the clinical exemplars.[12] In the following Schaffner clearly explains this view and this quotation offers some points for comparison with the principle of profile:

*"There   (in the clinical sciences, RV)the focus is the individual patient, and generalizations such as 'diseases' are utilized to assist in prevention, prognosis, and therapy. The individual patient is the **clinical exemplar** of a (often multiple) disease or pathological process. Clinicians bring to the examination of individual patients a repository of classificatory or nosological generalizations, as well as a grounding in the basic sciences of biochemistry, histology, physiology, and the pathological variants of the 'normal' or 'healthy' processes. A theory in pathology can be construed as a family of models, each with 'something wrong' with the 'normal' or 'healthy' process. Such a set of overlapping or 'smeared out' models is then juxtaposed, often in a fairly loose way, with an overlapping or 'smeared out' set of patient exemplars. This dual 'smearedness' - one being in the basic biological models and the other in the patient population - typically requires that the clinician work extensively with analogical reasoning and with qualitative and at best **comparative** connecting pathophysiological principles. Thus one can find fairly frequently in textbooks of medicine, generalizations that trace causal connections through a complex system that are written as:*

A ===   B   ===   C

indicating that an increase in variable A will produce a decrease in B that will in turn produce an increase in C. This is grosser way of articulating a generalization than, say, $f = ma$" [13]

It appears that Schaffner reduces the concept of exemplar to two levels: to that of the biomedical sciences (physiology, biochemistry, and pathology) on the one hand and the clinical sciences (and practice) on the other. In this respect he talks of "double-smearedness", that is at both levels families of exemplars are present. The involvement of these levels with each other, initiates the representative form which Schaffner discusses - although it is not clear how this form emerges.

Schaffner stresses the prominence of such schematic forms of pathophysiological connections in the medical literature, and discusses examples from cardiology (the formation of edema), pulmonary medicine (pathogenesis of chronic hypoxia) and endocrinology (aldosterone-renin-angiotensin system). This type of representation possibly plays an important role in medical science. Indeed, this form of representing knowledge was frequently encountered in the medical literature on angina pectoris, heart failure and heart rhythm irregularities during research for the present study. Also the representative forms similar to those described by Schaffner occur frequently in the literature on the mechanism of drug action.

Why therefore do medical scientists and clinicians use profiles as distinct from the schematic form of knowledge as proposed by Schaffner? The differences between both forms of representations are obvious. The most important difference concerns the cognitive structure: causal versus taxonomic. The crux of the matter seems to lie in Schaffner's scheme above. A normal situation in drug research (and also in clinical research) is that a causal relation can exist between A and B, but not between B and C, or not even between A and B.

None the less, the three characteristics are regarded as critical aspects of a certain disease or of a mechanism of action of a particular drug. The lack of knowledge about the causal relationships between these characteristics is compensated for by bringing presumably relevant items together in a profile. In other words, there are more or less large "gaps" in the causal chains which form the linking fabric between biochemical, pathophysiological and clinical knowledge. With the aid of profiles, in which presumed relevant items are taxonomically ordered, scientists try to circumnavigate these "gaps". Undoubtedly, this taxonomic form also relates to the practical goals in the scientific discipline. In order to develop a drug, a series of compounds and their related mechanisms of action have to be thoroughly and quickly compared. It is irrelevant which type of causal relationship exists between these items, whether it is to do with structural or functional properties of drugs. We can expect similar goals in clinical research or in medical practice where the recognition of a large series of (disease) patterns also plays an important role. Also by determining the prognosis or instituting therapy the doctor will be guided by the relevant features of the disease and therapy, and profiles form a useful instrument. Profiles also play an important role because they enable scientists to interrelate different forms of knowledge; biochemical, physiological, and clinical.

The fact remains that both forms of representation can be co-ordinated and scientists use both in an interrelated manner. The analysis in chapter 5 also used the schematic form of Schaffner as a starting point to relate the disease processes of angina pectoris and the mechanism of action of anti-anginal drugs. It is, however, outside the realm of this thesis to compare both schemes in detail. This does not mean that the epistemological role of profiles has been sufficiently clarified here but this study does give a general outline within which the answer can be sought.

The problem above, concerning the status of profiles sets a critical limit to the theory developed in this thesis. In addition, one can ask what is the sphere of influence of the concept of profile: it is not inconceivable that the role of the drug and disease profile remains limited to drug research and specific areas in medical practice. Even if this be the case, the model developed here should be applicable to other forms of technical and therapeutic development.

8.3.3. Is the discovery process explicable in terms of profiles and rules?

This point touches on the fundamental limits of the current theory. To examine these limits a model developed by Collins will be used to explore the results of artificial intelligence and the nature of knowledge.[14] Since Collins addresses the problem whether artificial intelligence, e.g. the creation of "knowledgeable machines" is possible, his treatise about the possible explication of knowledge is directly relevant to the present model.

Collins grasps the key to this problem in what he calls the "algorithmic/enculturational" dichotomy. The algorithmic model of knowledge implies that knowledge can be transmitted to *"members of society and the researchers alike in discrete bits capable of being written down, classified, and counted"*. [15] Conversely the enculturational model states that transfer of knowledge requires genuine understanding, skills and craftsmanship, and training or socialization into a culture.

On this basis he proposes a fourfold categorization of knowledge: (1) facts and formal rules; (2) heuristics; (3) manual and perceptual skills; and (4) cultural skills. The first two categories conform to the algorithmic model of knowledge, the second two to the enculturational model. This separation agrees with the crucial dividing line between explicable rules and facts and the non-explicable tacit component of knowledge.

Facts and formal rules include knowledge that is readily explicated; heuristics, though by artificial intelligence experts set apart from the first category, are still in principle open for definition. Manual and perceptual skills include *"such things as the ability to recognize the presence of shapes that suggest the existence of crystals within an otherwise undifferentiated lump of solid material, the ability to distinguish the different sounds that can be made within a prototype TEA-laser cavity, and the ability to take a throat swab and see relevant shapes under the microscope"*. [16]

Instead cultural skills conform to Polanyi's idea of tacit knowledge illustrated by the well-known example of the skill associated with bicycle riding. Without understanding the physics of riding the cyclist "knows" how to ride. Since Collins defines cultural skills as *"abilities required to understand and use facts, rules and heuristics"*, he uses the term to stress the fact that there is an "inexplicable component" of knowledge.[17]

Accordingly, Collins uses the model to explain how in the process of knowledge development pieces of knowledge are transformed from the one category into another. Collins shows for example, how Harrison, a laser expert, succeeded during the development of the TEA-laser in translating implicit knowledge into explicit knowledge and rules. Harrison knew, for example, that the distance of the electrical connections between certain components in the apparatus had to be "short", but he had no idea what "short" in this specific laser context was.

Only an expert like Harrison, initiated in the laser and electronics culture, was capable of performing this transformation. After this success similar apparatus could be built by less expert and qualified people. Collins points out that the interpretation of "short" - in electronic terms - can only be understood against the background of the wide spread distribution of "measurement skills" in our culture. Only then can we say that there is a successful transfer of expertise into the system that the user can utilize. If not then this knowledge remains within the culture of an esoteric circle of experts and would in all probability be resistent to explication.

Communicating and explaining knowledge depends on the ability to pass on knowledge to others. In other words Collins draws attention to the close inter-relationship of knowledge and culture and he contests the thought that there is one way traffic between the expert/ knowledge engineer - expert system - end-user: *"Unless, minimally, the end-user can interpret the symbols that the expert system uses to give its advice, nothing useful can be transferred".* [18] Certain skills such as measuring blood pressure or taking an ECG, once sophisticated procedures and restricted to the initiated, have now become everyday events. But these nearly commonplace skills do not mean that less competence is now required but reflect the fact that the skills have become so widely spread. This fact agrees with a conclusion from Artificial Intelligence research that *"some widespread abilities, such as speaking, writing, and interacting socially, are difficult to explicate and that the things we think of as the preserve of clever people, such as rapid calculation or playing good chess, are relatively easy to encapsulate in formulas. This is why we cannot think about the development of knowledgeable machines without thinking about how they are going to be used, or the way they will fit into the cultural ambience. A machine that can interact quite acceptably in one social setting may be unacceptable in another".* [19]

The manual and cultural skills make up the invisible part of the iceberg of knowledge, not able to be made explicit, but able to be used and understood. Explicit knowledge and rules make up the tip of the iceberg, a top that becomes ever larger, but which also shrinks when certain skills in our culture disappear. In this sense explicit knowledge and rules remain closely bound to the skills which lie hidden under the water. *"The role of the end-user is"*, as Collins writes, *"to insert that part of the iceberg of cultural knowledge that cannot be programmed".* [20]

The consequences of the above for the present model are clear. There is a fundamental limit to the ability to make knowledge and rules explicit. In this sense the current model does not describe the processes involved in drug discovery as "art", "craftsmanship", and "expertise", although these skills, as Collins shows, are crucial to the creative process. On the other hand, the boundary between explicit and implicit knowledge is not fixed; it moves constantly and these movements can be illustrated within the current model i.e. the changes involving profiles and rules.

The most important point which Collins raises is the inter-relationship of knowledge and culture.[21] Irrespective of how successful chemists are in explaining the lipophilic, electric and steric properties of molecules and in connecting them with the mechanism of drug action as understood by biologists, the knowledge produced remains dependant on the skills of the end users, i.e. the chemists who need to synthesize these compounds on a large scale, the pharmacists who have to check and deliver them, and the doctors who have to prescribe the drugs.

Collins provides a justification for the view held in this thesis that the end-users play an important role in the process of discovering new drugs. In other words the present model claims that we have to not only reconstruct the world of the experts and scientists but also that of practicing doctors and pharmacists. This role could be taken as "passive", i.e. as a supplement to what cannot be made scientifically explicit. However, it must also be regarded as active because the end-user also exerts a driving force in the discovery process. Culture - or rather "practice", i.e. application by the end-user - is no obstacle to scientific progress neither is it simply a centre of irrational activity that betrays the scientific norms. On the contrary, practice becomes the master-mind of discovery.

8.4. Practice - the contribution to drug discovery

8.4.1. Introduction

In this section an epistemological characterization will be given of the contribution made by medical practice to the development of drugs. By practice will be understood therapeutic treatment in the context of the doctor-patient relationship. This conforms to the majority opinion that the essence of medical practice is individual and patient centred. This study is not concerned with the treatment itself but with the cognitive characteristics that are of importance in the gaining of knowledge (8.4.3.). Further, the "accumulated experiences" in relation to therapeutic treatment (8.4.4.) will be examined, and finally the claim made here that medical practice is a source of new knowledge about drugs and disease will be further discussed (8.4.5.). Before examining therapeutic action as a source of new knowledge, it is necessary to characterize more specifically the process of gaining medical knowledge. For this purpose use will be made of the map which Toulmin developed (8.4.2.).

8.4.2. The conflict between controlled clinical trial and casual experience in therapeutics

8.4.2.1. Toulmin's epistemological map of medicine

The central goal of Stephen Toulmin's 1976' article "On the Nature of the Physician's Understanding" was to draw a first, rough map to locate the particular kinds of knowledge which are embodied in medicine.[22]
His natural taxonomy of knowledge starts from the distinction between **general** and **particular** knowledge. General knowledge encompasses the understanding of the relations between, for example, force, mass, and acceleration, or between molecular conformations and biological activity. Particular knowledge deals with particular objects such as a flying missile, an animal species, a disease entity or chemical compound. Both forms of knowledge regard their object differently. The first departs from the peculiarities of the object and looks for the rules and the regularities. Particular knowledge, on the other hand, examines the special characteristics of the object. With general knowledge the "exceptional cases" are only interesting in so far as they expose regular patterns; they are the exception to the rule. With particular knowledge they express the uniqueness of the object; deviation, idiosyncrasies, and paradoxes show the richness of individual variation. This knowledge directs itself to the

specific conditions of events and specifies time, place and circumstances in which special events occur.

Both types of knowledge are further sub-divided by Toulmin with the help of two pairs of epistemological terms. General knowledge can be pursued out of simple **theoretical** desire to improve our understanding **of** the world or, alternatively, with the aim of developing new **practical** techniques for producing results **in** the world. This is synonymous with the distinction between theory and practice. Theoretical knowledge is directed towards knowing, explaining and predicting events and practical knowledge to controlling and (re)creating the situation in reality.

Both theoretical and practical knowledge can be further sub-divided into **abstract** and **concrete** knowledge. Abstract knowledge goes back to Plato, and concerns the underlying mechanisms and lasting principles. These represent order in a world of chance and change. Concrete knowledge is the inheritance from Aristotle, and is concerned, as stated by Toulmin, "with natural kinds, life cycles, and other typical 'courses'".[23] Here too both forms of knowledge regard their object in a totally different way. Abstract knowledge directs itself to idealized systems, which as such, don't occur in reality (the Platonic idea). The guidelines for concrete knowledge are the "real-life exemplars": typical phenomena or processes which take place in reality. Therefore, in the case of concrete knowledge, a new experimental system to investigate new anti-hypertensive agents, is considered adequate when it represents hypertensive disease in a very realistic way. In the case of abstract (theoretical) knowledge one strives for a model that ideally looks like "hypertension" but may be satisfied with something that is far from reality.

This distinction between the abstract and the concrete can also be found in the area of technology and practical knowledge. When emphasis lies upon abstract knowledge, it is the general principles of the mechanism of action of antihypertensive agents, for example, that are relevant. In contrast, in the case of concrete knowledge, specific procedures and boundary conditions to control hypertensive disease are important.

Particular knowledge can be sub-divided into knowledge directed towards particular **collectives** or **individuals**. Collective knowledge directs itself to a certain group of patients, a country, or an   animal species; particular knowledge on the other hand is concerned with a specific individual. Roughly speaking this distinction is comparable with the work of an historian as opposed to a biographer. To use Toulmin's map, the understanding of the disease pattern in a group of patients must focus on relevant characteristics as perceived over a certain time period: age, sex, social-economic status, disease state, etc.; and not on all events that affected the life of these people. Collective knowledge requires a **selective** attention. By contrast, understanding individuals demands an **inclusive** attention: whatever significantly affects the life of a particular patient will be equally relevant for the general practitioner.

Finally, these two forms of knowledge can be further split, according to Toulmin: *"An understanding of particulars - whether individuals or collectives - may again be sought, either for its own sake, or, alternatively, in the service of advice and advocacy".* [24] The former I propose to call **detached**, the latter **concerned** knowledge. In case of detached knowledge the general practitioner explains the linking of facts and events that shaped the life history of a particular patient. This activity differs from getting information to intervene in the sick patient in the correct way. Even so, the epidemiologist in occupational medicine may provide a deeper understanding of the appearance and distribution of some occupational disease but this is quite different from the activity of developing measures to prevent this disease in a particular group of factory-workers by an occupational physician.

It is assumed that the following diagram approximately visualizes the map which Toulmin had in mind, though he did not actually draw one.

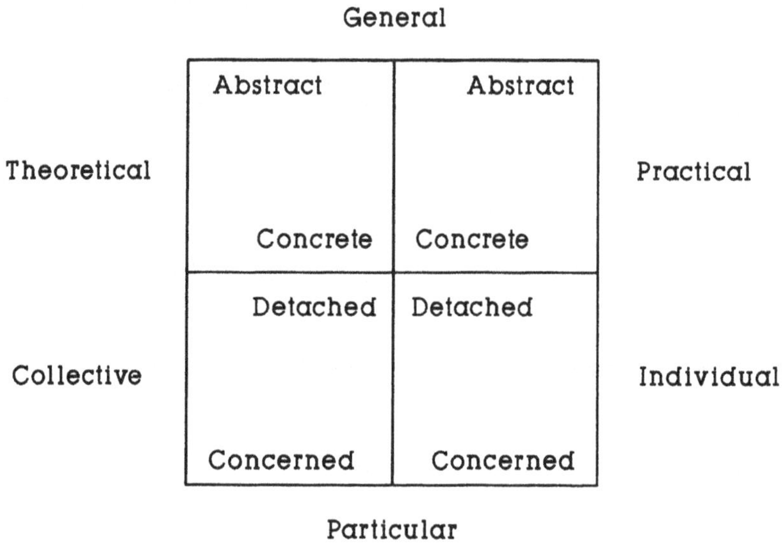

Figure 8.3
Visualization of Toulmin's map representing the types of gaining medical knowledge.

Some additional remarks are necessary. Firstly, the attractiveness of Toulmin's map lies in his combined use of dichotomies; medical knowledge is not reduced to a simple dichotomy; prime focus is on its complexity. Obviously, each of these dichotomies may be criticized but combined and properly used they are useful to discuss relevant epistemological issues in medicine and drug research. Secondly, the dichotomies are conceived of as reference points of a grid, not as absolute categories. Thirdly, the application to actual cases may cause difficulties, but is dependant upon the case under scrutiny and the purpose of the analysis.

8.4.2.2. Application of Toulmin's map on the conflict between controlled clinical trial and casual experience in medicine

Toulmin developed this map to explain the issue of epistemological pluralism in medicine.[25] For, *"the status of medical knowledge"*, as Toulmin notes, *"is a historical fact about the practice of medicine at the time in question".* [26] Throughout history the mix and distribution of the various ways of gaining knowledge in medicine shifted. This applies also to the conflict between controlled clinical trial and casual experience in medicine. Here Toulmin's map is used to perform a systematic analysis of this conflict.

Consider, for example, a medical discipline that merely consists of two epistemologies: "casual experience" and "controlled clinical trial" (figure 8.4).

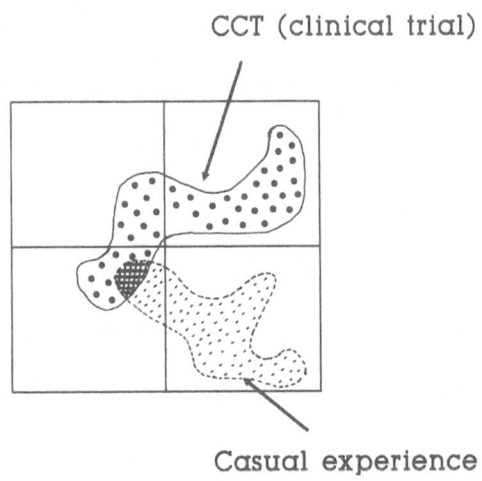

CCT (clinical trial)

Casual experience

Figure 8.4
The landscape of a medical discipline consisting of casual experience and controlled clinical trial as its basic types of gaining knowledge, drawn on Toulmin's map.

The aim of the controlled clinical trial is to validate the effectiveness of a new therapy. Hence, general knowledge is the issue, particularly of a technological, applied nature. Though the trial forms a test of the general principles of therapy, these principles are embodied in specific procedures to handle the therapeutic problem: route of administration, dosage regimen, duration of action, etc. Moreover, it treats its objects as real-life exemplars that actually exist in the world. Hence, the "density" of the controlled clinical trial is located in the area of practical, concrete knowledge. In addition it encompasses collective, detached knowledge because it collects information about patient populations. In contrast casual experience seeks particular knowledge. It focusses on individual cases with emphasis on advocacy and therapeutic concern. Moreover it reveals individual idiosyncracies, the signs and symptoms which are particular, time-bound and tentative. [27]

Both epistemologies make claims regarding the nature and justification of medical knowledge. These claims represent a spectrum between a weak and a strong interpretation. In the case of casual experience the strong interpretation maintains that the experience and observation of the doctor is central to the formation of knowledge in general and in particular about working principles and effectiveness. The weak interpretation, on the other hand, recognizes that general knowledge about therapeutic principles doesn't belong to its domain, but the application does.

In the case of the CCT-concept the weak interpretation restricts its claims to the evidence about the general principles embodied in the therapy and to the specific procedures appropriate to the handling of therapeutic problems. It then remains open, in particular cases, for physicians to decide to what extent this knowledge is pertinent to the therapeutic problem at stake. In contrast, the strong interpretation claims that the best information to assess whether a given treatment does more good than harm to individual patients is delivered by the CCT. This leaves no room for particular knowledge whatsoever.

In the following sections the analysis follows the line of the strong interpretation of the CCT-claim. Firstly, because the analysis gives insights which also apply to the other instances, and secondly because this strongly normative judgment is influential and popular.

8.4.2.3. Pragmatic attitude towards the controlled clinical trial

Before explaining this strong interpretation it is useful to put this claim in perspective because it has to be distinguished from the pragmatic attitude one encounters in practice. The claim doesn't deny that the choice of therapy depends on the context of the doctor-patient-relationship, nor that in choosing, the doctor has to decide what should be done for this patient. Further, the claim doesn't deny the fact, that in practice, doctors often decide on the basis of their own experience. However, this is regarded as undesirable because reliable knowledge is only obtainable from the CCT. In other words, the epistemological claim concerning the CCT has to be distinguished from the practical view which is motivated by pragmatic, economic or psychological factors. This attitude appears in different forms, six of which are mentioned here.

First, it is acknowledged that in particular situations the CCT is unfeasible or irrelevant. If, for example, the disease in question is rare or if it is invariably followed by death, then the CCT cannot be performed (too few patients) or is not required since any treatment effect is immediately obvious.

Secondly, for practical and economic reasons it is very often impossible to perform the required trials. Therefore, in practice, one has to take refuge in methods which produce less reliable information but with greater speed or lower cost. When no rigorously controlled studies are available, clinicians have to act in the face of incomplete information which is quite a common situation in medicine. Also every time a physician wants to treat a patient, he has to evaluate whether the patient concerned is recognizably similar to the patients studied during the trial.

Thirdly, it is acknowledged that controlled clinical trials are too small to detect rare but devastating side effects. Although such trials are the only way to assess the efficacy of a drug, other studies are required to determine its safety. But again, this is a matter of economics and energy, not of principle. For, when sufficient numbers of patients are enrolled and financial resources are available, the controlled trial is the ideal method. If, however, the principle itself is denied, we enter weaker interpretations of the CCT claim.

Fourth, the strong claim about the controlled clinical trial does not deny that therapeutic decision making is an inductive process which has as its input the specification of observed characteristics of the patient and as output a list of hypotheses each of which could explain the characteristics be they diagnostic, prognostic or therapeutic. That is, therapeutic decision making is an activity per se, but the truth of the hypotheses generated by the physician is determined by the controlled clinical trial.

Fifth, medical knowledge is probabilistic in nature, and so is the diagnostic and therapeutic process, but this is an expression of the present incapacity of medical knowledge. If otherwise conceptualized - for example, when it is claimed that medical knowledge is necessarily probabilistic by nature - weaker interpretations of the claim may come to the foreground. Sixth, the target of medical therapy is subject to the patient-doctor relationship. Though clinical trials determine the value of a particular therapy, physician and patient may jointly agree not to choose the therapy. Hereby norms and values enter the therapeutic and diagnostic process, a subject which will be left aside here.

However much these exceptions are acknowledged from the pragmatic point of view, they still prove the rule that the CCT generates the best information about therapy.

8.4.2.4. Dissection of the strong interpretation of the normative claim about the CCT

The strong interpretation of the normative claim implies two things. Firstly, knowledge of the efficacy of medical therapy is a mere matter of the CCT. Secondly, in prescribing the therapy the physician merely "applies" the knowledge generated by the CCT. Let us agree with the first aspect and examine the second in more detail.

The essence lies in the concept of "application", a very complex idea which has occupied many a philosopher.[28] In this context Toulmin notes: *"Though the physician's particular understanding of some individual patient may rely on general principles, whether physiological or psychological, the principles themselves will have a medical significance only so far as they can be related to a personal understanding of the particularities of clinical practice with actual patients, that is, individual human beings coming for professional advice. (...) Again, the general (technological) principles of diagnostics and treatment are one thing; the specific (craft) regimen appropriate to this or that childhood infection is something again".* [29] To mark this difference between general scientific principles and their "application" to actual cases Toulmin uses an obvious example drawn from physics: *"Scientists were rightly confident about the laws of gravitation, yet they are quite unable to say where a scrap of paper dropped from an upper window will finally touch ground".* [30] Thus, while the physician incorporates the body of scientific knowledge in therapeutic decision making, this knowledge enters a different world of concepts and relations. One way or other the physician specifies general knowledge, or juxtaposes it to particular conditions. In any case, he enriches the body of knowledge about medical therapy and he contributes to the growth of medical knowledge. Consequently, we have to reconsider our agreement with the first point, i.e. that knowledge about medical therapy is a mere matter of controlled clinical trials.

An important argument against this interpretation is that particular knowledge of therapy is not possible. Imagine for example that the doctor wants to treat a 50 year old, menopausal, woman with a muscle relaxant for tense back muscles - a legitimate therapeutic goal in case of back pain. A side-effect of certain types of muscle relaxants is orthostatic hypotension, an intermittent drop in blood pressure on getting up or other sudden changes in posture, through which dizziness can occur with a resulting fall. These side effects can be regarded as undesirable in this case. Through the possible presence of osteoporosis, a decalcification and weakening of the bone as a result of hormonal changes due to menopause, there is an increased chance of bone breakage on falling; and experience has shown that orthostatic hypotension often results in falls. The doctor decides to prescribe a muscle relaxant that does not cause orthostatic hypotension.

In this case, the physician takes account of specific characteristics - woman, 50 years, menopause, osteoporosis - in deciding to follow a certain therapeutic course. Even though these characteristics occur together in this particular case, they are not at all unique. There are more women of 50, in the menopause, who have an increased degree of osteoporosis. These are therefore characteristics of groups of patients which are attributed to individual patients but there is no question of uniqueness. This is perfectly illustrated by Lasagna's scathing opinion of the "no-patient-is-like-any-other-patient ploy" which according to him is maintained by the supporters of casual experience: *"We are, to be sure, all different from one another, and it is probably true that one could listen to hundreds of lungs during the pneumonia season and not find two that sounded exactly alike. But this is not the same as saying that there are no common features in such patients or that therapeutically one starts from scratch every time one faces a patient with pneumonia. If this were so, medical teaching would be impossible and the practice of medicine chaos, or at least anarchy"*. [31]

The argument is valid. For in therapeutic decision-making - and also in the diagnostic process -, the condition of the patient is, somehow, reduced to general categories or types, hence to the body of general medical knowledge. This argument even holds in cases of "uniqueness". Suppose that the pattern described above is indeed unique, then it still figures as a general account without which the physician is unable to decide whether it concerns a therapeutically significant pattern. Many other characteristics of the patient's condition can be considered in therapeutic decision making. One way or the other the physician "leaps" into a category. Though Lasagna's counter-argument is sound - mutatis mutandis the same holds true with respect to particular knowledge of collectives - it hinges upon the notion that the concerned pattern is part of the present body of general knowledge - which in addition is established by the CCT. However, it doesn't exclude the possibility that the pattern described is unknown, hence is "discovered" in this particular patient. But in agreement with the counter-argument, the physician inductively jumps to a general account of the therapeutic problem in question, e.g. that it is "typical" with regard to the patient's condition. Nevertheless, this account is distinct from existing categories, hence contrasts with the present body of knowledge. In specifying a particular set of characteristics or aspects of the patient's condition knowledge is particularized with regard to the body of general knowledge. From the perspective of particular knowledge the patient's condition is generalized (figure 8.5).

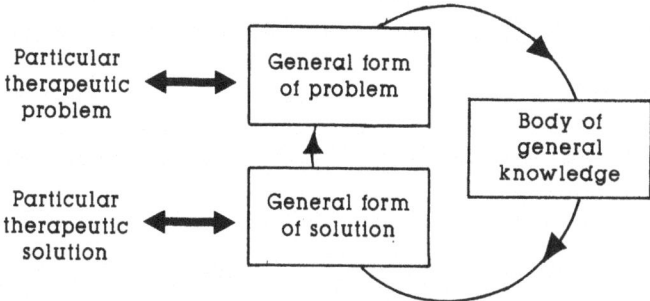

Figure 8.5
The circus movement of generalization and particularization in the process of creating therapeutic knowledge.
Adapted from Darden (1980).

When we distinguish between the therapeutic problem at stake, and the solution provided for it, we enter a sort of circular movement of creating therapeutic knowledge. The body of therapeutic knowledge is continuously nourished by different sources of medical knowledge. It is used to identify therapeutic problems, and to solve them. In this process generalization and particularization are intertwined. As a result the body of general therapeutic knowledge is used and applied, but also continuously enriched. The mechanisms through which this occurs, forms the subject of the next section.

8.4.3. Therapeutic treatment based on the individual patient

The way in which medical practice can be regarded as a source of new knowledge can be illustrated by reducing the diagnostic-therapeutic process to six basic steps. The first two concern the diagnosis and the last four the therapy.[32]

Step 1 Establishing the clinical picture CP(i) of patient i.

Step 2 Comparison of this specific clinical picture with the background knowledge, i.e. the domain of disease profiles: the clinical picture CP(i) is similar to the disease profile P.

Step 3 Establishing the desired therapeutic effect.

Step 4 Comparison of the desired therapeutic outcome with the background knowledge, i.e. the domain of drug profiles: choice of drug.

Step 5 Establishing the clinical picture CP'(i) after the therapeutic intervention.

Step 6 Comparison of CP'(i) with CP(i): evaluation of the intervention.

Firstly, the physician has to establish the clinical picture. This involves taking a medical history, performing a physical examination and possibly some laboratory tests. He then compares the clinical picture thus obtained with his background knowledge, and determines which disease pattern best matches that of this patient. During the third step the physician determines the desired therapeutic outcome, and in the fourth he compares this profile with the background knowledge, and he chooses the most suitable treatment from the range of available therapeutic possibilities. Finally he evaluates the intervention, for which he first establishes the clinical picture of the patient and compares this with his background knowledge: a repetition of the first two steps, and he then determines if the therapy is effective. In this step-wise scheme two events are concealed which are crucial with respect to the acquisition of knowledge:

A. (Step 2): $CP(i) = P$: the patient's clinical picture is considered to be the same as a known disease pattern.
When the doctor applies the rule in which $CP(i)$ is the same as the disease profile, he makes a dramatic decision. The deviation of the individual disease pattern from the model profile - which always exists - is regarded as irrelevant. This step implies a critical decision and can always result in a process of reconsideration. There are two possibilities:

1. Change in the disease profile P, mostly in the sense that a subtype of the sickness is created.[33]
2. Anomaly: the deviant nature of the patient's disease pattern is noted but no further action is taken.

B.   (Step 6): Comparison of $CP'(i)$ with $CP(i)$, in which there are two possibilities:
BI. $CP'(i) = CP(i)$: there is no change in the patient's condition.
        Conclusion: the drug is ineffectual.[34]
BII. $CP'(i) \neq CP(i)$: there is a changing clinical picture; the doctor now has to find out the cause of this change:
BIIa: $CP'(i) = N$, in which N is the normal situation: the doctor concludes that the drug concerned was effective.
BIIb: $CP'(i) = Q$, where Q denotes a disease pattern different from P $(P \neq Q)$:

$BIIb_1$: a side effect is produced.[35]
$BIIb_2$: a new disease has appeared in patient (i).[36]
$BIIb_3$: an unexpected effect has appeared in patient (i), that can result in a new therapeutic possibility for drug **x** (also indirectly via drug **y**).

A patient with two illnesses

Up to this point it is assumed that a patient has only one illness. However, it often happens that a patient has two or more complaints simultaneously. The following discusses only one specific situation which is important with respect to new knowledge: a patient has disease Q and R (P = Q ∪ R), he receives drug x for Q, which (unexpectedly) happens to be effective in treating R: a new indication is discovered for **x**.[37]

8.4.4. Accumulated experience and therapeutic intervention

In the previous epistemological analysis patient centred therapy was important. A medical practice, however, consists of a conglomerate of therapeutic interventions. Each treatment adds something new to the already accumulated experience and this experience exceeds that gained from the treatment of one patient. The most simple situation is the comparison of the therapy of two patients. If patient A and B have disease P, and drug x is effective in A but not in B, then the situation needs further examination. If patient A and B are treated with the same drug and both show a undesirable changed clinical picture that can be related to this drug, then these two patients show possibly unsuspected side effects.

In principle these situations don not differ from the observations of therapeutic intervention in the individual patient. At most one can say that two, three, or more of such observations are an extra indication that the background knowledge has to be modified. However, the act of comparison, and the intention to alter or consolidate the background knowledge shows already that a shift in the type of knowledge can occur.

The clinician - or a group of clinicians - could have the experience that in a certain group of patients with drug x, 70% of cases will be helped, while it is generally assumed that it will help in only 40% of the cases, and that the physician should resort to other forms of treatment in the remaining cases. Also a doctor may have experienced that a certain side effect of a drug rarely occurs in his practice or is at least less serious than indicated in the literature. The doctor may also notice that some drugs from a certain group are more effective than others or that some categories of patients respond better to therapy than others.

We can regard this knowledge as an extra layer between the generally accepted scientific knowledge and the diagnostic-therapeutic knowledge based on the individual patient (figure 8.6).

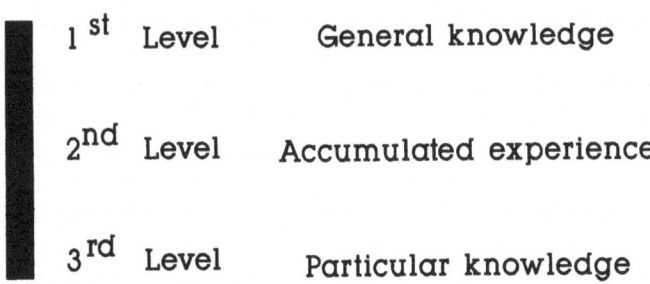

1st	Level	General knowledge
2nd	Level	Accumulated experience
3rd	Level	Particular knowledge

Figure 8.6
Three layers of knowledge in therapeutics.

The second layer is identified as a middle layer because it interacts between particular knowledge and the generally accepted scientific knowledge. Several additional comments are needed with regard to Toulmin's epistemological map. The term "accumulated" refers to the fact that the doctor accumulates experiences with his patients. This term is consciously used to distinguish it from collective knowledge, because he does not concern himself with a population of patients but gains experience with individual patients within this population. This involves particular knowledge; it is not concerned with the case but has a more remote character. One can speak of general knowledge when the accumulated experience is made explicit to illustrate phenomena of a general nature. This occurs also implicitly, because knowledge and experience is exchanged in the social interaction between doctors. Also doctors use this experience to adjust the scientifically determined standard for their practical needs. In this respect it also relates to general knowledge because it serves as a guideline for diagnosis and therapy.

This accumulated experience is the unwritten knowledge in practice, and includes the norms and standards which are generally known but which are not written down. This doesn't mean that this tacit knowledge is not able to be explained. This is contrary to the widely held belief that the very existence of tacit knowledge lies in the fact that it cannot be made explicit. However, there are limits in principle to the degree to which this can occur. There are three questions regarding this tacit knowledge.

(1) How does the doctor arrive at his knowledge in particular cases? Why does he regard one patient differently to another, i.e. why he applies drug x to patient y instead of drug z, which is generally regarded as the correct therapy?

(2) What are the reasons which the doctor can cite for his knowledge? Is the knowledge correct?

(3) What is the nature of the knowledge and the rules which the doctor applies?

The impression is that the uncertainty concerning (1) and (2) and thereby the rejection of "practical knowledge" as inferior to the scientific knowledge, is a barrier to the explication of (3). The same mechanism of gathering knowledge is involved in the accumulated experience, as in the individual-centered therapy. The content of this knowledge is however more elusive; rather we see slowly shifting patterns, i.e. changing knowledge about diseases and drugs. These changes can be characterized with the help of the present model. In addition certain ideas about the "effectiveness" and "ineffectiveness" crystalize out. These terms are put between inverted comma's to indicate the specific character of these ideas:

"In my experience, compound x works better with patients with disease y, if it is given at an early stage in the illness"; "my experience is that, that compound also has an effect on disease y, although it is said to be ineffective". In these opinions, two principles are operational: (1) making similar what was dissimilar before; en (2) making dissimilar what was similar before. These ideas concerning the effectiveness of drugs lead to new categories of knowledge that have not been identified up till now. This knowledge is produced on the basis of a mechanism that has been identified by Bignami under the heading "ex juvantibus logic" - the form of reasoning based on what helps.[38] Bignami gives the following two examples:

first example: *Clinically effective antidepressants modify monoamine metabolism via a blockade of reuptake at terminals, which enhances the availability of given neurotransmitters; therefore, depression may be the consequence of reduced neurotransmitter contents or availability.* **Second example**: *Effective antipsychotic (neuroleptic) agents are powerful dopamine antagonists; therefore, the cause (or primary pathogenetic mechanism) of schizophrenia may reside in a disturbance of dopamine metabolism"* [39]

Etiological or pathogenetic hypotheses are formulated on the basis of whether or not a drug is effective.[40] This form of reasoning plays an ongoing role. When new drugs are developed as an improvement of a known therapy, and have a similar mechanism of action to the original therapy then positive clinical results produce a strengthening of the formulated hypotheses. Another type of argument is also possible. When an etiological theory exists about a certain disease, and a new drug is found, then the evidence of effectiveness of this drug leads to hypotheses concerning the mechanism of action of the drug.

In contrast to the ex juvantibus logic one can also argue from the point of what doesn't help, because evidence of the drug's ineffectiveness can also lead to hypotheses regarding the drug's mechanism of action. In chapter 5 and 7, the simultaneous appearance of the above forms of reasoning have been extensively described, especially by the developments concerning nitroglycerine and dipyridamole. Both drugs, the first judged effective and the last ineffective, were used to decipher the important aspects of the mechanism of action of anti-angina compounds as well as the disease process. New hypotheses concerning the disease and treatment were formulated.

In summary, the following categories of acquiring knowledge in therapeutic interventions can be listed:
a. The discovery of new indications.
b. The discovery of new side effects.
c. The discovery of new aspects of disease: new classifications and the recognition of subtypes.
d. The discovery of effectiveness: responders/non-responders, idiosyncracies, paradoxical reactions, etc.
e. The generation of new insights in the mechanism of drug action.
f. The generation of new insights in the etiology and pathogenesis of the disease.
These categories of gathering new knowledge are not restricted to medical practice. Therapeutic intervention directed to the individual patient can occur in various medical situations, for example during randomized clinical trials or cohort-research; the same applies to accumulated experience. Also the accumulation of new knowledge is not only restricted to physicians. Patients, pharmacists, or scientists who experiment on themselves can arrive at these new discoveries.

8.4.5. Further explication of practice as a source of new knowledge

The classical model of drug development regards medical practice as the end-station in the development process. However, this model also assumes feedback from the medical practice to science. If a drug appears to be effective, then the underlying theories are correct; on the other hand, if the drug is ineffective then one questions the correctness of the scientific ideas.

In this way medical practice separates the chaff from the corn. This reciprocal influencing of science and practice is in conflict with the linearity of the discovery process which lies at the basis of this model. This conflict is solved, when one removes the measurement of effectiveness from medical practice and brings it within the realm of science such as recommended by the proponents of the randomised clinical trial. The practice is therefore the silent follower of science, and has the sole obligation of applying knowledge appropriately.

The dividing line between science and practice is created by the question of testing the effectiveness for a **group** of patients. From the viewpoint of the individual-patient-centred physician this dividing line is inadequate. Although such trials make powerful instruments for testing effectiveness they give no definite answer about the effectiveness of a certain drug in a particular case.

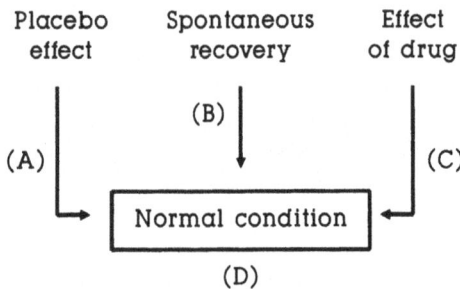

Figure 8.7
Three sources - placebo-effect (A), spontaneous recovery (B) and drug effect (C) - of restoring the pathological condition of the patient to the health state (D).

If the doctor - on the basis of the results of randomized clinical trials - can assume to be giving an effective drug, he can't exclude the possibility that spontaneous recovery or a placebo effect may bring about an improved condition in the patient: if (D), then not necessarily (C) but possibly also (A) or (B). If no improvement occurs in the patient's condition, then the conclusion is justified that giving the drug is not effective. In this case it concerns the knowledge deviating from the scientific standard. The doctor contributes directly to the development of new knowledge.

This conclusion contrasts sharply with the widespread view that the business of discovery lies outside the realm of medical practice. The biological psychiatrist Van Den Hoofdakker has contrasted this attitude in medical practice with that of the laboratory scientist: *"It is not the intention to discover something new in medical practice. It is expected that you recognize what your teachers have already seen. Anything new is a problem and dangerous for a young doctor. He wants a solution, a diagnosis. It is very difficult for him to say: I don't know, I've never seen this before, it's new. In the laboratory I had to search for what had never been seen before. Dare to look, as it were. That was tremendously fascinating...Of course, you cannot look with an untrained, naive eye. Basic knowledge and a pre-programmed vision are necessary. But the scientific approach consists of being able to adjust that vision: O.K. this is our diagnostic eye-glass for the present, but it is not eternal, it changes. It changes only because we dare to look in a different way. That is, after all, the power behind progress, that people dare to look at things differently and don't continue to think that they know it all. If you ask different questions, different truths emerge".* [41]

Medical practice has a negative attitude towards the "new", "unexpected" or "surprising"; and comforts itself with the "familiar" and the "ordinary". This attitude is also reflected in the physician's working methods. The physician makes a provisional diagnosis, a "probability diagnosis", evaluates this on the basis of the result of therapy, and when the treatment gives the desired result, it is concluded that the "correct" diagnosis was made.[42] This is a variant of the ex juvantibus logic. From whatever helps, i.e. in improving the patient's condition, it is concluded that the previously made diagnosis must have been correct. Bignami discusses this form of ex juvantibus logic, and cites the following two examples:*"first example: Patient A, but not B (both clinically depressed) have improved during treatment with drug X (a tricyclic antidepressant); therefore, it appears likely that A's depression is endogenous and B's depression is reactive. Second example: If a severely anxious patient fails to show improvement under a conventional anti-anxiety treatment, but responds well to a neuroleptic (i.e. to an "antipsychotic" agent), there may be a psychotic, rather than a neurotic state underlying the anxiety syndrome"* [43]

In this way, the therapeutic effect settles the diagnostic uncertainty which precedes the treatment. The diagnostic uncertainty is enclosed within step 2 of the diagram illustrating therapeutic treatment. During this step the doctor has to make a decision, based on one or other rule, that the individual patient's deviation from the general disease profile is irrelevant (figure 8.8 (a)).

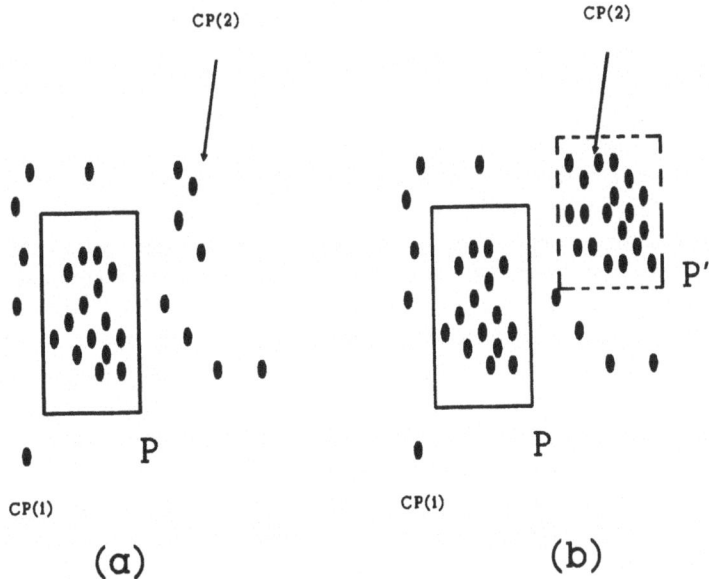

Figure 8.8
The diagnostic-therapeutic situation: a general disease pattern (open box) and the clinical pattern of individual patients (●).

The diagnostic uncertainty concerning patients (1) and (2) with a clinical picture CP is circumnavigated with help from the certainty concerning the therapeutic effect. The apparent certainty of this therapeutic assessment has already been shown. The point is that the deviation of CP(1) and CP(2) from the general disease profile P is not registered. Thereby no account is taken of the diagnostic situation, as shown in figure 8.8 (a), which in practice can appear as depicted in figure 8.8 (b). It appears here that patient (2) belongs to "another group" of patient - but not patient (1). The doctor can only trace P', when he takes deviating disease profiles into account.

This type of ex juvantibus logic does not therefore result in new knowledge. The doctor unconsciously adapts his observations to the background knowledge of known disease profiles. The practice of medicine remains caught in the network of scientific knowledge. Each attempt to escape, to look for "new phenomena" is curtailed. The above form of reasoning therefore, works against the principles of therapeutic practice, that is that each treatment is itself an **experiment**. Countless treatments are initiated by doctors daily. Each treatment implies the chance of deviation from generally accepted knowledge and could lead to new insights.

Here one must be careful because there are many definitions of the concept "experiment" in use. An extensive discussion of treatment and its place in the philosophy of experiment will not be covered here. However, it is useful to briefly examine several contrasting terms. A classic distinction, of course, is between "observation" and "experiment". In an experiment, the reality is consciously and actively manipulated and reduced, it is related to an artificial reality. Observation, on the other hand, focusses on the existing reality. For this reason discoveries in the clinic or general practice are called accidental observations. The term "accidental" then refers to the fact that there is no question of directed search or of a previously stated research goal. However, because in the clinic discoveries are elusive, they are not obvious to the casual observer, and require a receptive mind. Therefore, these clinical discoveries are also often called "serendipitous findings".

The suggestion here then, may be to regard the above examination of therapeutic intervention as a plea for conscious and goal-centered observation or serendipity. This is true, but the terms observation and serendipity are unfortunate. In the first place they carry too much the connotation of detachment and passivity. The gathering of exceptional cases and their possible grouping into new (sub)classes doesn't occur by itself. The doctor has to use criteria to decide which cases he will include and which he will exclude from the selected group. These criteria are partly established during the evaluation of the results of medical therapy. In this respect the term serendipity is preferable to observation. In another respect both terms are equally incorrect because of the passive connotation. These terms imply an "existing" reality, but in fact they involve a conscious action to artificially change this reality, i.e. the intervention in the pathological condition of the patient.[44]

In, what shall for convenience be called the "new philosophy of the experiment", this creative aspect of the experiment is emphasized. This means, as Hacking says, *"the purification and keeping stable of phenomena that in their pure state don't exist anywhere in the universe"*. [45] As an example he gives the transplantation of parts of the human immune system into mice, which was reported at the end of 1988 by two American research groups. This example illustrates the fact that experiments often do not work - many laboratories have tried to do the same -

and especially that a unique system is created: a human immune system that survives in another species has never existed in our universe before.[46]

Superficially, therapeutic treatment appears to differ from the above because it is meant to create a situation which has already been reproduced thousands of times in the laboratory. However, treatment itself creates a unique situation because the intervention in a particular patient induces a situation which has never before existed. In addition, as Wieland has shown, the essence of therapy is in fact, that it is a single event: it is irreversible.[47] Therapy, however, is directed to the individual patient, and is not aimed at generally occurring phenomena, which are central to the scientific experiment. However, if we look at therapeutic intervention at the level of the middle layer of knowledge - the accumulated knowledge - then this is the case. As already pointed out, the patient populations, with which doctors come in contact in general practice, differ from those in the hospital, and these differ again from those in the clinical experiment. In this sense all therapeutic intervention, individual and collective, breaks through all the scientifically established frames of reference.

Therapeutic intervention aimed at the individual patient is a journey through new and unknown territory with the help of a compass provided by science. The goal, of course, is to make a once only journey through this unknown landscape, not to make a map. But this territory is not an existing reality because it is partly created by the treatment. In the accumulated experience in relation to the therapeutic intervention, however, it is exploration of this unknown landscape that is important. Moreover, the compass of science becomes adjusted in order to adequately carry out the patient centred therapy. This adjustment implies an attempt to create a stable situation.[48]

8.5. Conclusions

The model in this thesis has been developed as an aid to the historical description of the development of the beta blockers and the calcium antagonists. In this sense it is a descriptive instrument, and the underlying theory can be regarded as a descriptive theory. In addition, it offers good possibilities for expressing conceptual problems in drug research. It can be used for example in the classification of disease and of (classes of) drugs; in describing the relationship between profiles and theories about the disease mechanism and the mechanism of drug action; in the role of therapeutic goals in the profiling of drugs and disease; in the profiling of diseases and treatment in practice; and in the further unravelling of the process of drug discovery. Finally, this current theory can be useful in the search for and development of expert systems in diagnostics and therapy.

Mention has been made of two critical limits to the developed model, that of the epistemological status of profiles and the (im)possibility of making knowledge fully explicit.

Further, the way in which medical practice, i.e. individual and collective therapeutic intervention, contributes to the growth of medical knowledge is discussed. Interpretations of discoveries in medical practice as "chance" events are incorrect. They don't do credit to the sense of curiosity and receptiveness which is necessary to recognise new phenomena concerning disease or drugs. In this respect the term "serendipitous findings" is more apt. But even this term denies the active and creative character of treatment. Each therapeutic action extends the scientific frame of reference and repeatedly shifts the limits of knowledge; a sometimes restrictive but usually expansive process. Therapeutically, intervening is like the sea which continuously changes the coastline of scientific progress. This may be very slight or suddenly very drastic; it may reduce the coastline or extend it. The recognition of these changing coastlines is a major task in the discovery of drugs. The changing frontier of medical progress depends not only on fundamental developments in the land of science but also on the changing tides of medical practice.

Chapter 9. The enigma of drug discovery

It is generally thought that we are on the eve of a new pharmaceutical revolution, and that the fundamental developments in molecular biology, genetics and biotechnology will soon bear fruit. In this sense it seems as though the "knowledge gap hypothesis" which attributed the decline in drug innovation in the 1960s and 1970s to a lack of fundamental knowledge may prove to be historically correct. The idea that complicated diseases can only be understood and treated at the bio-molecular level is becoming more widely accepted.[1] The quest for greater understanding in pathophysiology has led to increased molecular-level experimentation that should allow the drug designer and the biologist to make progress.[2] Considering the expansive growth in medical theory, the fundamental role played by medical-pharmaceutical practice in the drug discovery process might be regarded as in danger of becoming an anachronism. This view however is not only incorrect but also dangerous. It contradicts past events and misses the essence of the drug discovery process. It is also a threat to the development of new medical therapies. Because of the strong attractive power of this bio-molecular reductionist thought - in this respect there would seem to be a return of the classic view of drug discovery - it is worthwhile examining and clarifying anew the important role of medical-pharmaceutical practice.

The relationship of medical-pharmaceutical practice with fundamental developments in biomedical science

The claim that the rapid developments in the biomedical sciences throw benefits in the direction of drug research has often been made. However, this claim is vague and can be better understood through recent research in the philosophy of science. The following appraisal of scientific theory is based on Zandvoort and the Starnberg group.[3]

In the modern post-Kuhn philosophy of science the development of scientific knowledge is studied with the help of large analytical units, such as research programs and scientific paradigms rather than statements, hypotheses or simple theories.[4] The Starnberg group formulated a three phase model in which the developments in science are divided into a pre-paradigmatic, paradigmatic and post-paradigmatic phase based on Kuhn's paradigm theory.[5] In the first phase, the use of scientific concepts is tied to rules, there emerge fixed procedures for conducting experiments and the data is systematically ordered and evaluated. In this stage the definition of the research area is of major importance and fundamental theories are developed which compete with each other until one remains. In the second, paradigmatic phase in principle the fundamental problems in the area of research have been solved and work can continue on filling in the theory. The construction of Watson and Crick's alpha-helix model and the subsequent research into the structure of the human genetic material could be regarded as a paradigmatic period. This period includes a phase of "normal science" in which scientists work on recognizable problems which however require great resources of creativity and perseverance. In Kuhn's model this phase leads to many anomalies, in which the principle paradigm finally suffers its demise. Subsequently a crisis develops and after a stormy passage a new paradigm emerges. In the model of the

Starnberg group, the third, post-paradigmatic phase covers the period of so-called "mature" theories which can in principle be applied to practical problems. This maturity means that the fundamental theory on which scientists have worked has been found sufficiently adequate for the study and explanation of events in a particular area.

With the help of this three-phase model, the Starnberg group tried to give concrete form to their view that scientific development doesn't proceed autonomously, but that there are alternatives and the route chosen by scientists is partly determined by external, social factors. They point out a "third way" in science policy between the planners and the defenders of scientific freedom. At a particular moment, planning or guiding with a view to external goals has preference and at another, autonomous development is preferred, depending on the stage of development of the particular discipline.[6] In the pre-paradigmatic phase one can only profit from ad-hoc findings, in the following phase there is little to direct, because the development of the theory follows internally developed lines determined by scientists, and in the last phase the internal dynamics of science weakens and external goals determine the development of the theory. This last process is called finalization, and is literally "goal-directed".[7] External goals become internalised in the development of the discipline, in such a way that they form guidelines for the theoretical development within the discipline.

A standard example is plasma physics. When the crash program to use nuclear fusion for the generation of energy was unsuccessful in the early 1950s, scientists realised that greater insight into plasma physics was needed and research was stimulated. The developments initiated bore all the characteristics of fundamental research except that the direction was partly determined by the goal, i.e. to carry out controlled nuclear fusion. The inclusion of this goal into plasma physics generated questions of how to bring plasma to a sufficiently high temperature and how it could be stabilized. The subsequent theoretical and experimental investigations are automatically relevant for the stated goal.[8]

The criticism of this model, amongst others, must be that a too direct connection is imagined between internal and external goals. Armed with this criticism, Zandvoort has creatively reformulated the theory of the Starnberg group within a general model of scientific development, in which the interdisciplinary co-operation between research programs are taken as a starting point. Co-operation in modern science rests on the fact that some programs are directed towards problems which are provided by other programs. The first are the so-called **guide**-programs and the second the **supply**-programs. Examples of guide programs can be found in molecular biology which can be regarded as guides for the supply programs from chemistry and physics. Both sorts of programs have an internal development, but they are mutually interdependent. Supply programs rely partly on the problems found in other areas for their development, while the guide programs are dependant on specific concepts and instruments supplied by other programs for their further development.[9]

With this view, two goals are postulated in the discipline of science: intrinsic and extrinsic success. A research program has intrinsic success, when it is able to give an answer to self generated problems and to work out fundamental theories in a progressive series each being more successful than its predecessor. In addition the program has extrinsic success when it contributes to the development of other research programs. In this way Zandvoort solves an important philosophical problem, i.e. the justification of the scientists' decision to continue the research program, even if there is stagnation in solving the theoretical and experimental problems within this program. The development of the research programs can now be regarded as a sequence of intrinsic and extrinsic phases. In the intrinsic phase, the hard core of theoretical assumptions are formed and developed and, then the specific theories or experimental methods are supplied which contribute to the solving of problems elsewhere in the field of science.

The cognitive structure of scientific development can be described in more detail, and roughly two types of situations can occur (figure 9.1).

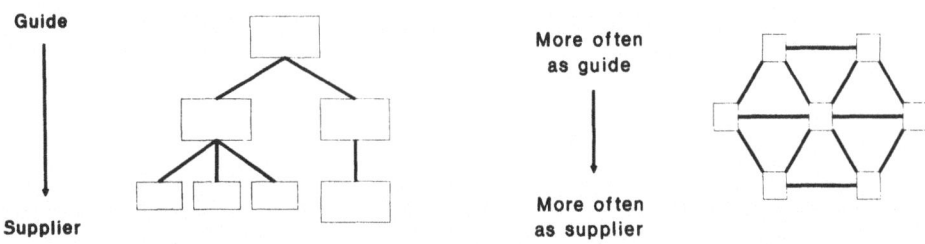

Figure 9.1
The relationships between supply and guide research programs in science: a hierarchical model (a) and an interaction model (b).
Reproduced with permission from Zandvoort (1986).

In the hierarchical model an asymmetrical guide-supply relationship occurs. In other words, one research program always serves as a guide for one or more research programs which in turn can become guide programs for others. In the interaction model research programs can function alternatively as guide or supplier for each other.

The claim that the fundamental developments in the biological sciences shall lead to new drugs in the near future can be more closely examined in the light of Zandvoort's model. The biomedical sciences have powerful theories which can serve as the starting point for the development of new drugs, for example in the disciplines of immune-modulation and gene therapy. The present day excitement in the pharmaceutical world, would seem to have a legitimate epistemological basis. The biological sciences function as a guide on the one hand for physics and chemistry and on the other for drug research. However, this claim is not tenable when proposed as such.

Although it may be true that research programs in molecular biology, immunology, and molecular genetics have an exclusive guide function for physics and chemistry - and even this has to be doubted - they simultaneously form supply programs for anatomy, biochemistry, physiology and clinical science. Also these research programs interact with each other but an absolute hierarchy in which one or several programs function as guide for all the others can't be shown. The present state of affairs in biomedical science is characterized rather by the interaction model. The advantage of Zandvoort's model is that the structural situation in the present biomedical sciences, such as included in the claim, can be specified, and also empirically investigated. In addition one can provide fundamental arguments why drug research will most likely remain structured according to the interaction model.

The biological sciences provide supply programs for industrial research. These industrial research programs can be taken as specific forms of research programs, i.e. **design**-programs.[10] In stead of describing, explaining and predicting events, the main concern of research programs is the development of drugs to alleviate disease. In this case "disease" and "therapy" are the orientation points. Not only medical theory but also medical practice changes these orientation points, as already shown in this study. For this purpose, the concept of "science" has been extended in order to explain the now anachronistic ways of gaining knowledge in medicine, such as casuistic and clinical experience in therapeutic intervention.[11] If the claim presented here and which currently enjoys popularity in the pharmaceutical sector should fail to recognize that medical practice moves with the times then this claim will itself become an anachronism.

Two additional comments are important. Firstly, the claim above includes a normative judgment; that medical theory should be a guide to the biomedical sciences. This implies an opinion about the development of knowledge which is untenable because the interrelationships between medical theory, experiment and practice are multiform. An argument against this is that rejection of a normative judgment on empirical grounds is not conclusive. However, if the judgment is also not realistic then such a judgment loses also its credibility and its right to existence.

Secondly, consider the fundamental point that medical practice sets the norm for what is understood by "disease" and "suitable therapy". Although medical science provides information for setting these norms, in fact it takes place in medical practice. Directly or indirectly, medical practice passes on an evaluation to medical science and that evaluation implies a judgment of which processes are healthy and which pathological, and in which processes intervention is required. Also from this normative aspect, practice functions as a guide for medical theory and drug research.[12]

Three Essentials of Drug Discovery

In the above, the nucleus of the discovery process has not been characterized in detail. For this, attention is drawn to the main principle behind the molecular-biological-reductionist claim, which can be stated as follows:

"For the development of new drugs it is necessary to uncover the secrets of human nature. The search has to penetrate deeper and deeper into the human organism to unravel the biochemical interactions at the cellular, intra-cellular and most importantly at the molecular level. In this way stronger and more selective drugs are developed"

The above appears to leave no room for the influence of medical practice. However, appearances are deceptive because with the aid of the philosophical knife this principle can be split into three essential elements of the drug discovery process and in each element medical practice is an essential component.

Fundamental theories such as the oncogen theory in cancer research and the antibody-antigen theory in immunology can lead to deeper knowledge and better explanations of the essential processes in the human organism. Such theories reveal deeper lying structures which are the basis for the observed symptoms, i.e. the diagnosed disease.[13]

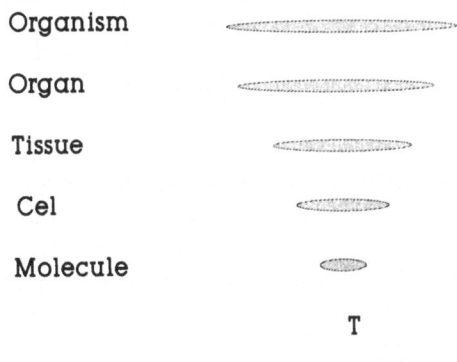

Organism

Organ

Tissue

Cel

Molecule

T

Figure 9.2   (Theory)
Hierarchical levels with respect to the human organism.

The above principle can now be reformulated: "For the development of new, powerful and selective drugs it is necessary to evolve theories which give a continually "deeper" explanation of the processes which take place at higher levels in the organism". If theory T_2 is more fundamental than T_1, then this reformulated principle implies that T_2 contains a longer and more complex chain of causal events than T_1 (figure 9.3).

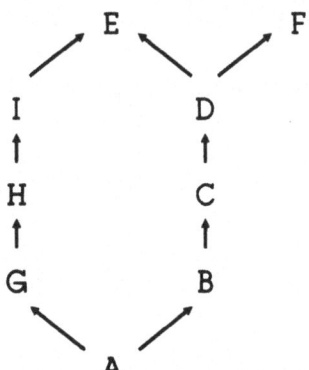

Figure 9.3
Chains of causal events in the human organism.

Theory T_1 explains the chain B - C - D·(E/F) and T_2 explains the chains A - G - H - I -(E) and A - B - C - D - (E/F). Link A involves a physiological mechanism at a deeper level, in which two series of physiological processes, which were previously regarded as independent from each other, have now received a common explanation. From the point of scientific explanation this can be called **convergence**.

At the same time the number of possibilities for intervention increases. If E represents a disease, then in principle the range of possibilities for intervention is increased because there is an increase from 3 to 7 possible points for manipulation. From the viewpoint of treatment possibilities, i.e. the number of possibilities to intervene in the disease process, the term **divergence** is used.

This explanation is actually too simple because **selectivity** also plays a role, which can be illustrated by a simple example. If drug **x** inhibits D and thereby blocks E (a pathological process), but also induces F through which an undesired effect appears, then **y** is a more selective drug than **x**, if **y** blocks E but doesn't induce F.[14] The new theory T_2 enables scientists via chain A - G - H - I to influence disease E without inducing F. There is thus no question of a simple increase from three to seven possibilities. None the less scientists possess more possibilities for intervention in the disease than before. The value of fundamental theories such as the hypothetical theory T_2, is that they can make clear why certain paths followed by drug researchers lead to a dead end. Theory T_2 explains, for example, why fundamental limits exist to the route of influencing disease process E via the chain of physiological events B - C - D.

However, there is also a dilemma in the fact that more fundamental theories explain more, but simultaneously offer more points of entry for the development of selective drugs. Although scientists know what they should no longer try, it is not clear what they should try. The juxtaposition of theory and therapy creates a solution to this dilemma. The drug functions as a reference point because judgment about the effects and side-effects offer points of contact for creating selective mechanisms of action. Where fundamental theories lead to completely new working principles the process often turns out to be aimless, until a new therapy with clinical relevance can function as a point of reference. Until such a therapy is found, existing treatments function as reference points in the investigation.

The above epistemological comment gives only a general idea of the contrast between convergence and divergence. However, numerous examples from drug research suggest that it is useful to think further along these lines. The discovery of dopamine as a neurotransmitter enabled scientists to explain psychiatric and neurological complaints and to develop suitable therapies. Subsequently dopamine regulated systems have been shown to be the basis of communication processes in more places than was originally supposed. The development of interferon shed new light on complaints such as flu, colds and cancer. In the meantime more than 20 types have been discovered and appear to be involved in more than two hundred biological processes, e.g. regulation of inflammation, interference with cell growth and differentiation, immune-modulation, etc. In both examples one can see convergence on the theoretical side and divergence on the practical side, i.e. the therapeutic aspect. This mutual tension between convergence and divergence is the first essential of drug discovery.

The examples of dopamine and interferon reveal a second essential of drug discovery. Dopamine and interferon are not only valuable points of contact for influencing pathological processes but they are also involved in a large number of normal events in the organism. The deeper researchers delve into the organism, the more vague becomes the distinction between "normal" and "pathological". The development of the oncogen theory illustrates this.

In the regulation of the growth of animal and human cells, certain protein hormones, called growth factors, play an important role. Specific genes are responsible for the production of these growth factors for the regulation of cell growth and are therefore called "regulatory genes". Mutations or other lesions of these regulatory genes ("proto-oncogens") lead to disturbed regulatory genes ("oncogens") which transform the normal cell into a cancer cell. The oncogen-theory reduces the question "What is the cause of cancer?" to "How do regulatory genes change into oncogens?". The discovery that very small pieces of DNA could cause unlimited cell growth was a breakthrough in cancer research and the oncogen theory was a driving force in that field of investigation. An obstacle to the further development of this theory is the fact that the steering role of these regulatory genes and their products, the growth factors, takes place within a complex cascade of biochemical and physiological processes both in and outside the cell.[15] To unravel these complex cascades it is necessary to distinguish between normal and deviating regulatory mechanisms at various levels.

Looked at as a reduction-problem - reduction is when processes at one level are explained with the help of knowledge and principles from a lower level - the following can be seen, i.e. that the oncogen-theory offers fruitful perspectives to explain pathological processes at higher levels, but it cannot "reduce" these in its own terms; in other words, this perspective cannot yet be verified.[16] There could be two reasons for this. Firstly, the formulated theory is inadequate, and secondly, the theory is adequate, "mature" in terms of the Starnberg group, but it has to be applied to complex processes at higher levels. Most likely, scientists would say that elements of both were involved but for the present it is assumed that the theory is sufficiently adequate. This then, implies that the theoretical knowledge collected at the deepest level has to be transferred to the higher levels.

The Starnberg group has proposed two types of transfer mechanisms, i.e. **coincidence** and **transfer** research.[17] Coincidence research means use is made of suitable experimental systems - relatively simple, intensively studied and providing penetrating insights - in which fundamental and specific problems can be worked on simultaneously. An example is the virus system, e.g. phages, which negotiate between cell biology and tumour virology. Other examples are certain tumour cells or systems of blood forming cells in cancer research, and the special cell systems of the immune defense system. In transfer research on the other hand, use is made of more "complex" or "dirty" systems, e.g. cell cultures of epidemiologically relevant tumors or in vitro cultured tumour cell lines from individual patients. Such systems are imminently suitable for transferring the results of fundamental research to clinically relevant phenomena, and to determine experimental parameters necessary for the development of specific therapeutic methods or in which to place fundamental concepts into the clinical setting.

The importance of these distinctions is that between the opposing poles of "fundamental" and "applied" a stepwise system of transfer mechanisms is spread out.[18] In walking this ladder, fundamental forefront research changes gradually via the interrelated development of fundamental and applied research questions to applied research. Research moves from the theory to become more and more involved in the practice. This account encompasses an ingenious proposal to conceptualize science, at least along certain rungs of this ladder, as a process in which theory and application oriented research proceed hand in hand.

However, the disadvantage of this view is that the fundamental theory acts as the centripetal force. But there are other possibilities. The major flaw is the assumption of the presence of such a fundamental theory. The **genesis** of a fundamental theory in which completely different transfer mechanisms can occur remains outside this discussion. Most probably, the transfer mechanism is an iterate process in which scientists send information collected at one level through to theory and concept forming at another level and back again. Scientists refer to this situation. To unravel the cascade of physiological events the critical difference between normal and pathological has to be continually (re)interpreted. The stepwise system as sketched by the Starnberg group, functions therefore more like a two-way street.[19]

Looked at from this development perspective the transfer of knowledge between the different levels plays a crucial but undervalued role in the biomedical sciences. This is certainly true for the drug discovery process. Who ever develops a new drug, whenever a new theory is developed, is too late. Therein lies the essential tension of drug discovery. In such a situation industrial scientists should close the "gaps" in the causal chain of pathological processes by drawing together the available information regarding the mechanisms at different levels. A good example is the development of zimelidine, an anti-depressive drug, described by Carlsson.[20]

At the end of the sixties and beginning of the seventies Carlsson and his group developed new in vivo methods for measuring norepinephrine (NE) and 5-hydroxytryptamine (5-HT) re-uptake in the brains of intact animals. In this manner they discovered, according to their report, that tri-cyclic anti-depressants not only blocked NE-re-uptake as already known, but also the 5-HT-re-uptake which was not known. Also they made the remarkable observation that within the group of tri-cyclic anti-depressants the tertiary group differed from the secondary group. The tertiary group showed a stronger effect on the 5-HT-re-uptake than on the NE-re-uptake, while the opposite was true for the secondary group.

This discovery, a distinction in properties of compounds at the biochemical and pharmacological level, enabled the group to link the chemical distinction, i.e. between tertiary and secondary amines, to profiling in clinical practice. An important aspect of this clinical profiling was that tertiary tri-cyclic amines were preferred in the clinic. Although the reason was not completely clear, this preference was possibly due to the lower degree of psychomotor activity of the tertiary amines.[21] As Carlsson notes: *"Based on the different biochemical and clinical profiles of the tricyclic antidepressiva, we suggested that norepinephrine might be especially involved in the control of psychomotor activity and 5-HT in the control of mood. We were of course aware of the fact that such a statement necessarily is an oversimplification; nevertheless, it may have heuristical value".* [22]

The zimelidine story illustrates that a link in profiling occurs in the development of a drug in research as well in the clinic. In this two way traffic, the transfer of knowledge cannot take place directly such as is the case in coincidence research. An important means of transfer is the drug itself. Drugs are not only a suitable means for selectively blocking or stimulating a certain process at a certain place in the organism, and for gathering new knowledge about the normal and pathological processes. They also enable scientists to pinpoint the induced effects within a working pattern. From this pattern the significance of new effects can be seen, and the effects in turn help explain the pattern. Differences in working patterns, e.g. which were previously not understood, can now be interpreted. These distinctions played a significant role in the history of zimelidine. Also "practical" knowledge concerning the different effects of the anti-depressants proved to be very important.

These distinctions originate on the dividing line between general and particular knowledge. This brings us to the third essential of drug discovery: the drug as general technological principle and as therapy for the individual patient.

The previous chapter contains a discussion of how new distinctions arise and how new knowledge is created through reflection on therapeutic intervention. Treatment takes place in a field of tension in which the knowledge goal of theory and practice meet each other. In the theory patient and drug appear as objects of general knowledge, in the practice as object of particular knowledge. While in the theory the general event appears as departure and end point, in practice it functions as starting point, or rather, as orientation point. Because the doctor during consultation pays attention to all the factors which can influence the patient's condition, he deviates from that orientation point, but he returns in two ways. Firstly, he comes back to it by reducing the patient to a "type", to a general pattern stored in his background knowledge. The general event then serves as orientation point in evaluating the therapy, in which the doctor again reduces the patient to a type.

In this twofold movement, the drug is of equal importance. During the first movement, the doctor establishes which changes in the patient's world, which is in turn reduced to the general world, are desirable. Afterwards he determines if the desired changes have indeed occurred. It is true that the drug then appears as a general object, i.e. as a type of technical means, which is thought to induce the desired pattern, though in the particular case ("casus") itself it is this particular drug, which here and now, in its special form, and with its peculiarities that produces its effect.[23]

During this double movement the orientation point itself is adjusted and the related new experiences are stored in a separate layer of knowledge. In this way the doctor gains experience with the chosen orientation points, the disease as well as the drug.[24] It is known that a conceptual framework precedes therapeutic intervention. It is however not well recognised that this framework for medical thinking and treatment is not only supplied from the theory but also as a result of practical experience. That the adjusted compass often appears aimless, that it directs treatment in the wrong directions does not detract from it. Against this background the concept of selectivity has a different meaning. This concept is stretched out between the general and the particular object which form poles supporting the thread on which the dance of drug discovery occurs. At one pole, is the drug which is the most suitable general pattern that scientists can conceive. At the other is the particular pattern which is most suitable for that individual patient. If this second pole is extended to its limit, then the goal of drug discovery is the development of the best therapy for the individual patient. This goal, however, forms a hypothetical point. In reality, one has to proceed from a general type in the discovery process. The practicing physician finds himself in this vacuum between the real and the hypothetical. He floats between reality and utopia. The result is however that the physician continually judges selective working patterns, and tries to modify them. At one extreme, selectivity means that in a general way drug A sufficiently blocks process **p**, but then not too strongly, and gently adjusts process **q**; without interfering with the other processes at this level, etc. At the other end of this spectrum selectivity implies that compound A in a particular case sufficiently blocks **p** in this patient, etc. Here selectivity implies a never to be realized goal, and the doctor judges this working pattern in a concrete case. Related experiences lead to a new categorization of the group of patients who are eligible for treatment.

Knowledge about selective patterns comes from activity at both ends. At one end, a general principle is created, and one speaks of **generalization**, while at the other the principle is applied and specified and may be called **particularization**. This tension between generalization and particularization is the third essential of drug discovery.

The diagnosis of Gross can also be understood in this light when he states *"that progress in medicine and in understanding the pathogenesis of disease is far behind our knowledge in biology. We have also to accept that the diagnoses made often refer to quite heterogeneous types of disease, but we do not know how to differentiate them, so we have big baskets in which we put together all possible types of regulatory disturbances. This is one of the shortcomings of clinical medicine".* [25]

The growing discrepancy between biological and clinical research does not come from a lack of fundamental knowledge but from the lack of directed application of it. In other words, there is no lack of theories, i.e. of generalization, but of serious practice, i.e. of particularization. Through the universal pretensions of clinical research and the large scale operations in the pharmaceutical sector, the importance of this fundamental activity in medical practice has been lost.

If one claims that the clinician is too occupied with techniques instead of the patient, too much with signs instead of symptoms, and too much with biochemical and physiological parameters instead of clinically relevant data such as the natural course of the disease and the effect of the subsequent treatment, then of course one is right. Generally, one creates the contradiction that the "technical" pole of the above dichotomies - techniques, signs and parameters - is interesting from the scientific point of view, but that the "clinical" pole is of direct importance for the clinician himself, and for the patient. The clinician as researcher is best for scientific research as the doctor is for the patient. The dilemma for the clinician is, as Barber stated *"to be a discoverer in science and to be a physician who treats his patients humanely".* [26] This common distinction between the role of scientist and physician signifies the field of tension in which the clinician operates. The epistemological structure of this field, however, is much more complex. Right across this field run three trails which have been called here the essentials of drug discovery.

The basic structure of gathering knowledge in medicine exists in the transferral of knowledge along these trails, not from point to point but in both directions. Penetrating deeper into biochemical processes produces insights, but also more chaos, in terms of treatment possibilities and in the critical ratio of signal to noise, with respect to what should be interpreted as normal or pathological. Clinically and in general practice, the compounds relevant for intervention in pathological processes have to be determined, each with its own mix of physical-chemical, biochemical and pharmacological properties. In this way medical practice not only creates order in the growth of medical knowledge, but also chaos. Through the unobtainable goal which medical practice has set itself, i.e. to choose the best treatment for the individual patient, it exceeds the limits of knowledge. In this way, medical practice is lost without the compass supplied by research. However, this compass is itself adjusted by therapeutic experiences which give rise to new orientation points for medical theory.

The key lies therefore not in the medical theory or in practice, but in their relation to one another. To paraphrase Immanuël Kant: "The growth of medical knowledge is empty without theory and blind without practice, and it is just as empty without practice as blind without the theory".

The role of practice in drug discovery reviewed

The concept of transmission of information lies at the basis of the classic view of drug discovery. Until the 1950s, direct testing of the imagined clinical relevance of biochemical, physiological and pharmacological drug profiles was always possible in the clinic. In this fertile climate in the 1940s and 1950s the "Golden Age of Drug Discovery" grew to full glory. The process of innovation consisted of a limited number of links; the distance between laboratory and clinic was short. The value of this system is that the exchange of information between laboratory and clinic is so rapid. From this angle one can understand present day developments in the pharmaceutical sector. The criticisms of the rules regarding clinical research are basically that the process of innovation should be shortened or speeded up. The common practice of introducing new drugs in categories of seriously ill patients should be regarded in the same way. These groups of patients are an important sluiceway in the system of rules and ethics, through which the development of a new therapy can become accelerated. Furthermore, the specific regulations for introducing new drugs from recombinant-DNA technology, immunology and biotechnology into the clinic as fast as possible are also based on the speedy exchange of information.[27]

The excitement about the nearby emergence of a new pharmaceutical era creates a climate in which the shortening or speeding up of the development process becomes the main goal. Then there is a danger of a return to the classic vision of the discovery process, in part due to a romantic longing for the glorious past. This is a threat, not only because the classical vision disguises the commercial driving force - large investments have to be recovered - as a result of which ethics and the patient have to make way for new products of research and technology the value of which are unknown. But also, because it doesn't recognize the far-reaching epistemological changes which are taking place in present biomedical research. Three fundamental changes can be listed.

1. The distance between the laboratory and the clinic, and from there to general practice has become larger because of the set of regulations and ethical standards relating to clinical-

experimental research. However, it is also due to the explosive growth of the discipline and the structural changes in the industrial research process. In addition, the chronic diseases present structurally different problems to medical science. This has been so often stated that it is almost a commonplace, but something of importance cannot be repeated often enough. The point is that the course of these diseases is spread over a long time period. This causes difficult problems with respect to the end points of prognosis and therapy: they are complex and difficult to measure. Also it takes the time period of a generation of doctors and patients to study the natural course of these diseases.

In view of the expansive growth of the chains of medical knowledge, shortening or speeding up the knowledge process should not be the main goal, but rather the control of the quality of the information. Admitting new results of biomedical science too quickly or not well thought through leads to a disruption in the critical balance between signal and noise in medical research. As long as one interprets the setting of standards as holding back science, as protecting patients against the dangers of medical technology or as embanking the unchecked growth of industrial research, one forgets the enormous importance for the growth of knowledge itself. The present discussions about the standards set for clinical-experimental research should therefore not take place outside the discipline but at the centre of it. Moreover, when these discussions are restricted to the limits of the research centres, which are supposed to function as "testing ground" and "passage way" for medical practice, one fails to see not only the essence of therapeutic intervening but also the practice as a rich foundation of research. One doesn't catch fish by closing one or two holes in the net but by throwing out a strong and large net at the right place, and medical practice is a rich fishing territory.

2. The classical vision fails to appreciate that the nature of medical therapy changes. More powerful and selective compounds possess a broad working spectrum, and in principle are considered for ever more indications. The fact that a drug is developed and marketed for a certain indication, simply means that one specific working pattern, i.e. one compound, has been selected from a large number of possibilities. In other words, from a large selection of working characteristics, the wished for effect, the main effect is selected out from the other undesirable effects, the side effects. Mutatis mutandis the same applies to the wished for structural characteristics of the therapy. The compound is the result of a research process in which the desired properties are achieved and the undesired eliminated as much as possible. One should not be surprised that the same compound later appears to be also suitable for indication B, C or Z, but in fact this continues to create a surprised reaction. Very many "discoveries" - and many more than reported in the literature - occur after the drug is already on the market. The beta blockers and the calcium antagonists are an example of this.

This is the reason this thesis is titled "Drugs Looking for Diseases". The title refers to the fact that we increasingly have the situation where drugs are searching for the right indications. The development of the drug doesn't stop the moment it appears on the market but in fact is just beginning. There are also critics who regard current research in the clinic as a world wide "human pharmacological" experiment; and they are correct.[28] But this "human pharmacological" experiment takes place on a much larger scale than most people realize because it stretches to include medical practice itself. Recognition of this phenome-non and the striving for an improvement in patient-bound and practice-orientated research offer a more realistic solution than the attempt to force drug research back into the laboratory or the specialized clinical research centre.

3. The classical vision leaves insufficient room for the far-reaching changes in clinical and general medical practice. These are the fast and widespread introduction of computerized information systems, data bases, algorithm procedures and decision-making techniques in medical-pharmaceutical practice. The fact that dichotomies such as science-art, qualitative-quantitative, ratio-intuition and objective-subjective repeatedly spring up, betrays the fact that the available epistemological vocabulary is too limited to indicate the far-reaching changes. On Toulmin's map they are to be seen as new relationships between theory and practice. Undoubtedly information science, data bases and new research approaches in post-marketing-surveillance create new possibilities for unravelling patterns of knowledge concerning disease and therapy which are created in the practice itself.

This study attempts to show how clinic and general medical practice provide an important contribution to knowledge of pathophysiology and the mechanism of action of drugs. This contribution comes not only from experimental research but also via the clinical-epidemi-ological and patient-bound research and in the therapeutic application itself. Following from this one can expect that patient-bound research in practice, drug utilization studies (pharmaco-epidemiology) and post-marketing-surveillance studies will lead to new insights in disease mechanisms, working patterns and side effects.

In this sense, practice reclaims that which it had lost, the generation of knowledge while therapeutically intervening in the pathological condition of the patient. It goes without saying that this therapeutic intervention remains imprisoned in the no man's land between general and particular knowledge, between the real and the hypothetical. And that this no man's land sets a critical limit to medical research. During their journey doctors will find other answers at different times and in different places. This cultural variation is no obstacle to research, rather a source of inspiration for new ideas. It also forms a contact point of new research. This chapter ends therefore in wholehearted agreement with Payer's conclusion about wide cultural differences in treatment:

> "..the different ways that different countries treat the same disease constitute a
> sort of natural experiment; yet because most people are unaware of the
> experiment in the first place, they are unable to draw the conclusions that might
> result. For example, French doctors have widely prescribed calcium for a number
> of years, and a closer examination of osteoporosis rate there might help illuminate
> the role of calcium in this disease. As a corollary, a greater understanding of
> medical culture bias might predict the country in which side effects will first
> surface - or will be hidden" [29]

Notes

References

Appendices

Notes

Notes Introduction

1. Comroe (1978), p. 933.
2. Rosenberg (1977), p. 485. Recently, however, therapeutics is increasingly becoming a subject of interest to the historian; see Warner (1986).
3. Kuipers (1988).
4. Mol and Lieshout (1989). See also the approach followed by Vos and Willems (1988), (1989); this is in accordance with the "empirical turn" in the philosophy of science.
5. De Jong (1988).
6. This also requires the interdisciplinary co-operation between philosophers, historians and scientists which is realized in the foundation of the International Institute for Theoretical Cardiology in 1984. The institute has organized several symposia and studies on topics of interest to cardiology. This has formed a source of inspiration and a fertile intellectual climate for this project.
7. See Hunter (1989) for the term science of individuals. See for references with respect to the other terms Hucklenbroich (1981).

Notes Chapter 1.

1. Quoted from Mulrow et al. (1984).
2. A placebo is an inert substance such as a sugar pill or a saline injection.
3. Lasagna (1973), p. 92.
4. Lasagna (1973), p. 94.
5. Lewis (1930), p. 479.
6. MRC (1948). The field seemed to be ripe for an intervention because D'Arcy Hart reported the emergence of "a general and probably healthy reaction among clinicians against drugs in tuberculosis, apart from a few valued symptomatics. The lack of a scientific basis for most of the traditional empirical 'specifics' ...had won more or less general acceptance among the medical profession, with their consequent virtual disappearance from therapeutics" (D'Arcy Hart (1946), p. 809). See further Green (1954).
7. Cf. Hill (1983).
8. Several reports, e.g. on PAS and isoniazid appeared in the early 1950s in the British Medical Journal.
9. Cf Fletcher et al. (1981); Hill (1983); Horwitz (1987); Lilienfeld (1982); Mulrow et al. (1984).
Though precise data about manpower, economics and the number specialised institutions are not available, this area dramatically expanded during the past decades. Controlled clinical trials, as Lilienfeld comments, "now constitute a major research area with its own methods and problems. The extent of their importance is indicated by the fact that, in 1979, a Society for Clinical Trials with its own scientific journal was established in the United States" (Lilienfeld (1982), p.1).
Hill labeled the evolution of the controlled clinical trial as a "clinical trials industry": "There is no doubt that this is a real phenomenon. In North America alone, the funding of clinical trials by industry, government and charitable foundations probably exceeds $100 million a year. A plethora of multi-centered research groups, with specialized expertise, and of journals devoted to methodology has arisen. The growth has been most evident where treatment is most institutionalized (e.g. cancer therapy), and where large scale trials are obligatory (e.g. in secondary prevention)" (Hill 1983, p. 29).
10. The development of research areas can be studied by using indicators such as numbers of scientists, institutions, articles/citations and journals. The typical pattern is represented by a S-shaped curve (Mulkay (1980). See also appendix II.
11. Juhl et al. (1977); Mulrow et al. (1984).
12. The authors' comment on their own finding is that the sample might not be representative but that, since the most widely circulated and prestigious journals were included in the study, it is reasonable to expect the research reported in other journals being of lower, not higher quality (Fletcher et al. (1981)).
13. The comparison of the findings of Juhl et al. (1977) and those of Fletcher et al. (1981) - assuming that the criteria used by both groups are the same - would indicate that the amount of controlled trials performed in gastroenterology is lower than average. Therefore other medical areas must score higher.

14. Cf. Hill (1983).
15. Hemminki and Falkum (1980).
16. Quoted from Payer (1988), p. 28; see Cochrane (1971).
Juhl and co-workers found that more than half of all controlled trials in gastroenterology reported during 1964-1973 were from Great Britain (27%) and the United States (25%); the others came from Italy (5%), West-Germany (5%), Japan (4%), Denmark (4%), South Africa (3%), Australia (3%), France (2%) and Norway (2%). Cruickshank once commented on the CCT as "this essentially British method for the assessment of drugs" (Cruickshank's comment was referred to during the Symposium on Clinical Trials (quoted from Anonymous (1958), p. 1057)).
17. Juhl et al. (1977).
18. Ross (1951).
19. The majority of these studies were published in Anglo-American journals, particularly in the Journal of the American Medical Association and the Journal of Clinical Investigation; articles also appeared in the New England Journal of Medicine and British Medical Journal (see Haas et al. (1959)).
20. Charlier (1961), p. 55.
21. This was put as a question in the Annual Report of 1928-29 of the Medical Research Council: see Armstrong (1977).
22. Hutchison (1930); quoted from Armstrong (1977), p. 799.
23. Casual experience, or clinical sense as Armstrong calls it, forms a distinct system of knowledge connected with a particular system of education and control. Clinical observation gave the doctor a dominant position in the doctor-patient-relationship; the educational system was authoritative, based on a tutor-trainee relation; and knowledge was personally based. This particular system was undermined and threatened by the controlled clinical trial: "Whereas in a series of 500 appendectomies, for example, only the operating surgeon can claim to know the signs of impending complications, in a clinical trial the results can be generally known and debated both within and outside the medical profession" (Armstrong (1977), p. 799).
24. Ethical concern pinpoints basically the dilemma of healer and scientist. As healer, the physician is bound by various professional codes to act in the patient's best interest. As scientist, the physician's main concern is to respect the scientific canons of valid experimental design. The latter role may require that the physician sacrifices the goal of individualized best treatment for statistical efficiency. This dilemma has been labeled by Lellouch and Schwartz as the clash between "ethique collective" and an "ethique individuelle".
See for discussions on this topic The Journal of Medicine and Philosophy, Theoretical Medicine, and The Journal of Medical Ethics.
25. Ambrose (1950).
26. This finding was based on the analysis of research descriptions during the period from 1953 to 1965 submitted as abstracts for the annual meetings of the American Society for Clinical Investigation, the American Federation for Clinical Research and the Association of American Physicians. These medical organizations constituted the major portion of American clinical investigators and medical educators.
The percentage of projects containing human material progressively declined from 88% to 62%: the percentage of disease-oriented projects fell from 79% to 58%, and that of patient-centered projects from 40% to 15%. During the same period, the percentage of research activities that had neither human material or a disease orientation rose from 6% to 26% (Feinstein et al. (1967); see also Feinstein (1967).
27. Feinstein et al. (1967), p. 403.
28. Ruesch (1962), p. 111.
29. "The clinical scientist is in the ascendant and the scholar-consultant is becoming a rare species: the two are much less in communication with each other than ever before" (Pellegrino (1974), p. 41). However, more recently the inverse trend is noticed and Wyngaarden patronized the clinician with a firm footing in basic science as "an endangered species" (Wyngaarden (1979)).
30. Mulrow et al. (1984), p. 116.
31. Dukes (1985).
32. Schmidt (1981), Temin (1980).
33. Schmidt (1981), 241-242.
34. Thalidomide was developed, and first and most extensively marketed in West-Germany. Total incidence of the birth malformation induced by the drug (phocomeli) was on the order of 10 times greater in West-Germany than elsewhere, being about 4 per 1000 live 1961 births and 4000 West-German cases in contrast with the over 7.000 world-wide cases attributable to thalidomide (Peltzmann (1963), p. 196).
See for national differences in drug licensing, Dukes (1985), (1986); Klaes et al. (1982), Burley and Binns (1985).
35. Quoted from Dukes (1985), p.20.
36. Dukes (1985), p. 20.
37. Jölndal (1984); Dukes (1985).

38. Dunlop (1973), p. 235.

39. Cf. Burkhardt and Kienle (1974), (1978); Bodewitz and Denig (1986). In the late 1950s and early 1960s a series of articles appeared in the German journals such as Therapiewoche, Therapie der Gegenwart, and Die Medizinische criticizing the controlled clinical trial as the base of therapeutic evaluation.

40. This is supported indirectly by several professional ethical codes, for example, by The Declaration of Helsinki: "Biomedical research involving human subjects must conform to generally accepted scientific principles and should be based on adequately performed laboratory and animal experimentation and on a thorough knowledge of the scientific literature".(WMA, 1964); see further Hill)1983) and Lilienfeld (1982).

41. See for this description Burley and Binns (1985).

42. See for a description of regulatory systems in USA and Europe Burley and Binns (1985).

43. Talalay (1964), p. 271. Goodman, coeditor of the authoritative drug compendium Goodman & Gilman's "The Pharmacological Basis of Therapeutics", stated that it was not possible to separate efficacy and safety in viewing "side-effects, toxic effects, and all other effects of a drug, wanted or unwanted, as part and parcel of the total response to that drug" (Goodman.. (1964), p. 51).

44. Talalay (1964), p. 271.

45. Clymer (1975), p. 151.

46. Presentation at the American Cancer Society's Writer's Seminar, St. Augustine, Florida, March 1974 (quoted from Clymer (1975), p. 151). From another address: "But all of these are bits and pieces of a bigger problem. The bigger problem is the need for new knowledge of the basic mechanism of disease of aging, and even normal physiology. New drug development will follow advances in bio-medical science" (presentation at the PMA meeting, Boca Raton, Florida, April 1974; quoted from Clymer (1975)).

47. Cf. Leufkens (1982).

48. ibidem.

49. Clymer (1975), p. 151.

50. Idänpään-Heikillä (1985), p. 126.

51. Burley and Binn (1985), p. 107. However this criticism does not necessarily affect the principle of the clinical trial. Two interpretations can be distinguished. Firstly, the principle of the clinical trial is extended to medical practice, not criticized. In recent years, general practice trials have received much attention (see Good (1976), particularly Chapter 9 (Statistical Aspects of Trial Design, K.D. Macrae) and Chapter 14 (Statistical Analysis of Trial Results, J.J. Grimshaw). Secondly, the artificiality of general practice trials is emphasized as a matter of principle, for example by taking the view that an experiment never really corresponds to medical practice. Then, the principle of the clinical trial is contested from an epistemological point of view.

Though both interpretations of the artificiality of the controlled trial underlie contemporary discussions about post-marketing-surveillance programs, the author's impression is that the first interpretation prevails. See for a criticism of the controlled clinical trial from both perspectives as well as a proposal for developing alternative strategies Hansen and Launso (1987).

52. A representative of the FDA declared "the generation of new biomedical knowledge" as a major objective of PMS-systems (FIP congress 1987). Thus, the FDA reconsidered the prominent place of the controlled clinical trial in its regulatory decision process, and challenged the basic view on drug innovation that basic biomedical science preceded medical practice to which it so strictly adhered.

53. Oates (1982), p. lxxix-lxxx. Crout, FDA commissioner, said in 1975: "The issue isn't whether regulation cuts down on innovation. Indeed it does. It must. There's hardly any way that regulation can stimulate innovation. Those are cross-purposes. The issue is whether regulation accomplishes some higher-purpose and does so with minimum inhibition of research" (quoted from Leufkens (1982). See for discussions about drug regulation Dukes (1985); Helms (1975); Wardell (1978a), (1978b), (1981).

54. Oates (1982), p. lxxix.

55. An additional point is the distinction between clinical investigation and clinical trials. The critic of Oates focusses on the former while preceding the clinical trial and following on basic and applied research as perceived by the NHLBI report (Oates (1982), p. lxxx-lxxxi).

56. Oates (1982).

57. Schaffner (1980).

58. Sackett et al. (1985).

59. Sackett et al. (1985), p. 176-177.

60. Sackett et al. (1985), p. 176.

61. Schaffner (1985), p. 29.

62. Schaffner (1980), p. 198. Philosophers and cognitive scientists working on a logic of discovery have come up with different notions such as "provisional field" or "domain" to denote the relevant background of scientific activity (see Schaffner (1980), (1985).

63. Cf. Fletcher et al. (1981).

64. These articles were published particularly in Circulation, the Journal of the American Medical Association, and American Journal of Medical Sciences.

65. See chapter 8.

66. The internal development of the controlled clinical trial paradigm and its relationship with the social and cultural environment has been left out from the analysis.

67. The controlled clinical trial might be included in a subjectivist account of hypothesis testing, for example based on Bayes theorem. Such an account can be related to an acceptable view of the discovery process.

Notes chapter 2.

1. Smith (1985), p. 3.

2. Spilker (1988), p. 11.

3. Different terms are used to describe the various stages a drug passes such as lead compound, candidate compound, project compound, project drug and marketed drug. Cf. Spilker (1988).

4. Spilker (1988) distinguishes four sources of drug discovery:
1) the source of the intellectual idea that led to the drug's discovery; 2) the source of the material that is the drug; 3) the business source from which the company obtained the drug; 4) the type of institution in which the drug was discovered. With respect to the second source the compounds belong to the following three classes: a) natural products: compounds occurring in and isolated from micro-organisms, plants or animals; b) derivatives or close analogues of natural products, made by partial or total synthesis; and c) synthetics: artificial compounds.

5. Hahn (1975).

6. Bartholini (1983).

7. Cf. subsequent editions of Trends in Pharmacological Sciences.

8. "Rational approaches to drug design still depend on the availability of suitable prototypes which can be structurally modified to produce more selective compounds. The most fruitful source of these prototypes has been that combination of chance and sagacity which Horace Walpole described as 'serendipity'. He coined this term more than two hundred years ago after reading a poem about the three princes of Serendip (Sri Lanka) who repeatedly made discoveries they were not seeking" (Sneader (1986), p. 13); see also Neiss and Boyd (1984).

9. Schwartzmann (1976).

10. Maxwell (1984), p. 377.

11. Cf. Spilker (1988); Comroe and Dripps (1976).

12. This does not imply that it cannot be improved. Particularly with respect to the interaction between academic sciences and industrial research, philosophy makes a good case to rationalize this interaction: cf. Zandvoort (1985); see also chapter 9.

13. Spilker (1988); Comroe (1977).

14. The science-technology spiral concept of Casimir (1983) for example; see also Zandvoort (1985) for discussions by scientists in the natural sciences on this topic.

15. Spilker (1988); Comroe and Dripps (1976).

16. Cf. Jolles and Wooldridge (1984).

17. Pellegrino (1983); Warner (1986).

18. Biel and Martin (1971). In this quotation the vocabulary of art is also incorporated which will be discussed in the text later on.

19. Lasagna (1964), p. 91.

20. Hamner (1982), p. 55; Craig (1980), p. 331.

21. Hamner (1982); Craig (1980); Gross (1983).

22. Hamner (1982).

23. Cf. Spilker (1988); Jolles and Wooldridge (1984).

24. See Jolles and Wooldridge (1984), p. 241.

25. The subject of art in drug discovery is left out from the analysis here but reappears in chapter 8.

26. Langley et al. (1987).
Cognitive science is presented here as the discipline pre-eminently dealing with the creative processes in science. However, this not to deny the active involvement of philosophers. Particularly in the American philosophy the discovery process has always received attention originating from the work of Hanson, Toulmin and other in the 1950s and 1960s; see in particular Hanson (1969), (1972). This philosophical tradition influences the concepts developed in this thesis while using the intellectual work of Schaffner (1980), (1985), (1986) as the reference (see chapter 1, 2 and 8).

27. Langley et al. (1987), p. 4-5.

28. Langley et al. (1987), p. 45-47.

29. This expression is used by Langley et al. (1987).

30. The example presented is meant to clarify the concept of inductive problem solving.

31. The example is typical for data driven discovery, that is, from data bases rules are taken to seek patterns in the data which are further manipulated. In case of theory driven discovery the origin of the heuristic rules lies in the theoretical framework.

32. Langley et al. (1987), p. 306-307.

33. Francis Bacon wrote in the Novum Organum: "Those who have treated the sciences were either empirics or rationalists. The empirics, like ants, lay up stores, and use them; the rationalists, like spiders, spin webs out of themselves; but the bee takes a middle course, gathering up her matter from the flowers of the field and garden, and digesting and preparing it by her native powers" (quoted from Langley et. al (1987), p. 25).

34. Langley et al. (1987), p. 305-306.

35. Hacking (1983), p. 246.

36. Hacking (1983).

37. Hacking (1983), p. 162.

38. Probably, the term "art" used by workers in the pharmaceutical sector when asked to define the essence of the discovery process partly refers to this creative aspect of science: experimental skills, getting the apparatus working, calibrating and improving the signal-noise ratio, and solving technical problems.

39. Hacking (1983), p. xii.

40. It falls outside the scope of this section to discuss the philosophical issues related to observation.

41. Hacking (1983), p. 167.

42. The basic assumptions of the approach of cognitive science as exemplified by the work of Langley and colleagues will not be criticized here. The claim of Langley and colleagues that the creative process can be simulated, is criticized by Van der Veer, Miedema and Ijzendoorn (1983) with emphasis on five issues: 1) a set of data is presupposed; 2) the input of the set of potential solutions precedes the search process; 3) data driven discovery only yields descriptive generalizations; 4) the search process is only applicable to "well-structured" problems; and 5) the use of primitive notions, e.g. "same", "similar", "next" which require clarification.

43. Zsotér and Church (1983).

44. There is some ambivalence in the sense that drugs may have variable effects or that there is a lacuna in scientific knowledge.

45. Taking the term remedy in its broader sense, including in it apparatus and procedures this will not alter the present interpretation of structural characteristics.

46. This distinction is valuable in all cases of designing apparatus, compounds or procedures.

47. Feinstein (1967), p. 73.

48. Morris (1975), pp. 108-120.

49. Engelhardt (1975).

50. This example comes from Engelhardt (1975); see also for an extensive discussion on clinical judgment Engelhardt et al. (1979).

51. Wulff et al. (1986).

52. Fleck (1983).

53. Prinzmetal et al. (1959).

54. The first aspect of the concept of disease profile leads us to the key-concept of set theory, namely "is element of" ("is a member of", "belongs to"). The notation $x \in A$ denotes: "x is an element of A"; in contrast, $x \notin A$: "x is not an element of A". As a rule capitals A, B, C, ... represent sets, and lower case characters a, b, c, ... represent elements of sets. At several places definitions and other expressions drawn from naive set theory are formulated informally. Cf. Suppes (1966).

55. Example derived from Harrison's principles of internal medicine (1974).

56. Disease characteristics are conceived of in a broad sense: properties, relations between properties, processes, and structures.

57. If A and B are sets such that every member of A is also a member of B, then we call A a **subset** of B, or say that A **is included in** B. The sign ' $\subseteq$ ' is used as an abbreviation for "is included in". In this case the possibility is not excluded that $A = B$. When $A \subseteq B$ but $A \neq B$, A is called a **proper subset** of B, in which case the sign ' $\subset$ ' is symbolically used. By the **intersection** of A and B (in symbols $A \cap B$) we mean the set of all things which belong both to A and B. If A is the set of all drugs, and B is the set of all toxic compounds, then $A \cap B$ is the set of all toxic drugs. By the **union** of A and B (in symbols $A \cup B$) we mean the set of all things which belong to at least one of the sets A and B. If A is the set of all human males and B the set of all human females, then $A \cup B$ is the set of all human beings. Finally, the symbol ø denotes the empty set.

58. Cf. note 57.

59. In case of comparing disease profiles this appears to be an arbitrary or inadequate way of putting things. However, in case of comparing drugs (i.e. drug profiles) it will become clear that this decision problem is realistic. Sometimes rules have to be introduced to provide a more satisfactory comparison. If so, we exceed the limits of the model and drop into the domain of heuristics and statistics.

60. These values might be numerical, nominal, ordinal or symbolical. For example, it is common to label complaints of patients as "mild", "moderate" and "severe". Medical language is full of such, from the quantitative viewpoint vague classifications. However, clinicians also use very often symbols to group "ranges of numerical values", for example, with the help of arrows pointing upwards or downward, and of the "=" symbol. When c denotes the disease characteristic "cardiac output", that is the volume of blood pumped by the heart per minute into the circulation, there are three possibilities: c ↑ , c ↓ , c=. Heart failure might be characterized by c ↓. Other types of symbolical representations such as "+"- and "-" are also possible. Medical terminology is ambiguous, but serious problems will not rise.

61. An ordered couple consists of two objects given in a fixed order. The concept of ordered couple can be generalized into that of ordered n-tuple which expresses that n objects are ordered in a fixed order.

62. This product represents the set of all ordered 5-tuples which can be formed from the five sets (in a fixed order), and is called the **Cartesian (or cross) product**. Considering two sets A and B, the Cartesian product of two sets A and B (in symbols: A **x** B) is the set of all ordered couples <x,y> such that $x \in A$ and $y \in B$.

63. N, X, Y en Z can also be defined "in a direct way":

Definition:

$$X =: \{<v_1, \dots , v_5>\mid \text{ for all i: } r_i < v_i\}$$
$$Y =: \{<v_1, \dots , v_5>\mid \quad ,, \quad : s_i < v_i \leq r_i\}$$
$$Z =: \{<v_1, \dots , v_5>\mid \quad ,, \quad : t_i < v_i \leq s_i\}$$
$$N =: \{<v_1, \dots , v_5>\mid \quad ,, \quad : v_i \leq t_i\}$$

Further, it is true that

. Disease profile P: $P =: \{<v_1, \dots , v_5>\mid \text{ for all i: } t_i < v_i\}$.

. $P' =: X \cup Y \cup Z$.

. $N \neq V - P'$; in other words: N is not exactly the complement of P' because P' is incomplete. N is even a proper subset of V - P.

64. The profile P and the elements p_i can be reinterpreted as the result of, in this case of maximally coarsening of the space of values. If P^+ denotes this profile, then:

Definition:

$$p_i := (t_i, \infty)$$
$$d_i := (-\infty, t_i]$$

$P^+ := \{<v_1, \dots , v_5> \mid \text{for all i: } t_i < v_i\}$.

65. To be exact, "coarsened" specific profiles are the point of issue; this is omitted, and the term specific profiles will be used. From the formal viewpoint the procedure is that each patient will be attributed a specific profile from V. From this follows a specific profile in terms of V'. Finally, the clinician is able to determine, on the basis of some rule, whether the specific profile "matches" the category-profiles X, Y, Z or N. These four category-profiles belong also to the set of 1024 specific profiles.

66. Another objection is that this misses the important point that profiles in combination with rules play a role on different levels. Dissatisfaction merely increases when considering the fact that distinct types of ranking of order are possible; the pathognomonic sign is merely one type.

67. Here the suggestions are followed which have been provided by Kuipers (1988), (1989) to improve the model developed at the Science Studies Unit at the University of Groningen to study R&D processes. This model (Bodewitz, De Vries and Weeder (1988)) conceives the process of research and development (R&D) as an attempt to match the set of materials with certain relevant properties with the set of intended applications, or demands. This matching process is represented in a lattice model, and R&D processes can be reconstructed by tracing the changes in the properties/demands lattice. In the course of the development of a lead to a product, the lattice evolves from a network of loosely connected sets of properties and demands to a tightened cluster of connections between properties and demands which is no longer susceptible to improvement without rigorous change. During this process of evolvement difficulties in

matching properties with demands may arise, and different heuristic strategies are available to solve the problems. See for a review of models developed to study the intra-firm innovation process, Saren (1984). Saviotti and Metcalfe (1984) have proposed a model of technological development distinguishing between technical and service characteristics. The improvement proposed by Kuipers is to reformulate the model in terms of set theory, in particular by assembling factual (operational) and desired properties (demands) as subsets of the set of relevant properties. When, in joint cooperation, applying this improved model to drug research, it seemed convenient to project this pair of concepts on the distinction between structural and functional characteristics of drugs hereby generating the concepts described in the text. The model has been adapted to connect it with the cognitive structure of biomedical knowledge about diseases and drugs, i.e. disease and drug profiles.

68. In the text qualitative definitions are given but quantitative definitions can be formulated analogously.

69. This solution is based on the assumption that there are two categories of properties: desirable and undesirable. This dichotomy implies that all properties considered not undesirable, i.e. not as side-effects, are seen as desirable characteristics. An objection is that the distinction between therapeutically desirable properties and side-effects becomes obscured. Another objection might be that some properties, either explicitly or implicitly, are considered desirable nor undesirable.

The former objection is not decisive because the evaluation of a novel drug encompasses both "positive" and "negative" aspects. The latter objection however, is fundamental but can be removed by the following modification of the model. For this purpose a tri-partition of relevant characteristics of a drug is appropriate: wished for, indifferent, and not wished for. Desirable properties are therapeutically beneficial effects, undesirable properties side-effects while indifferent properties are those characteristics which presumably are not important with respect to the disease concerned, nor in a positive sense, nor in a negative way. This category of indifferent properties has to be introduced because in each stage not all possible relevant properties are determined as desirable or undesirable.
Then:

K: domain of conceivably relevant functional properties
W: set of desirable properties
U: set of undesirable properties
I: set of indifferent properties
of(x): factual, i.e. operational (functional) properties of drug x.

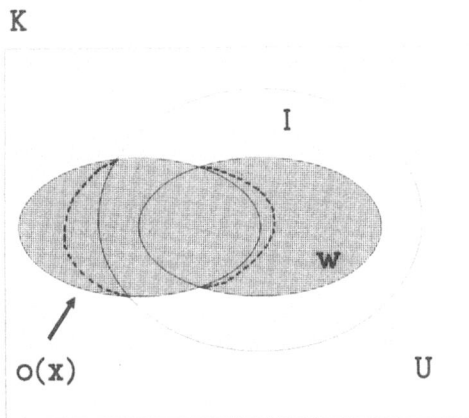

figure

Further, we assume that W, U en I do not intersect each other, and exhaust K.
Now the following qualitative definitions hold true:

1)x_2 is an improvement of x_1 in view of W/I/U:=

of(x_2) Δ W$\subset$ of(x_1)ΔW **and** I $\cap$ of(x_1) = I $\cap$ of(x_2)

2)W_2/I_2/U_2 is a concession to x with respect to W_1/I_1/U_1:=

of(x) $\Delta W_2 \subset$ of(x) Δ W_1 **and** $W_1 \subseteq W_2$ **and** $U_1 \subseteq U_2$ (hence: $I_2 \subseteq I_1$)

The second and third term in the definition above explicitly indicate that the alterations are confined to reconsider, positively or negatively, one or more indifferent properties that belong to I_1. In other words: I forms in general the **primary** space of negotiation for extension of W and/or U. This does not alter the fact that properties belonging to W and/or U can be eliminated or changed, or that properties can be interchanged between W and U.
This revised model can replace the version elaborated in the sections 2.7.2. - 2.7.4.
70. Again, coarsening of the space of values of the characteristics e and c occurs, and the procedure can be treated in the same way as described in section 2.6.3.
71. From the clinical point of view this is not an adequate interpretation of the term "exercise tolerance". This term expresses the extent of exercise a patient suffering from pain in the chest tolerates before getting this complaint. The paragraph in the text implies that any human being, also the healthy and trained subject, reaches a level of exercise where pain in the chest occurs. This is by no means implied by the term as used by cardiologists.
72. Otherwise than described in the text, it is possible that in case of the simultaneous occurrence of two diseases the clinician uses different criteria to divide the space of values of the characteristics of both diseases respectively. Thus, he "descends" to the original space of values in order to start over again coarsening this space.
In both cases, i.e. as described in the text and in this note, it is assumed that the characteristics of both sets are not interrelated. If so, then a characteristic representing the relation between e and c has to be added to AP.
An interesting case is found in chapter 7 about the German medical views of angina pectoris, i.e. "Verkettungsangina". This disease entity concerns the specific combination of a particular affliction with an atypical form of angina pectoris in which the one affliction modifies the manifestations of the other. In part this concerns the manifestation of **new** signs of angina pectoris distinct from the typical form, and partly the alteration of values (and/or priorities) of characteristics of the classical pattern of angina pectoris, i.e. angina of effort.
73. This perfect drug in view of the wished for profile might be one compound, but also a combination of two or more compounds, or of one or more compounds and other forms of medical therapy.
74. The question whether or to what extent heuristic principles are explicable, is not answered here but will be dealt with in Chapter 8.

Notes chapter 3.

1. Langley (1905).
2. Dale (1906).
3. Ahlquist (1948).
4. Powell and Slater (1958).
5. Biel and Lum (1966); Barrett (1972); Carrier and Shlafer (1984).
6. Moran and Perkins (1958).
7. Ahlquist (1982).
8. Black and Stephenson (1962).
9. Prichard (1964); Clark (1976).
10. Barger and Dale (1910).
11. Nickerson (1949), p. 27.
12. Dale (1906).
13. Nickerson (1949).
14. Fildes (1940).
15. Martin (1951).
16. Martin (1951), p. 477.
17. Cavallito (1968).
18. Bloom (1970).
19. Albert (1960), p. 147.

20. Carrier and Shlafer (1984); Ahlquist (1958), (1973).

21. Cavallito (1973).

22. Carrier and Shlafer (1984). See for this criticism of Ahlquist's experimental work also Kalsbeek (1969), a Dutch clinician who questioned at the time the relevance of Ahlquist's alpha and beta receptor theory for the the clinician.

23. Ahlquist (1948), p. 587.

24. Ahlquist (1948), p. 588.

25. Furchgott (1959).

26. Dresel (1960); Lucchesi and Hardman (1961); Moore and Swain (1960); Moran et al. (1962).

27. Nickerson (1959).

28. Winbury (1964), (1984).

29. Winbury (1964), p. 21.

30. Black and Stephenson (1962), p. 311.

Notes chapter 4.

1. Black, interview.

2. Black, interview.

3. Black, interview.

4. Raab (1940); see further Raab (1953), (1962), (1971).

5. Black, interview; see also Charlier (1961), (1971).

6. Black (1959).

7. The project delivered one of the screening tests being used by Black in the early phase of the ICI project to find anti-adrenergic compounds (Black, interview).

8. These stressful events could also be mimicked by injecting adrenaline. Injecting adrenaline was used for some time as a diagnostic test for angina pectoris but it had many risks and became obsolete.

9. Black (1976), p. 12.

10. Dollery, Prichard, interview. Guanethidine, an adrenergic neuron blocking drug, has for some time been the leading antihypertensive drug in the United Kingdom. The discovery of the class of adrenergic neuron blocking drugs with TM 10 (xylocholine) and subsequently bretylium took place in the British context. Bretylium was quickly thereafter challenged by guanethidine (cf. Sneader (1985)) which became a popular drug in British medicine.

11. In angina pectoris the situation is much more complex. For many years, the view was widely held that the nerves that transmit cardiac pain and accompany the sympathetic nerves of the heart, if cut, would relieve the pain, but not the disease. However, this view was replaced by the notion that cutting the sympathetic drive improved the patient's condition. Resection of the anginal pathway, i.e. by cutting the sympathetic nervous system to the heart, was advocated and introduced by White in 1940. Various surgical procedures were described of which the bilateral thoracic sympathectomy in which the upper three or four dorsal ganglia of the sympathetic chain are excised, had been found most satisfactory (cf. Burnett and Evans (1956).

12. Drill (1954); see Ahlquist (1958).

13. Black (1967), p. 120.

14. Shanks, interview.

15. Shanks (1984), p. 49-50.

16. Powell and Slater (1958); Moran and Perkins (1958).

17. Black, interview.

18. Cotten et al. (1957).

19. Shanks (1984), p. 50; see also Black (1967).

20. In the course of 1959 Black changed the test-system. Instead of the Langendorff preparation he used the isolated rat papillary muscle preparation. In this preparation the contraction of cardiac muscle induced by isoprenaline was assessed and hence the activity of potential blocking compounds was measured. It was a difficult test-system. The recording of the muscular contraction response requested much of the ingenuity of Brian Horsfall, the technician, who got involved in the project. Continuity on the technical level, however was that the heart rate remained the key parameter (Black 1967).

21. The ICI Research Report noted: "**Isolated heart muscle** 112 compounds tested, of which 10 are active, none as much as DCI. This is a disturbing result, because it was reported that 32, 278 (DCI) did not block the action of adrenaline on guinea-pig hearts, and that compound itself was a potent cardiac stimulant" (Woodbridge (1981); also interview Black).

22. The ICI Research Report noted: "A new compound, 38,174, appears to possess most of the properties that may be

necessary to protect the heart in coronary muscle artery disease. It has not yet been shown that 38,174 is a candidate for clinical trial, and much work on toxicity and particularly on pharmacological side-effects including hypertensive action will be necessary before its suitability for trial can be assessed. The new work will be given very high priority, as will the evaluation of new analogous, and this will probably involve a much reduced effort on potential hypertensive compounds" (Woodbridge (1981), p. 164); also Black (1967).

23. Full quotation: "that analogues of ICI 38, 174 (pronethalol) were being tested to find a compound which (was longer acting, had greater resistance to catecholamino breakthrough and) showed less penetration of the central nervous system" (Shanks 1984, p.54).

24. Alleyne et al. (1964); Fulton and Green (1963).

25. Shanks comments to this: "The laevo isomer was 40 times more potent than the dextro isomer in blocking beta adrenoceptors, but the two isomers were equally effective in producing effects on the central nervous system (and had the same acute LD_{50} in mice)"
(Shanks (1984), p.55).

26. Robinson, interview.

27. Robinson, interview.

28. The criteria for assessing the therapeutic ratio shifted over time.

29. Shanks (1984), p. 54.

30. Howe, pers. comm.

31. Obviously this was not the only reason. The ICI team realized very early its unstable position. For example, in a series of 76 analogues of pronethalol 41 compounds proved to be as potent as pronethalol whereas 7 compounds exhibited an even much stronger beta blocking activity. Cf. the two series of three articles published in the Journal of Medicinal Chemistry of 1968 and 1969 that provided some insight in the stock of numerous compounds synthesized and screened, albeit in retrospect (see for references Howe et al. (1970)).

32. Gill and Vaughan Williams (1964).

33. Moreover this concerns both experimental and clinical profiling (chapter 2 and 3).

34. Vaughan Williams, interview; Barrett, pers. comm. Gill and Vaughan Williams had obtained the supplies of pronethalol by chance. However, the similarities in chemical structure between quinidine and pronethalol were already recognized by Gill.

35. The latter term concerned the effect on cell membranes that can be measured in the frog sciatic nerve using procaine as the standard (Barrett (1972).

36. Stock and Dale (1963). The authors describe the issue in technical terms, but basically they state that the sympathetic system has a significant role to play in the maintenance of circulatory hemodynamics, particularly in patients with (incipient) heart failure. Two mechanisms of aggravation or precipitation are proposed, one focussing on the contractile state of the heart, the other on the heart rate. These two parameters structured research at ICI and in the field at large.

37. Another important toxicological problem concerned the hypotensive activity of pronethalol, an unexpected finding. During a trial at the University College Hospital Prichard and his colleagues observed that pronethalol produced small but nevertheless significant hypotensive effects. Black reported: "In anaesthetized cats and dogs, rapid intravenous injection of pronethalol produced an abrupt fall in blood pressure, whereas slow intravenous infusion produced a significant, steady decline in blood pressure. (..) A satisfactory explanation for this vasodilation was never found" (Black (1967), p. 112-113). This problem initiated research into the vasodilator properties of beta blocking compounds (see the section about the development of practolol).

38. Paget (1963).

39. Barrett, interview.

40. Shanks (1984), p. 56.

41. Howe et al., interview - interviews were held with Dr. R. Howe and Dr LH Smith together with other chemists; i.e. Dr. D.J. Le Count, Dr. B.J. Main and Dr. H.Tucker involved in later stages of research at ICI: Dr. DJ Le Count has been deeply involved in the atenolol project (Count, Le (1981). Henceforth this interview will be referred to by Howe et al.

42. Shanks (1984), p. 59.

43. Barrett (1972), p. 223.

44. Barrett, interview.

45. Howe et al., interview; Barrett, interview.

46. Shanks, interview.

47. Fitzgerald, interview.

48. Dornhorst, interview; Robinson added that Dornhorst was much more likely to be asked to make such a decision being the senior (Robinson, interview).

49. Robinson, interview.

50. Robinson, interview.

51. Robinson, interview.

52. Black, interview; Fitzgerald, interview.

53. Academic scientists showed that the effect of adrenaline upon fatty acid mobilization was mediated by the beta receptors. The action of adrenaline on glucose mobilization did not seem to be mediated by either alpha or beta receptors. Human studies confirmed this pattern (cf. Pilkington and Lowe (1962)). Thus, it matches the typical pattern of the expansion of pharmacological methodology into the various therapeutic fields.

54. Barrett (1972), p. 213.

55. Cf. Black (1967).

56. This was shown in the syrosingopine treated rat which is devoid of sympathetic control; this test system is similar to the reserpinized cat used by the Hässle team (see 4.5).

57. Howe et al, interview.

58. Cf. Shanks et al. (1966). Rightly or wrongly these differences might have been explained by the fact that ICI 45763 exhibited intrinsic activity while propranolol did not. But I presume that this type of explanation did not play a major role and the participants did not suggest this when interviewed; neither had this explanation a prominent role in literature.

59. Shanks, interview.

60. Prichard, interview; Dollery, interview.

61. Illustrative is the following quotation that refers to the dramatic effects of pronethalol and simultaneously illustrates the clear-cut effects of the drug on the heart: "(..) I should like to tell you briefly about my first experience with them (beta blockers, RV). In 1961/62 I was an intern working in an intensive care ward of a surgical thoracic unit. One day, while I was doing internal cardiac massage on a heart with ventricular fibrillation, a research assistant gave the patient some pronethalol intravenously. The effect was staggering. The small, coarsely fibrillating heart suddenly became a dilated sac, quivering like a jelly, for which nothing further could be done" (Gau (1974), p. 135-136).

62. The Buxton Symposium in November 1965, the first symposium on propranolol, attracted about eighty British clinicians, representing about 45 hospitals, infirmaries and clinical institutes in the United Kingdom. Half a year later a British invasion in the American Journal of Cardiology (1966; see Shanks (1966c) took place when more than twenty of these "Buxton" articles were published - in the form of full articles and abstracts.

63. Dollery, interview.

64. This interesting sketch of the connection between the development of the beta blockers and the discipline of clinical pharmacology, within the fold of British cardiology, I owe to professor Dollery (Dollery, interview).

65. Barrett, pers. comm.

66. Black (1967), p. 116.

67. Shanks, interview.

68. Shanks, interview.

69. Stephen (1966).

70. Fitzgerald (1969), p. 297.

71. Goodwin quoted from Stephen (1966), p. 468. To a great extent the discussion focussed on the quantity per ampoule; for example, Dornhorst stated: "I would like to suggest that the ampoule size be reduced. It is 5 mg. at the present, and junior hospital staff are rather apt to assume that one ampoule is a safe dose" (Stephen (1966)). Similarly Rosenheim noted: "I would like to emphasize again the need for a smaller ampoule, and I would quite agree with Professor Dornhorst that if one puts 5 mg. in an ampoule, it is an invitation to give 5 mg." (Stephen (1966), p. 472).

72. Cf. Gillam and Prichard (1965).

73. Later on it was discovered that propranolol showed considerable variance in metabolism thus resolving much of the confusion about the dose variation.

74. Barrett, interview.

75. Dunlop and Shanks (1968).

76. Dr. Howe and Dr. Smith, chemists, as well as Dr. Barrett and Dr. Fitzgerald, biologists, confirmed that such a broad project was going on (interviews).

77. See Black (1967). This effect was initially noticed in anaesthetized cats and dogs, but became urgent when the hypotensive action of pronethalol during clinical trials was noticed.

78. For example, propranolol, ICI 45.763 and pronethalol produced a marked increase of hind-limb blood flow in the dog, whereas MJ 1999 produced an increase that was dose-independent and much less than the maximum produced by the former compounds. This difference was explained by the fact that MJ 1999 probably lacked the local anaesthetic property. This explanation seemed to be valid especially since the optical isomers of propranolol - the (+)isomer possesses less than one-twentieth of the ß-blocking action of the (-)isomer - increase blood flow to the same extent having the same degree of local anaesthetic activity whereas MJ 1999 is devoid of the latter activity (Shanks (1967)).

79. The experiments are marked by three key articles.

The first is received September 13, 1966 and concerns the peripheral vascular effects of propranolol and other related compounds as described (Shanks (1967)). The second article was received October 3, 1967 and discusses the selective blockade of the beta receptors in the heart by practolol and concerns animal experiments, as indicated before (Dunlop and Shanks (1968)). The third article was received April 25, 1968 and concerns studies in healthy volunteers (Brick et al. (1968)). The timing of the publications shows the neat sequence from laboratory to man. Yet the time course is much more complex because the latter two articles were published as short communications simultaneously (Barrett et al. (1967/1968; Brick et al. (1967/1968)).

80. Shanks, interview.

81. Glover et al. (1062); Brick et al. (1966);Brick et al. (1967); Brick et al. (1968) and several other articles in the domain of physiology.

82. VanDeripe et al. (1964), (1965); Levy and Wilkenfield (1969).

83. N-isopropylmethoxamine blocked beta receptors in the rat uterus (Levy 1964); moreover it blocked beta receptors mediating the metabolic actions as the marked rise in free fatty acids, blood glucose and blood lactic acid produced by the catecholamines (Levy (1966b).

84. N-tertiary butylmethoxamine (Levy 1966a); other scientists such as Burns, Lemberger and Salvador came to the same results) and dimethylisoproprylmethoxamine (Levy, 1966b) blocked beta receptors in the rat uterus, canine intestine and peripheral blood vessels.

85. Similar differences in patterns of response were noticed when testing beta receptor stimulating agents in particular experimental systems, particularly in relation with metabolic effects (Cf Lands et al. (1967) and many other references in the field).

86. Levy (1965), p. 413.

87. Other terms like "certain", "not properly" and "only" denote the extent to which scientists were certain of their case.

88. See for the review of the state of affairs in the field Moran (1967).

89. Furchgott (1959); Nickerson (1965).

90. Cf. Anonymous (1966).

91. It is interesting to note that at the time that Ahlquist formulated his theory of α- and ß-receptors, Lands proposed a classification in which he distinguished the receptors in the heart as a separate subcategory. When elaborating his classification of β_1- and β_2-receptors Lands worked at the Sterlop Winthrop Institute, i.e. in an industrial setting.

92. Moran's definition was in accordance with Ahlquist's functional definition of the receptor. The hypotheses described fitted pharmacological methodology (as described in Chapter 3).

This methodology dominated the 1960s and firmly linked academic and pharmaceutical research. "Receptor hunting", e.g. the biochemical attempt to identify and to trace the molecular configurations that made up "the receptor", which rapidly emerged during the 1960s, did not fundamentally affect the course of academic and industrial research on beta blocking compounds until the 1970s.

93. Cf. Bartholini (1983) and many short accounts of the development of beta-blocking and beta-stimulating agents in medical literature; the participants involved however, emphasize the development of the selectively acting compounds rather than the theory (see also Sneader (1985)).

94. The Science Citation Index started in 1961 while the compound was launched in 1958.

95. Cf. Idänpään-Heikillä (1985) for references or standard references such as Inman's textbook on monitoring for drug safety.

96. More sophisticated techniques such as co-citation-analysis methods may provide a better understanding.

97. This is not an universal pattern per se. Some articles concerning methods rank very high on the list of "citation classics" published in Current Contents.

98. Moran (1966); see further Dornhorst (1966).

99. Moran (1966), p. 507-508.

100. This definition reflects the growing influence of biochemistry on receptor research.

101. Moran (1966), p. 509 -510: "New information, such as that discussed above with respect to α-methyl DCI, suggests the possibility of using modifying designations to describe the receptors, such as the tissue involved, e.g., $beta_{heart}$ and $beta_{blood\ vessels}$ to differentiate the cardiac and vasodilator beta receptors. Although this terminology is cumbersome, evidence does not justify adding to the complexity of classification by introducing completely new types whenever a new drug is found which interferes with an adrenergic response". Illustrative for Moran's position is his paraphrase of Robert Frost's couplet ("We dance round in a ring and suppose/But the Secret sits in the middle and knows"; "We dance round the cell and suppose/But the Receptor sits inside and knows" (Moran (1966), p. 511).

102. Braunwald (1966), p. 307.

103. Interview Jack: the same history was sketched by Brittain.

The initial target was a metabolically stable long-acting beta-stimulant and this was sought by replacing the catechol group in adrenaline by a variety of disubstituted phenyl substituents and increasing the size and complexity of the N-substituent. Salbutamol, the saligenin analogue of N-t butyl noradrenaline, was found to be more active on respiratory smooth muscle than on heart muscle in the guinea pig and other species, results which were consistent with Lands' beta-1/beta-2 classification of beta-adrenoceptors. Jack & Brittain explained the selective action of salbutamol by supposing that the physiological receptor proteins for adrenaline were different in detail and that this allowed the receptors for salbutamol to be different in respiratory and heart muscles (Brittain, pers. comm.; see also Brittain, Dean and Jack (1981)).

104. Engelhardt, interview: ["Ich habe nie viel davon gehalten, dieses starrer System von beta-1 und beta-2 zu verfolgen weil nach meiner Erfahrung von Substanz zu Substanz die Übergänge fließend sind und es keine so scharfe Differenzierung eigentlich gibt. Wenn sie einige Prototypen herausnehmen, denn ja aber wenn sie jetzt größere Substanz Serien betrachten, dann geht das fließend ineinander über. So hab ich also dieses Konzept oder die Bezeichnung dieses relativ starre Kästchenbezeichnung ß1 und ß2 nie gern gemocht. Aber die Differenzierung, natürlich daß das möglich ist, daß hatten wir schon in einem Beispiel hier befor Lands und die anderen aufgetreten waren. Da hatten wir nämlich das Berotec (fenoterol, RV) bereits hier in den Hand, nicht. Das ist vom 1964 glaube ich. Das war die erste Agonist die diese Differenzierung deutlich zeigte"].

105. Carlsson (1983), p. 36.

106. These compounds were the result of improving the separation of desired actions from undesired effects and were picked out from a whole array of compounds synthesized for different purposes: for profiling desired therapeutic actions; as tools for inside comparative analysis in animals and men; for class exemplification in filed patents; for calibration of technical apparatus and validation of experimental systems. The compounds were selected for various reasons including therapeutic reasons.

107. The distinction between these three levels is arbitrary but expresses the view that the creation of compounds and experimental systems is an innovatory activity per se.

108. Cf. Moran (1966).

109. Carlsson et al. (1972).

110. See chapter 2 for the discussion about the differential relationships between theory and experiment; cf. Hacking (1983).

111. Cf. Dunlop and Shanks (1967); Shanks (1968).

112. See Shanks (1984).

113. Shanks, interview.

114. Shanks, interview.

115. Robinson, interview.

116. Howe et al., interview.

117. Barrett, interview.

118. Fitzgerald, interview.

119. Davies, interview.

120. Around 1968 ICI started a project to provide such a theoretical basis but the project failed (Davies, interview).

121. This is also the case in man, particularly in patients with a decreased heart function (Shanks (1984); Shanks, interview).

122. Robinson, interview.

123. Barrett, interview. From the pharmacological point of view it was recognized that oxprenolol was an effective beta blocker and that there was little the ICI scientists could do from laboratory data to offset Ciba claims against propranolol. Barrett suggested that the main benefit Ciba had might have been their avoidance of an intravenous preparation thereby allowing justifiable claims for greater safety in clinical practice, i.e. most of the deaths from propranolol at that time followed intravenous administration (Barrett, pers. comm.).

124. As was explained by Pfizer's Medical Director to Fitzgerald (Fitzgerald, interview).

125. Howe et al, interview.

126. Barrett, interview.

127. McNeill (1966); Stevens (1966).

128. Braunwald (1966), p. 307.

129. Furthermore, the American situation stimulated the development of practolol. Leading cardiologists in the United States, and among which the renowned clinical scientist Braunwald, were very sceptical about the dramatic effects of propranolol on the cardiac output (Fitzgerald, interview).

130. Interview Fitzgerald: "Of course, patients have died on the needle, there is no question about that. That was horrible. But I think the great sort of attraction that practolol had on people was they felt that they could shoot it in and nothing would go wrong".

131. Shanks, interview. This mystery lost its attraction when the toxic effects of practolol were revealed.

132. Powell and Slater first presented their results at the Federation Meetings (1957). Their full report appeared in 1958 (Powell and Slater (1958)).

133. Moran, pers. comm. (quoted from Shanks (1984), p. 41).

134. Moran and Perkins (1958).

135. This quotation is taken from their comment on Moran and Perkins' paper at the symposium on Catecholamines (Bethesda, Oct. 1958); cf. Powell and Slater (1958b).

136. "Thus DCI can be considered an useful tool for the qualitative separation of alpha and beta receptor sites, but for the present it must be used with caution for the quantitative aspects are not clear" (Powell and Slater (1958b)).

137. Cf. Dresel (1960); Moran and Perkins (1961); Biel and Lum (1966). Thus, it was shown, for example, that beta blocking agents were more specific than the alpha blockers which exhibit also other types of activity, e.g. anti-acetylcholine and antihistamine activity.

138. Dresel (1960).

139. In this early phase the hypothesis emerged in the field that DCI might be beneficial in clinical conditions associated with an excessive adrenergic stimulation. Hence, its use in the surgical removal of phaeochromocytoma, a catecholamine producing tumor releasing excessive amounts of catecholamines when manipulated, was suggested as a possibility (cf. Dornhorst and Laurence (1963); Barrett (1972); Biel and Lum (1966).

140. This concerned, for example, the coronary ligation method; see Furchgott (1959); Dresel (1960); and Lucchesi and Hardman (1961).

141. Slater, pers. comm. quoted from Shanks (1984), p. 41.

142. Lilly investigated DCI clinically (Werko, Ostholm and Ablad, interviews).

143. Cf. Shanks (1984), p. 44: "(...) Lilly filed a United States patent on nethalide (pronethalol) which was withdrawn because of an earlier filing date by Imperial Chemical Industries".

144. Lish et al. (1960), p. 129. Unlike the opening sentences suggest, the article does not cover cardiovascular problems.

145. The proprietary designation Vasodilan was applied to the compound (Lish et al. (1960).

146. Sneader (1985).

147. Larsen and Lish (1964), p. 1283. Larsen had considerable experience in the synthesis of sulphonamides, and joined Mead Johnson around 1960. Attempts were made to incorporate sulphonamide-groups into the benzene ring of the phenethanolamines. This was supported by experiences with extensive modification of these amines, the phenolic hydroxyl groups being replaced by a variety of substituents but without any success. According to Larsen these failed modifications shared a common characteristic: the substituents exhibited no acidic character. Therefore, Larsen searched for substituents with an acidity comparable to that of the phenolic groups.

However, another sequence of events might have taken place. Perhaps, Larsen just replaced the phenolic groups by the sulphonamide-groups with which he was so familiar, then found a reasonable activity subsequently providing an ex-post-facto explanation in terms of this acidity. Alternatively, the polar structure of the phenethanolamines, represented by the phenolic groups, had to be remained to avoid entrance into the central nervous system. Ephedrine, for example, an important remedy against asthma attacks, caused central side-effects; phenethanolamines did not. Furthermore, the polar structure was of interest for increasing the biological stability of these compounds against catecholamine destructive enzymes. This was also related to the duration of action.

This episode in asthma therapy research falls outside the scope of this study.

148. Larsen had synthesized MJ 1999 (sotalol) in October 1960. Since the various compounds containing a sulphonamide-group are numbered in order, this series of compounds has presumably been synthesized around the same time.

149. Inside information collected by Shanks supports this conclusion (personal communication with Stanton, one of the researchers at Mead Johnson from the early beginnings): "As it was noted that MJ 1999 resembled DCI, tests were established to examine this activity further. On 22nd March, 1962, it was observed that MJ 1999 (0.01 - 0.1 μg) blocked both the isoprenaline and adrenaline induced relaxation of the pitocin stimulated rat uterus in vitro (..). Lish commented on the test sheet that MJ 1999 (sotalol) was "probably the first known and most potent drug capable of blocking beta stimulants in the uterus (..)" (Shanks (1984), p. 68-69).

150. Howe et al., interview.

151. Lish et al. (1965).

152. This supports the conclusion of the ICI chemists that Mead Johnson was poor in developing MJ 1999 as an cardiovascular drug (interview Howe et al.). Undoubtedly, the taking over of Mead Johnson by Bristol Myer at the time must be taken into account. Another hypothesis, however, would be that the search for **antispasmodic** drugs prohibited Mead Johnson from entering the cardiovascular field. The search for antispasmodic drugs was firmly linked with the concept of coronary vasodilation which was on strained terms with the objective of beta blockade (cf. chapters 5 and 7). However, the material presented is not sufficient to substantiate this hypothesis. Neither did I intend to do so. However, to some extent the issue will reappear when discussing the beta blocker project of Boehringer.

153. Dr. Ivan Östholm is working on a book about the beta blocker project at Hässle. He has provided much of the material presented in this section and has made many comments. I am very grateful for his efforts.

154. Östholm, pers. comm. Roberts had done research in this area at the Department of Pharmacology during the

1950s (cf. Roberts and Baer (1960).

155. Roberts and Baer (1960).

156. Östholm, interview.

157. Östholm, pers. comm.

158. Östholm, pers. comm.

Carlsson commented: "They explained what they were searching for. I saw the structures of the compounds, and I told them: "If you want to do anything you must go into the beta-adrenergic field". It was new to them. Nothing was known about beta receptors..." (interview, Carlsson).

According to Östholm the collaboration with Arvid Carlsson can be looked upon as one of the most important crossroads in the development of a new approach in the Astra-group. Not only the beta blockers, i.e. alprenolol and metoprolol, and the beta agonist terbutaline, but the whole CNS-research program at Astra aiming at new classes of psychopharmaca may be considered as the result of his ideas and approach (Östholm, pers. comm.).

159. Following a sabbatical leave in 1955-56 at the Laboratory Heart Institute in Bethesda, Maryland, Carlsson performed studies about the effects of reserpine on the adrenergic system (Carlsson, pers. comm.). He was among the first to show that reserpine depleted the storage vesicles of noradrenaline.

160. Carlsson, interview.

161. Carlsson, interview.

162. Östholm, pers. comm.

163. Carlsson, interview.

164. Moran worked at the Dept. Pharmacology, Emory University, Atlanta and was deeply involved in the field of adrenergic receptors (cf. Moran (1958), (1962), (1966); VanDeripe et al. (1964); VanDeripe and Moran (1965).

165. VanDeripe and Moran (1965), p. 712.

166. Shanks (1984).

167. Barrett, interview; and Howe et al., interview.

168. The sheer fact that several companies succeeded in synthesizing propranolol-like compounds at about the same time doesn't provide evidence for either version of the story. From the chemical point of view it is a creative step to proceed from compounds with an ethanol-amine side chain to compounds with an oxypropranolamine side chain.

169. The origin of the idea is described by Brändström et al. (1966).

The synthesis of beta blocking compounds with the propranolamino-side-chain at ICI and Hässle even occurred along different chemical routes. It is interesting to note that the ICI team refers to O. Stephenson, working at British Drug Houses, whereas the Hässle team refers to Fourneau.

170. Berntsson, pers. comm.

171. Ablad, interview; Ostholm, interview.

172. The code numbers of H 29/50 and H 56/28 show wide margins. However, the Hässle numbering system is not a purely chronological one. The numbers to the left of the slash is the number of the laboratory notebook used by a certain chemist and the numbers to the right are the page number in that notebook (ranging from 01-99). The numbers show only which book the chemist has happened to take from the bookshelf when he had finished his old one and needed a new one. Since all pages are signed and dated there is no problem of telling when a certain compound was made. Compound H 29/50 was made on the 3rd of April 1963; this is only one year and 3 months before the synthesis of H 56/28 (alprenolol), synthesized on the 27th of August 1964 (Berntsson, pers. comm.).

173. Carlsson, interview.

174. Ablad et al. (1967a), (1967b). Somewhat earlier some results were published in the Swedish journals.

175. Werkö, interview; Sannerstedt, interview.

176. Ostholm (1972), p. 22.

177. Östholm, interview.

178. Folkow (1952), (1955); Folkow and Hamberger (1956); Folkow et al. (1956); Folkow et al. (1967). This experimental work of Folkow can be seen in the wider context of Swedish physiology and the successful research tradition in the field of catecholamines. The experimental work of Von Euler, laureated with the Nobel prize for establishing noradrenaline as the true neurotransmitter of the sympathetic system, exemplifies this tradition.

179. See for references note 178.

180. "It is now fairly well established that in animals the correlation between stimulation frequency and the effector response of sympathetically and parasympathetically innervated structures forms hyperbolic curves, reaching nearly maximal values at frequencies around 8-10 impulses/sec. with a definite maximum approximately at 20 impulses/sec. Animal experiments show that the tonic discharge rate of autonomic fibers under 'resting' conditions is only about 1/3 impulses/sec., and rarely exceeds 10 impulses/sec., even on extreme excitation of central structures" (Folkow and Hamberger (1956), p. 268).

181. Different test-systems existed and also the species used differed.

182. Reserpine perfectly illustrates how therapeutics are powerful investigational tools. This drug had a tremendous

impact in biomedical research.

183. Werkö, Sannerstedt, Ablad, interviews.

184. From these results it was concluded: "1) propranolol reduced cardiac output by inhibiting endogenous sympathetic tone on the cardiac ß-receptors, 2) H 56/28 inhibited endogenous sympathetic tone on the heart to the same degree as propranolol, 3) the hemodynamic consequences of this action of H 56/28 was compensated by a cardiac stimulation due to the slight "intrinsic" ß-receptor stimulating action that this agent possesses" (Forsberg and Johnsson (1967), p. 1153).

185. Ablad, pers. comm.; Östholm, interviews; see also Ablad et al. (1970).

186. Ablad, interview.

187. Werkö, interview.

188. Ablad, pers. comm.

189. The observation in 1966 gave a hint as to the structure activity relationship of cardio-selective beta blockers, which was pursued in more intense chemical-synthetic work at Hässle from 1968 (Ablad, pers. comm.).

190. Ablad et al. (1973).

191. Ablad et al. (1973).

192. The idea of the Hässle team was that H 93/26 would not block the peripheral vasodilator effects of circulating catecholamines and therefore it would not potentiate the hypertensive effect of adrenaline. Non-selective agents as alprenolol and propranolol as well as cardio-selective beta blockers **with** intrinsic activity potentiate this hypertensive effect. This was considered disadvantageous in some clinical conditions (Astra (1972)).

193. This was suggested by Dr. Enar Carlsson, and has subsequently been confirmed in many laboratories (Östholm, pers. comm.); see also Carlsson et al. (1972).

194. Hässle was not supported by the mother company Astra. When in 1970 the merger between Ciba and Geigy took place, Hässle had to provide access to Geigy to its research portfolio in danger of loosing the distribution rights of the Geigy products for the Scandinavian countries. Together with two other interesting compounds in Hässle's research pipeline, the compound H 93/26 (metoprolol), was selected by a Ciba-Geigy investigational team. Metoprolol entered a co-marketing project and arrangements were made with respect to market sharing and distribution.

Ciba-Geigy's participation in the development of metoprolol was limited. They did not perform long term toxicology and clinical trial studies. Ciba-Geigy contributed by synthesizing large amounts of metoprolol which enabled the Hässle team to start clinical studies on a large scale and much earlier (Östholm, pers. comm.). The limited interest of Ciba-Geigy's medical department is reflected in: "... this cardioselectivity is only relative and offers little if any real advantage..." (Imhof (1974), p. 41).

When practolol unexpectedly had to be redrawn from the market because of serious side effects, the market was open for this new compound metoprolol. The strange and extraordinary phase of one and the same drug but two **differently profiled therapeutics** started (Bodewitz et al. (1986)).

195. Brunner, pers. comm.

196. Brunner, pers. comm.

197. In 1968 the CIBA group published that oxprenolol possessed no intrinsic activity: Also the lack of a positive inotropic and chronotropic effect in the isolated guinea pig heart and a bronchodilator effect of Ciba 39'089-Ba (oxprenolol, RV) indicates that this substance does not match ß-stimulating effects ["Auch das Fehlen einer positiv inotropen und chronotropen Wirkung am isolierten Meerschweinchenherzen und einer bronchodilatatorischen Eigenwirkung von Ciba 39'089-Ba (oxprenolol, RV) deutet darauf hin, daß dem Präparat keine ß-stimulierende Effekte zukommen"] (Brunner et al. (1968), p. 169.

198. Brunner et al. (1971), p. 222; see also Imhof (1974). See for the results of the experiments with oxprenolol also Brunner et al. (1970) and Meier (1970).

199. Brunner interview; and pers. comm. The other paticipants interviewed where Dr. M. Meier and Dr. F.Ostermayer.

200.Burley, interview.

201. Silk, interview.

202. Cf. Gross (1981).

203. The role of university contacts for the successful development of new drugs in a R&D-organization so small as Hässle is important as Östholm commented: "When I visited ICI in Alderley park in 1962 they had well over 700 people in medical-pharmaceutical research while we at Hässle had only 35 people. Without the guidance of scientists at the medical faculty in the University of Göteborg we could not have achieved what we did. Folkow, Carlsson and Werkö all participated in research conferences when our projects were evaluated and criticised" (Östholm, pers. comm.). This collaboration with university Gross referred to as unique and deserving to be copied by other firms (Gross (1983), p. 237).

204. Barrett, interview.

205. Quoted from Talalay (1964), p. 267.

206. Fitzgerald, interview.

207. Barrett, interview.

Notes chapter 5.

1. Follansbee and Shaver (1986).
2. Schwartz and Taira (1983); see also Van Zwieten (1985).
3. Pfennigsdorf, pers. comm.
4. Pfennigsdorf, pers. comm.
5. Verapamil was defined as a **benign** coronary vasodilator in dilating the coronary vessels and therefore increasing blood and oxygen supply to the heart without increasing the demands of the heart. In constrast, malign coronary vasodilators dilated coronary vessels and increased total coronary blood flow at the expense of an increase in cardiac work; see for this distinction also chapter 7. See for experimental research on verapamil at Knoll: Haas and Härtfelder (1962), (1964a), (1964b), (1964c), Haas and Busch (1967), Haas (1968), Haas and Igarashi (1968), Haas (1970); Haas and Gokel (1970). Further: Schlepper and Witzleb (1962), Melville et al. (1964). With respect to clinical studies: Anonymous (1963), Tschirdewaahn and Klepzig (1963); Hoffmann (1964); Strässle and Burckhardt (1965); Hoffbauer (1966); Wette et al. (1966); Zimmer (1966); with respect to the use of verapamil in cardiac arrhythmias in German medicine: Bender et al. (1966); Bender et al. (1968); Bender et al. (1969); Bender (1970); and Bender (1971).
6. See also appendix III.
7. Charlier (1971).
8. This author's analysis of the retrieved articles confirms this pattern.
9. Mignault, de L (1966), p. 1253, and further: "Therefore, one must explain the clinical improvement experienced by patients taking the drug by mechanism that is independent of any change in coronary blood flow".
10. Luebs et al. (1966), p. 540.
11. Neumann and Luisada (1966), p. 552.
12. Engelhardt, the pharmacologist at Boehringer commented: "That verapamil had to be something different from Persantin was in fact already obvious from the whole activity spectrum, in particular because verapamil has a strong cardial effect which is totally absent in Persantin" ["Daß Verapamil etwas anderes sein müsste als Persantin, war eigentlich schon klar aus dem ganzen Wirkungsspektrum besonders deshalb, weil Verapamil eine starke kardialen Wirkung hat die ja beim Persantin total fehlt!"] (Engelhardt, interview).
13. Haas commented: "And I remember that I was at Hoechst and I said to Härtfelder, who had already left me at that time: "I have discovered something new about Isoptin; it is a beta blocker". And he said: "You don't say!". It is a great development if it can be done like that. That's how new it all was" ["Und ich erinnere mich das ich bei Hoechst war und dem Härtfelder die damals schon von mir weggegangen war, habe ich gesagt: 'Ich habe was neues von Isoptin entdeckt; das ist ein Betablocker'. Und er sagte: 'Donnerwetter'. Eine tolle Entwicklung wenn man das so machen kann. So neu war das alles"] (interview Haas).
14. Haas commented: "That would have been an advantage at the time, because in fact only propranolol existed. We would then have been so to speak the second to be clinically relevant. So in that respect it would have been an initiative that would have been already very rewarding at the time. There wasn't this abundance of beta blockers yet" ["Das wäre damals vielleicht ein Vorteil gewesen, weil eigentlich nur Propranolol existierte. Wir wären dann so zu sagen der Zweite gewesen, der klinisch relevant gewesen wäre. Also insofern war das schon ein Ansatz der sich damals gelohnt hätte. Es gab ja noch nicht diese Fülle von Betablockern"] (interview, Haas).
15. According to Haas the view held at the pharmacology department of Knoll was that verapamil possessed beta blocking properties which was somewhat later rejected (cf Haas (1964); Haas, pers. comm.). However, the issue to what extent and in what way verapamil differed from beta blockade was elaborated by Fleckenstein.
16. Gebhardt and Büchner (1967).
17. Melville et al. (1964); see also Melville and Benfey (1965).
18. Fitzgerald and Barret (1967).
19. ibidem.
20. Bateman (1967).
21. ibidem.
22. ibidem.
23. Shanks (1967).
24. Robinson, interview; see also the description of the development of propranolol (4.2.4.1).
25. Fitzgerald and Barrett (1967).
26. Bateman (1967).
27. ibidem.
28. Anonymous (1968).

29. Anonymous (1967).
30. Anonymous (1968).
31. Anonymous (1967).
32. Anonymous (1969a); see further Anonymous (1969b); Grant et al. (1968); Thompson and Letley (1968).
33. Sandler (1968), p. 226; see further for a negative judgment Phear (1968).
34. Anonymous (1968).
35. Shanks (1967).
36. Anonymous (1968).
37. Wilkinson (1967).
38. See for references Fleckenstein (1964). Further it is interesting to note that clinicians were also involved in research on this topic; cf. Nägle (1970).
39. Fleckenstein (1964).
40. Cf. Fleckenstein (1964).
41. For the effects induced by these compounds mimiced the symptom complex of utilisation-insufficiency.
42. Cf. Later we also included Isoptin and Segontin in our research; since, according to the producing firms, these two substances have - apart from the direct coronary vasodilator main effects - beneficial sympatholytic effects in the manner of beta receptor blockers. As a matter of fact, we could fully confirm these assertions" ["Später haben wir dann auch Isoptin und Segontin in unsere Untersuchungen mit einbezogen; denn nach Mitteilung der Herstellerfirmen besitzen auch diese beide Stoffe - neben direkten coronarerweiternden Hauptwirkungen - günstige sympatholytische Nebeneffekte nach Art der Beta-Receptorenblocker. Tatsächlich konnten wir diese Angaben voll und ganz bestätigen"] (Fleckenstein (1964, p. 92-93).
Cf. also: "Because Isoptin also exceeded the sympatholytic effect of Alderlin on the hearts of guinea pigs by five or six times, it may probably be regarded as the strongest - hitherto known - sympatholytic antagonist for the myocardium" ["Da Isoptin am Meerschweinchenherzen auch den Herz-sympatholytischen Effekt von Alderlin um das Fünf- bis Sechsfache übertraf, darf es wahrscheinlich überhaupt als der stärkste - bisher bekannte - Sympathicus-Antagonist für das Myokard gelten"] (Fleckenstein (1964), p. 93).
Fleckenstein's brother B. Fleckenstein, a clinician, worked at Knoll BV.
43. This figure is taken from Fleckenstein (1968a). Before that the scheme had been published in German medical literature (e.g. Fleckenstein et al. (1967c), p. 11).
44. Fleckenstein related this biochemical and physiological explanation of cardiac insufficiency to the concept of coronary vasodilation in the following way. The diastolic tone is a major factor in the regulation of the coronary circulation. When during hypoxia or exercise high-energy phosphates are broken down, the diastolic tone decreases and consequently the resistance of the coronary circulation increases thus improving oxygen supply to the heart and the increased synthesis of high-energy phosphates; and this physiological cycle could start again (Fleckenstein (1964).
45. See Fleckenstein et al. (1967a), (1967b); title in German: ["Zum Wirkungsmechanismus neuartiger Koronardilatatoren mit gleichzeitig Sauerstoff-einsparenden Myokard-Effekten, Prenylamine und Iproveratril"].
46. The criteria used by Fleckenstein were still incomplete in comparison with the full set of criteria proposed by the ICI scientists (Fitzgerald, Barrett (1967); Shanks (1967)).
47. The latter were determined by using the ratio of CP to Pi as the index, the former by using the inhibition of isoprenaline induced tachycardia as the standard.
48. Fleckenstein (1967a), p. 726: ["Der Gedanke ist naheliegend, daß die Hemmung von Kontraktilität und Frequenz durch ß-Rezeptoren-Blocker, Segontin und Isoptin auf einem Ausfall des sympathischen Antriebs infolge einer spezifischen Blockierung der im Myokard gestapelten und am Myokard angreifenden sympathischen Überträgerstoffe beruhen könnte. Wir selbst haben zunächst ebenfalls zu dieser einfachen Erklärung geneigt"].
49. Fleckenstein et al. (1967a), p. 727: ["Infolgedessen ist das Ausmaß der Herabsetzung der Herzkraft und der Frequenz am Herzen in situ nicht streng mit dem Ausmaß der ß-Rezeptoren-Blockade korreliert"]. The question is put as subheading of the section (p. 726): ["Ist die Hemmung von Kontraktilität und Frequenz durch ß-Rezeptoren-Blocker, Segontin und Isoptin Folge einer Herzsympathikolyse?"]
50. Fleckenstein et al. (1967a), p. 730: ["Man kann aus allen diesen Ergebnissen folgern, daß eine ß-rezeptoren-Blockade nicht unbedingt mit einer starken Herzhemmung und umgekehrt eine starke Herzhemmung nicht zwangsläufig mit einer ß-Rezeptoren-Blockade vergesellschaftet sein muß"].
51. After the second quotation the authors immediately continue as follows: "Incidentally, this is confirmed by later findings by Levy and Richards (1965); they report about a beta receptor blocker (MJ 1999) with only very little negative inotropic effect" ["Im gleichen Sinne sprechen übrigens auch neuere Befunde von Levy und Richards (1965), die über einen ß-Rezeptoren-Blocker (MJ-1999) mit nur sehr geringer negativ-inotroper Wirkung berichteten"] (Fleckenstein et al. (1967a), p. 730).
52. The German terms are: ["nicht streng ... korreliert" and "nicht unbedingt .... nicht zwangsläufig .... vergesellschaftet sein muß"].

53. The following quotation is characteristic: "It is of particular interest that Segontin and Isoptin have also shown certain beta receptor blocking properties in the frequency-test with Aludrin (isoprenaline, RV), as has been described by Lindner (Segontin, 1964) and by Haas (Isoptin, 1964)" ["Von besonderem Interesse ist, daß auch Segontin und Isoptin im Frequenztest gegen Aludrin (isoprenaline, RV) gewisse ß-Rezeptoren-blockierende Eigenschaften besitzen, so wie dies schon von Lindner (1964) für Segontin und von Haas (1964) für Isoptin beschrieben worden ist"] (Fleckenstein et al. (1967a), p. 729).

54. Huxley (1969); see also Singh (1980).

55. It is interesting to note that the latter possibility is explicity referred to in the article (e.g. Fleckenstein et al. (1967b), p. 853) but not mentionned in the conclusion and English summary.

56. Fleckenstein et al. (1967b), p. 853: ["Letzlich entscheidend für die Zügelung der mechanischen Myokardfunktionen ist vielmehr ein hemmender Eingriff in die "elektromechanische Koppelung", wobei die spezifischen ß-Rezeptoren-Blocker sowie Segontin und Isoptin vor allem auch als Ca++-Antagonisten wirken, indem sie die physiologische Mittlerfunktion der Ca++-Ionen zwischen dem elektrischen Erregungsprozeß und dem Kontraktionsakt beeinträchtigen"].

57. Fleckenstein et al. (1967b), p. 853: ["Alle diese Befunde weisen darauf hin, daß die negativ-inotropen Myokardeffekte von ß-Rezeptoren-Blockern sowie von Segontin und Isoptin auf einer komplexen Hemmung der Myofibrillen-ATPase beruhen, indem sich (a) die unspezifische Ca++-Verdrängung sowie (b) die spezifische Auschaltung der endogenen Catecholamine infolge ß-Rezeptoren-Blockade jeweils im Endeffekt addieren"].

58. Fleckenstein et al. (1967a), p. 734: ["daß sich hinter dem wenig präzisen Begriff der 'elektromechanischen Koppelung' wohldefinierte Reaktionen verbergen (...)"].

59. ["Segontin und Isoptin wirken offenbar an der Myofibrillen-ATPase in erster Linie als Ca++-antagonisten und erst in zweiter Linie als Catecholaminverdränger an ß-Rezeptoren"] (Fleckenstein et al. (1967b), p. 856.

60. Cf. Fleckenstein et al. (1968b), p. 344: "..because basically the art of therapeutic application to human beings of beta receptor blockers and related substances consists for the most part of manoeuvring between the Scylla of non-effective doses and the Charybdis of an immanent insufficiency of the heart" ["..denn die Kunst der therapeutischen Applikation von ß-Receptorenblockern und verwandten Stoffen am Menschen besteht im Prinzip hauptsächlich darin, sich zwischen der Scylla einer unwirksamen Dosierung und der Charybdis der drohenden Myokardinsuffizienz hindurchzuwinden"].

61. Cf. Fleckenstein et al. (1967b), p. 855: "Moreover, the possibilities of sympathetic regulation of the cardiac function are preserved in a somewhat mitigated way under the influence of Segontin and Isoptin, so that the danger of a sudden circulatory collapse is smaller than that which is to be feared with the application of specific beta blockers" ["Darüber hinaus bleiben die sympathischen Regulationsmöglichkeiten der Herzaktion unter dem Einfluß von Segontin und Isoptin mäßig abgeschwächt erhalten, so daß die Gefahr eines plötzlichen Kreislaufzusammenbruchs weniger als bei Anwendung spezifischer ß-Rezeptoren-Blocker zu befürchten ist"].

62. Moreover, the direct mechanical effects had to be separated from secondary changes in the cardiovascular system as the fall in arterial and venous pressure that indirectly result from these mechanical effects. These problems were assessed by continuously registering the cross-section of the heart and relating it to both the time of onset of the dilation and the changes in the electrical system.

63. Fleckenstein, pers. comm. See for the early reception of Fleckenstein of the role of calcium in the bio-electrical processes in the heart, for example: Antoni H, Engstfeld G, Fleckenstein A. Inotropic effects of ATP and epinephrine on hypodynamic frog myocardium following excitation-contraction uncoupling by Ca withdrawal. [In German] Pfluegers Arch. Gesamte Physiol. Menschen Tiere 1960; 272: 91 - 106. An extensive survey on this matter is given by Fleckenstein (1983), particularly Chapter IV, pp. 165-185, and Chapter V, pp. 186-208. See for fundamental research on verapamil Nayler (1967); Nayler et al. (1968).

64. Vaughan Williams, pers. comm.: his hypothesis was, for example, ignored in the computer construction of the cardiac action potential in 1962, performed by Noble. In the late 1950s and during the 1960s Vaughan Williams and Singh developed a classification system of anti-arrhythmic drugs (e.g. Singh and Vaughan Williams (1970), (1972); Singh (1980), and the references in these articles). When the anti-arrhythmic properties of verapamil were reported, Singh and Vaughan Williams reported that the drug was not a class 1, 2 or 3 agent, and thus suggested that it had a new "class 4" action in restricting the second inward current revealed as persisting in the presence of quinidine (Vaughan Williams, pers. comm.). See for a review of this sequence of these events Vaughan Williams (1989a) (1989b), i.e. Chapter 1 (Cardiac Electrophysiology) and Chapter 2 (Classification of Antiarrhythmic Actions).

65. Fleckenstein et al. (1967b), p. 848: "All these findings show that the coronary vasodilator effect of Segontin and Isoptin is an exceptional property which appears independent of the other cardiac effects of this substance" ["Alle diese Befunde zeigen, daß die koronardilatatorische Wirkung von Segontin und Isoptin eine besondere Eigenschaft ist, die unabhängig von den sonstigen Herzeffekten dieser Substanzen in Erscheinung tritt"].

66. E.g. Fleckenstein et al. (1967b), p. 851: "The discharge of the heart as a result of blood pressure fall is considered by some authors as the therapeutically more decisive factor in the nitroglycerine treatment of an anginal attack. At the same time however, the true coronary vasodilator actions of nitroglycerine and erythroltetranitrate should not be

depreciated too much (cf. Bernsheimer and Rudolph (1961); Klensch and Juznic (1964)" ["Die Entlastung des Herzens infolge Blutdrucksenkung ist von einigen Autoren als der therapeutisch wichtigere Faktor bei der Nitroglyzerinbehandlung eines Angina-pectoris-Anfalls angesehen worden (vgl. Bernsheimer und Rudolph (1961); Klensch und Juznic (1964). Gleichwohl sollte man die echten koronardilatatorischen Wirkungen von Nitroglyzerin und Erythroltetranitrat nich zu gering einschätzen (..)"]. This implies that the German authors referred to above by Fleckenstein disagreed with the concept of coronary vasodilation (see for the references Fleckenstein et al. (1967b).
67. Fleckenstein (1967b), p. 855: "Since, however, Segontin and Isoptin can, in addition, also increase the coronary flow, they have a preferential position with which no specific beta blocker can compete" ["Da jedoch Segontin und Isoptin auch noch zusätzlich die Koronardurchblutung steigern können, besitzen sie eine Vorzugstellung, mit der kein spezifischen b-Rezeptoren-Blocker konkurrieren kann"].
Some ambiguity about the coronary vasodilator concept needs to be noted. On the one hand he argues - in an Anglo-American way - that coronary vasodilators are often used although probably the coronary vessels during hypoxia are dilated maximally and that the sclerotic vessels can hardly be expected to dilate. In this sense he considers the coronary vasodilators as the classic approach, the beta blockers as the new approach; "classic" comes close to meaning an outdated approach. On the other hand he approves verapamil and prenylamine because they include both therapeutic principles.
68. Thus, Fleckenstein represents the typical German view that beta blockers were dangerous drugs: "However, beta receptor blockers are dangerous in all cases in which the necessary heart minute volume and the arterial pressure can only be maintained with stronger aid of sympathetic heart and circulatory regulations (immanent myocardial insufficiency, inclination to peripheral circulatory collapse, acute loss of blood and others)" ["Dagegen sind ß-Rezeptoren-Blocker in allen Fällen gefährlich, in denen das erforderliche Herzzeitvolumen bzw. der arterielle Druck nur noch unter stärkerer Zuhilfenahme der sympathische Herz- und Kreislaufregulationen aufrechterhalten werden kann (larvierte Myokardinsuffizienzen, periphere Kollapsneigung, akute Blutverluste u.a.)"] (Fleckenstein et al. (1967b), p. 855).
69. Fleckenstein et al. (1967b), p. 857.
70. Fleckenstein et al. (1969a), p. 227: ["Iproveratril, D600 und Prenylamin können als die ersten hochwirksamen Vertreter einer neuen Klasse von Pharmaka gelten (..)"] and ["Gaben von Extra-Calcium oder Sympathicomimetica (speziell Isoproterenol) heben die Effekte der Ca++-Antagonisten prompt wieder auf"] (this was a short communication delivered at the 10 Frühjahrstagung der Deutschen Pharmakologischen Gesellschaft (Mainz, 16-19 März, 1969); see also Fleckenstein et al. (1969b). See for research on prenylamine Lindner (1960a), (1960b); and nifedipine Bossert and Vater (1971) and the proceedings of the series of nifedipine-symposia (cf. Lichtlen and Ebner (1986)). The references regarding research on verapamil have been given throughout this chapter; D600 has received relatively little attention.
71. Fleckenstein (1971).
72. According to "This Week's Citation Classics" - Science Citation Index, 1988; 31 (nr. 23 June 6): 19 - the 1977 paper of Fleckenstein has been cited in over 1.380 publications (making it the most-cited paper from the journal Ann Rev Pharm Toxicol). This number differs from that presented in this study because of the period covered and the methodology used; see also appendix II.
73. Mulkay (1980); see further Moravcsik and Murugesan (1979).
74. Since research into calcium antagonism is built up of a highly complex mixture of theory- and technique-based specialities and evolved in response to the requirements of pharmaceutical-industrial and medical research, it is very unlikely that curve D reflects the same patterns as those which evolve out of largely autonomous research networks. This falls outside the scope of this analysis. Furthermore, it has to be stressed that the scientometric data shown are not corrected with respect to various factors; for example, the increase in the total number of medical publications over past decades.
75. Cozzens (1985); Dolman and Bodewitz (1985).
76. Fleckenstein, interview.
77. Bender, Kaltenbach, interviews.
78. Refsum and Landmark (1975), p. 374.
79. Newman et al. (1977), p. 723.
80. Lively et al. (1973).
81. So, for some time profiling of verapamil by clinicians in angina pectoris concurred in two ways. Firstly, the determination of the efficacy of the drug without reference to its mechanism of action. Secondly, the profiling of the drug on the basis of cardiovascular characteristics that were not yet connected to the concept of calcium antagonism.
82. Bender, Huijbers, interviews.
83. Pfennigsdorf, interview. In Anglo-American medicine it was particularly Melville (Melville et al. 1964; Melville and Benfey (1965)) who initiated this area of interest (see also Britchard and Zimmerman (1970; Zipes et al. (1975); Zipes and Troup (1978)). In the German context Bender elaborated the anti-arrhythmic activity of verapamil and discovered the beneficial effects in supraventricular tachycardia; the work performed by Bender and co-workers during the 1960s

(Bender et al. (1966); Bender et al. (1968); Bender et al. (1969)), was unknown to clinicians in the English speaking world.

84. Singh (1980).

85. Singh (1980).

86. Fleckenstein, interview. Lichtlen and Ebner (1986) point out that at the first Nifedipine meeting "(..) the word "calcium antagonist" was used only by Fleckenstein. At that time, clinicians still had to get acquainted not only with this term but also with the whole concept of calcium antagonism". See also Kroneberg (1975, p. 9) where he proposes a different mechanism of action to explain the complex effects of nifedipine; and in this proposal the concept of calcium antagonism plays a minor role.

87. Lichtlen and Ebner (1986), p. 9.

88. Parodi et al. (1979); Maseri et al. (1979); Pfennigsdorf, pers. comm.

89. See for references Lichtlen and Ebner (1986).

90. The following procedure was performed to achieve the figures depicted in the table. Using verapamil and nifedipine as key words the number of articles indexed by MEDLARS during the period 1966-1987 (november 1987, i.e. the time of the research performed) was retrieved by computerized search. Subsequently these sets of articles were further restricted by using the selection procedures "Find x and PY<1971", "Find x and PY<1976", etc. until the numbers of the articles indexed could be calculated for the periods represented in the table; where x denotes a specific item in the computerized search, e.g. the set of articles about verapamil. The same procedure was repeated for the sets of articles achieved by using the names of the drugs and "angina pectoris" as the keywords. The term "clinical" was defined as CT=Human in MEDLARS; this implies that articles reporting on both experimental (animal, in-vitro) and clinical aspects are also classified as clinical.

91. Pfennigsdorf, pers. comm.

92. In earlier times coronary blood flow was considered from the perspective of increasing blood flow whether or not at the expense of energy. The concepts of benign and maligne vasodilation denoted compounds which increased coronary blood flow without increasing demand (benign vasodilation) and which increased flow at the expense of demand (maligne vasodilation); see also Chapter 7.

93. Preload is a determinant of afterload and as such a determinant of myocardial oxygen demand, hence (A)—(P)—(I)—(O). Furthermore, decreased afterload decreases demand but with secondary decrease in supply, hence: (A)—(I)—(O); (A)—(C). Considering the effects of nitrate therapy, for example, both effects have to be taken into account with a clear-cut net effect of decreasing demand over decreasing supply. Confusion may also rise because of the present use of variables. The variable intracardial tension is nowadays divided into diastolic and systolic wall tension. It is known that decreased diastolic wall tension facilitates coronary perfusion while it is at the same time a principle determinant of myocardial demand. The same applies to systemic venodilation which is divided into end-diastolic volume (preload) and end-diastolic pressure. Other examples may be given as well (Follansbee and Shaver (1986).

94. See for the present views about the major and minor determinants of myocardial oxygen demand, Follansbee and Shaver (1986).

95. The drugs X,Y and Z are "unrealistic" drugs, because the sets denoting these drugs contain also elements other than a, v, i, m, h, o, s or c.

96. This is not to say that nitrites have no effect on coronary vessels, that is, dilation of larger resistance vessels, collateral channels as well as stenotic vessels. Nowadays the view is held that these effects lead to the net result of a redistribution of flow towards ischemic areas (which are perfused by stenotic vessels). In the late 1960s and early 1970s however, a spasmolytic effect (s) was attributed to nitroglycerine but an increased coronary flow (c) was doubted. For this reason of(nit) contains characteristic "s" but not "c". See for a research article in which the comparison between nitroglycerine and dipyridamole served the purpose to unravel the mechanism of action of antianginal agents, Bousvaros et al. (1966).

97. Scientists are ambivalent in classifying a compound or a class of drugs. For example, sometimes the profile of verapamil includes the antianginal effects, then its antiarrhythmic drug action; and at other times its general profile is depicted. Furthermore, in some cases scientists use the operational (functional) profile of a drug, in other cases they refer to the overlap between the operational functional profile and the wished for functional profile.

98. This differentiation of two profiles of cardiac dysrythm is an idealized representation of the actual developments in the 1960s.

99. Vaughan Williams, interview. See figure 5.1; the actual reference Vaughan-Williams has in mind is: figure 7 on page 233 in Fleckenstein A, Döring HJ, Kammermeier H. Experimental heart failure due to inhibition of utilization of high-energy phosphate. In: Marchetti G, Taccardi B (eds). Coronary circulation and energetics of the myocardium. Basel, Karger: 1967: 220-236 (Vaughan Williams, pers. comm.).

100. This expression arose during the interview with Prof. Bender.

101. This term came from Dr. Pfennigsdorf during the interview when confronting him with Bender's opinion that verapamil was a dying drug.

Notes chapter 6.

1. Heberden, 1772, quoted from Matthews (1977), p. 3.
2. See Charlier 1971, p. 95: Symposium on the Diagnosis of Thoracic Pain.
3. Friedberg (1956), p. 449-450.
4. Friedberg (1956), p. 472.
5. Friedberg (1956), p. 451.
6. Robinson, Dollery, Prichard, Chamberlain, interviews.
7. Wood (1952), p. 376.
8. Paul Dudley White (1951) was interested in the interaction of 'the psyche and the soma' in heart disease. He pointed out that emotion might cause angina not only in patients with coronary artery disease but also in humans with normal coronary arteries; and rarely, even death in a person with a healthy heart (White (1951)). Presumably this was a defendable position from the viewpoint of the theory of coronary spasm prevalent at that time. During the 1950s this became 'unthinkable'.
9. Friedberg (1966), p. 713; see also Preston (1977) and Schaefer (1980).
10. Friedberg (1956), p. 376.
11. Wood (1952), p. 376.
12. Friedberg (1956), p. 470.
13. Dexter (1981), p. 13.
14. Wood (1952), vii.
15. Anonymous (1960), p. 1063.
16. ibidem. There was no need for technical measurement to differentiate angina pectoris from other conditions because in "practically every instance the typical history is sufficient to distinguish the anginal syndrome from those diseases simulating it".
17. Anonymous (1960), p. 1064.
18. Wood (1952), vii.
19. Cf. Preston (1977), particularly Chapter 2: "Historical Development of Operations for Coronary Artery Disease".
20. Vineberg, Walkers (1957); quoted from Preston (1977), p. 18.
21. Preston (1977), Schaefer (1980).
22. Preston describes how the Vineberg operation that remained highly controversial, received a boost from the work of Sones and Shirey in Cleveland in 1962. With the help of coronary angiography they documented definite connections between the internal mammary artery and the coronary circulation. It was thus shown that surgeons indeed provided "fresh blood to the ischemic myocardium" as Vineberg claimed (quoted from Preston (1977), p. 18).
23. Preston (1977). This is also reflected in the clinical taxonomy of angina pectoris; see further this chapter.
24. See Preston (1977), particularly pp. 153-171; international comparison yields important differences for the various countries. About 28 operations per 100.000 population were performed in the United States while this number for Britain and West-Germany amounted 2.5 and 1.4 operations per 100.000 population respectively. The fact that in the USA ten times more operations are performed is explained by Preston in terms of economic, social and psychological factors.
25. Silber, Katz (1953), p. 1075-1076.
26. Beecher (1953), p. 44.
27. Charlier (1971).
28. Silber and Katz (1953), p. 1075.
29. Russek, Urbach and Doerner (1953), p. 207.
30. Wood (1952), p. 378.
31. Friedberg (1956), p. 470.
32. Cf: "The exercise and other test must definitely be regarded as of accesory value to the clinical history, and not as the decisive factor in the diagnosis of angina pectoris" (Friedberg (1956), p. 470).
33. As encountered in the samples of, for example, therapeutic evaluations of verapamil and dipyridamole (chapter 5 and 7).
34. Robinson, interview.
35. I asked for this because of my impression that Circulation was characteristic for this hemodynamic approach.
36. Chamberlain, interview.
37. Swales (1985), particularly his introduction, p. ix-xviii.
38. Quoted from Swales (1985), p. xiv.
39. Quoted from Swales (1985), p. xiv. One of Platt's opinions made during his Harveian Oration, might have been taken straight from Ryle as Swales commented: "Clinical science has shown an unfortunate tendency to follow only the

methods of physical science, which try to prove everything by contrived experiments to the neglect of discovery by deliberate and relevant observation and the kind of evolutionary or if you like teleological thinking necessary to the study of biology". (Quoted from Swales (1985), p. xvii).

40. See for the formation of British cardiology in the early decades of this century Lawrence (1985). The journals in which this second group of clinical researchers published were particularly Clinical Science (founded by Lewis), Circulation and Circulation Research, as well as the general medical journals (e.g. British Medical Journal) and the general scientific journals (e.g. The Lancet).

41. Cf. Swales (1985).

42. Silk, interview.

43. Screening the British Heart Journal over the period 1951 - 1959 using as key words the terms "angina pectoris", "hemodynamic", and "(cardiac) catheterization" yielded few articles, i.e. 6, 5, and 11 respectively - the average number of articles of a volume (including 4 numbers) amounts to a little more than 60 articles (counted for the 1959' volume and excluding editorials, comments, etc).
In the 1960s the British Heart Journal published various articles including therapeutic evaluations, on the beta blockers. However, the British Medical Journal formed the platform for exposing the new way of thinking.

44. Chamberlain, interview; Silk, interview.

45. Dollery, interview.

46. Robinson, interview.

47. This concept of coronary insufficiency has been variously defined. This means in the author's terminology that the three patient profiles intersect to a greater or lesser extent or that the sets of characteristics vary.

48. Raab (1953), p. 291.

49. ibidem.

50. Raab (1953), p. 295.

51. Maseri (1980).

52. Monroe and Chung (1976).

53. Friedberg (1972), p. 1037.

54. Preston notices the first aspect regarding coronary surgery. The other aspect is discussed by Lawrence (1985).

55. Friedberg (1972), p. 1038.

56. Friedberg (1972), p. 1038.

57. See Preston (1977) and Schaefer (1980).

58. Friedberg (1972), p. 1038.

59. Yet another feature contributed to this renewed interest for clinical symptomatology. Due to the rapid expansion of angiography, angina pectoris had become a symptomless disease. Not the symptoms of the patient, but the anatomic lesions of the coronary vessels played the active role in establishing the parameters for the therapeutic and prognostic outlook of heart disease. In a sense this offended professional identity in cardiology. It is striking to see that particularly in this period, late 1960s and early 1970s, the symptom of pain and physical signs observed with simple bedside techniques reappeared in cardiology. However, they were considered as too vague and too uncertain for exact diagnosis (e.g. Proudfit and Hodgman (1968)).

60. Cf. Maseri et al. (1979), Maseri (1980), (1983), (1985).

61. Kübler and Tillmans (1985).

62. Maseri (1985); Kaltenbach, interview.

63. Hillis and Braunwald (1985).

64. Lichtlen (1986), p. 11.

65. This implies that the gap between structure and function is great and variably filled up: "A century has passed since the hypothesis of coronary arterial spasm was first proposed. It remains a pathophysiological and clinical enigma. The incidence of the phenomenon may be quite small and its penalty even more inconsequential. But, in the present state of knowledge, the gap that separates anatomic structure from function is great and it underscores the many determinants regulating the balance between coronary perfusion and myocardial metabolism that fall beyond our understanding. Coronary artery spasm may be among the more significant of them" (Likoff (1976), p. 245).

66. Cf. Dhurandhar et al. (1972), p. 902.

67. Venn-diagrams are not suitable for representing the (logical) relationships between sets when the number of sets exceeds three or four. However, the purpose here is to mark the major shifts in relationships between the sets which can be visualized. No intersection is meant to be empty.

68. Vakil (1961); Beamish and Storrie (1960); Papp and Smith (1960).

69. In another article a few clinical and therapeutic differences between the forms of angina pectoris were discussed (Prinzmetal et al. (1959b)).

70. Prinzmetal et al. (1960).

71. Gazes et al. (1973).

72. Gazes et al. (1973), p. 331.

73. Maseri (1980); further he lists five lines of research to elucidate the characteristics of this form of angina: 1. continuous electrocardiographic monitoring; 2. stress testing; 3. continuous haemodynamic monitoring; 4. regional myocardial perfusion studies; and 5. coronary arteriography.
See for an extensive discussion of the two major classes of angina, i.e. classic angina and variant form of angina, from the perspective of two fundamentally different pathogenetic mechanisms (Fuchs and Becker (1980)).

74. Selzer et al. (1976).

75. To mark the difference in using Venn-diagrams for the cognitive and social dimensions of medical knowledge, the **circles** represent the cognitive features; the **squares** the social aspect: the **size** of the square is crucial, not the intersection.

76. Friedberg (1966).

77. Further, to cover Anglo-American cardiology and cardiovascular research the British Journals were studied including: British Medical Journal, Nature, The Lancet, British Heart Journal and Clinical Science; as well as the American Journals: American Journal of Cardiology, American Heart Journal, Circulation, Circulation Research, JAMA, American Journal of Medicine. All Journals were screened on the same key words over the period 1955-1970 systematically whereas with respect to the periods 1950-1955 and 1970-1980 the snowball-method was used.

78. Bruce (1964), p. 290.

79. Gorlin (1965).

80. This is especially because angina of deglutition denoted a pre-infarction state which is also depicted in figure 6.2.

81. Gorlin (1965), p. 145.

82. Elsewhere he stated: "In addition, during active coronary vasoconstriction, an "inappropriate" sympathetic nervous system response, may be a major factor in many attacks of angina" (Gorlin (1965), p. 147).

83. In this way MacAlpin (1973) summarized the prevalent opinion in the field. At that time MacAlpin helped to set through this concept (cf. MacAlpin et al. (1973); MacAlpin (1976). Just like MacAlpin (1973) Aisner (1970) summarized: "Many current textbooks still emphasize the fact that, if the pain does not occur with effort or emotional stress or cannot be reproduced by physical exertion, the diagnosis of angina pectoris is suspect". Silber and Katz (1975) stated that "vasomotor changes" (i.e. coronary vasospasm) were considered by several authors as the cause of anginal attacks at rest; and they admit that temporary occlusion of the great coronary vessels had been established. However, their opinion was: "It is likely, however, that these vasomotor phenomena in architecturally normal coronary arteries are of no importance". Thus, Silber and Katz considered atherosclerotic occlusions of the coronary vessels as the most important cause of angina pectoris, also in case of spontaneous or nocturnal angina. The period 1970-1975 shows therefore a variety of positions intermediate between enthusiast acceptance and total rejection. See further Schrenk (1967); Whiting et al. (1970); Griffith (1971); White (1974); Meller et al. (1976); Hillis and Braunwald (1978); Maseri et al. (1979).

84. Scherf and Cohen (1974).

85. For example, by asking around. The interviewed Anglo-American clinicians suggested that Gorlin's classification, though Gorlin himself was a well-respected clinical investigator, certainly was not as influential as the ones proposed by Friedberg or Wood. Sophisticated scientometric techniques are available to investigate this problem.

86. In 1951 Pickering criticized the theory of vascular spasm: "At the present time the idea that vascular spasm produces the manifestations of disease is entertained too freely and too uncritically. It is my purpose here to try to show how closely organic vascular narrowing or occlusion may mimic vascular spasm, and to show that true spasm is a rare rather than a common condition" (Pickering (1951), p. 845).
He therefore condemned the theory of coronary spasm as an unnecessary hypothesis (with respect to all types of vessels and corresponding pathological conditions): "Before closing, one point should be made abundantly clear. There is no contention here that vessels do not contract and expand, for such indeed is their essential function in ministering to the wants of tissues that vary in their activity and hence in their requirements from minute to minute, from hour to hour, and from day to day. What is claimed is that many of the manifestations of disease that have been ascribed to abnormal contraction of a single artery, or group of arteries, are in fact due to other circumstances, of which the chief is organic arterial occlusion or obstruction. In other words these phenomena can be interpreted in terms of known pathological or physiological processes, without assuming that arteries behave like whimsical children (as children were understood before contemporary psychology) and react violently to a perfectly ordinary stimulus or to none at all" (Pickering (1951), p. 850). It is interesting to note that the claim of Pickering was picked up by the German physician Hoffman who wholeheartedly disagreed (cf. the description of the German medical views in chapter 7).

87. Kübler and Tillmans (1985).

88. Prinzmetal et al. (1959a), (1959b), (1959c), (1960), (1961).

89. See chapter 7.

90. Cf. Goodman and Gilman's textbook (1970).

91. Combination therapy of nitrates and beta blockers in exertional angina was established; hence their profiles

intersected considerably. The additive efficacy is the result of one drug blocking the adverse effects of the other on net myocardial consumption. Cf. Goodman & Gilman's textbook (1985).
92. Cf. Lie (1987).
93. Anonymous (1960a), p. 291.
94. Interview Silk.

Notes chapter 7.

1. Matthews (1977).
2. Matthews (1977); see for the quotation of Brunton in the text Goodman and Gilman (1941, p. 548), (1955, p. 730).
3. MacAlpin (1980).
4. Goodman and Gilman (1941), (1955).
5. Goodman and Gilman (1965), (1970) and (1975).
6. Lie (1987).
7. Cf. Lie (1987).
8. Lie (1987).
9. This theoretical pluralism with respect to angina pectoris - not described in many historical accounts as Lie rightly argues -is to set the scenery for the development of the coronary vasodilator concept in the post-Second-World-War period.
10. Lie (1987); Leibowitz (1970); Burch and DePasquale (1964).
11. This "ischemia" theory of angina pectoris was constructed on the analogy of the widely accepted view that muscular pain was caused by an impaired blood flow due to arteriosclerotic stenosis of the blood vessels (cf. Goodman and Gilman (1965), (1970). Anginal pain became synonymous with muscular pain.
12. See chapter 6.
13. Braunwald (1981), p. 299.
14. See for history of coronary theory and theory of coronary spasm: Amsterdam and Mason (1981); Lichtlen and Ebner (1986); Likoff (1976); MacAlpin (1973); Maseri (1983), (1980); Friedberg (1972); Lie (1987); Leibowitz (1970); White (1974); Braunwald (1981).
15. However, the spasm theory underlied views about these disorders as well.
16. For example, Pickering (1951); see for other references MacAlpin (1980).
17. MacAlpin (1980), p. 302.
18. MacAlpin (1980), p. 302.
19. MacAlpin (1980).
20. This study takes a global contextual analysis as point of departure but regional variation figures prominently in therapeutic change and drug prescribing. The spasm theory, for example, must have been influential in several parts of Anglo-American medicine since some influential textbooks referred to it till the seventies: see for example Krantz and Carr (1965).
21. This is not say that there is no disagreement. Cf. Silber and Katz: "We have relied solely upon relief of pain as a criterion of the efficacy of a particular agent. We have rejected exercise tolerance or hypoxemia tests because response to these procedures varies spontaneously in patients and requires repeated testing over long control periods to make their use at all worthwhile. More important, these tests are artificial and are not comparable to the clinical situation that evokes anginal pain" (Silber and Katz (1953) p. 1076; see chapter 6.
22. Silber and Katz (1953), p. 1075.
23. Traks et al. (1959).
24. The famous article by Gregg and Sabiston is dated 1956 but the differentiation was formulated earlier. This is exemplified by Silber and Katz (1953): "(..)it must always be established that drugs that increase coronary flow do not at the same time increase the metabolism or work of the heart proportionately or disproportionately and thereby nullify the anticipated benefits" (Silber and Katz (1953), p. 1075).
25. Gregg and Sabiston (1956).
26. Quoted from Lichtlen (1972), p. 193.
27. A systematic analysis of the state of affairs in the various European countries was not performed.
28. Kreuzer (1969), p. 186: ["Es gibt wohl kein therapeutisches Prinzip, bei dem trotz der zahlreichen experimentellen Ergebnisse die klinische Beurteilung so unterschiedlich ist, wie bei der medikamentösen Coronardilatation. Die Angaben über die klinische Wirksamkeit bei Angina Pectoris schwanken zwischen 0 und 90%. Besonders in der

deutschsprachigen Literatur finden sich zahlreiche Arbeiten, die über erstaunlich gute Resultate in erstaunlich kurzer Zeit und mit erstaunlich geringen Dosen berichten (..). Demgegenüber stehen negative Urteile nicht zuletzt aus dem angelsächsischen Schrifttum, die bis zur völligen Ablehnung dieser Substanzen reichen. So schreibt Fisch in einem Übersichtsreferat, daß keines dieser Präparate (er bezieht sich auf Persantin, Segontin und Amplivix) zur Behandlung der Angina Pectoris empfohlen werden können"].

29. Lichtlen (1972), p. 205: ["Entsprechend sind die klinischen Resultate - in der Regel auf Doppelblindversuchen beruhend - bezüglich der antianginösen Wirkung ebenfalls widersprüchlich. Während die meisten angelsächsischen Autoren, mit einer Ausnahme, über negative klinische Ergebnisse bei Angina Pectoris berichten, liegen von deutschen und französischen Autoren zahlreiche positive Resultate vor"].

30. Kaltenbach, interview: ["Und ich kann mich noch erinnern wie ich mit den Freiburgern mal diskutiert habe und dann meine Einwände eingebracht habe. Die sagten: 'Ja, aber Kaltenbach, hör doch mal. Wenn jetzt Deine Mutter Koronarbeschwerden hat, wollen Sie dann ihr die Koronardilatatoren vorbehalten? Das kann man doch nicht tun"].

31. Kaltenbach, interview.

32. Bender, interview: ["(..)muss man sagen daß in Deutschland anders als in den USA ein starke Trennung ist ins allgemeine - hier nicht in Münster - zwischen Experiment und Klinik und so daß der eine nicht weißt was der andere macht und sich das sehr auseinander entwickelt hat"].

33. Kaltenbach, interview: ["Vielleicht waren auch die Ärzte die zu der Zeit in den führenden Positionen waren, einfach nicht Ärzte denen das naturwissenschaftliches Denken ganz besonders nahelag, die eben groß geworden waren in einer Medizin die anders eingerichtet war"].

34. Kaltenbach, interview: ["Belastungsuntersuchungen waren ein Stiefkind in vielen Kliniken. Beispielsweise hatte man in Düsseldorf frühzeitig mit der Herzchirurgie begonnen, sich aber diagnostisch ganz auf den Herzkatherismus konzentriert. Dies lag nahe weil vorwiegend Patienten mit Vitien und Mißbildungen nicht aber Koronarkranke behandelt wurden"].

Furthermore Kaltenbach referred to an anecdote: "A man who has been a co-operator in my department for as long as twelve, fourteen years told me just the other week that until 1972 he used to work in a German university hospital. In that hospital an exercise-ECG-test which showed a coronary insufficiency was a sensation that occurred only twice or three times each year" ["Ein Mann der schon zwölf Jahre mein Mitarbeiter ist in meine Abteilung, vierzehn Jahre, der hat mir gerade vorige Woche erzählt, er war in einer Deutsche Universitätsklinik bis 1972. In diese Klinik war ein Belastungs-EKG das eine Koronarinsuffizienz anzeigte, eine Sensation die im Jahre nur zwei, drei Mal vorkam"].

35. Kaltenbach, interview: ["Und speziell in Zusammenhang mit der Prüfung solcher Medikamente wurden immer wieder Studien vorgelegt mit klassische Koronardilatatoren wie Persantin. Und dann musste ich immer wieder sagen: 'Was definieren Sie eigentlich als Angina Pectoris? Wenn man alle Brustbeschwerden als Angina Pectoris bezeichnet, kann schon Luminal ein wunderbares Mittel sein, um zu wirken; aber das hat nichts damit zu tun, daß die Koronarinsuffizienz beeinflußt wird"]. Kaltenbach was very much involved in developing exercise ECG tests in Germany; cf. Kaltenbach and Klepzig (1963); Kaltenbach and Zimmermann (1968); Kaltenbach (1970); Kaltenbach et al. (1971).

36. This applies to Klinische Wochenschrift, Deutsche Medizinische Wochenschrift and Münchener medizinische Wochenschrift, and particularly to Therapiewoche and Therapie der Gegenwart (cf Klever (1966); Kolodzig (1966); Dornaus (1967); and Hirsch und Woschée (1967).

37. Pfennigsdorf, interview: ["Die Durchführung einer plazebokontrollierten doppelblinden Crossover-Studie bei Angina pectoris bedeutet in der Regel, daß der Patient mindestens 10 - 12 Wochen an der Studie teillnehmen muß. Da die meisten deutschen Kliniken nicht über ein eigenes ambulantes Krankengut verfügen, können die Patienten zum Biespiel für Wirksamkeitsuntersuchungen von Koronarmitteln in der Regel nur mit Zustimmung des behandelnden Hausarztes rekrutiert werden. Hierbei ergeben sich Probleme, da der behandelnde Arzt nich selten befürchtet, seinen Patienten zu 'verlieren'"].

38. Kreutzer (1969), p. 193: ["Es ist deshalb verständlich, daß bei der Anwendung von Coronardilatatoren in der Klinik große Unsicherheiten bestehen. So reichen die Ansichten von der völligen Ablehnung bis hin zur großzügigen Medikation auch bei funktionellen Beschwerden. (...) Trotz der häufig enttäuschenden klinischen Wirksamkeit der Coronardilatatoren und trotz der Schwierigkeit, ihre Effekte zu objektivieren, erscheint es vorläufig nicht gerechtfertigt, auf ihre Anwendung generell zu verzichten. Die experimentelle Ergebnisse über die Kollateralenentwicklung sind so eindrucksvoll, daß es angezeigt ist, Coronardilatatoren mindestens so lange zu geben, bis zweifelsfrei feststeht, daß sie beim menschlichen Herzen die Kollateralenentwicklung nicht begünstigen. Dieser Nachweis wurde jedoch bis jetzt nicht geführt"].

39. Typical is, for example: "It must be assumed that the regulating function of adenosin in such a situation (i.e. the occurrence of disturbances of the oxygen supply of the myocardium) not only exists in an increase of the blood flow but also in the passage rate of the most important substrates" ["Es muß angenommen werden, daß die regulierende Rolle von Adenosin in einer solchen Situation (i.e. Auftreten von Sauerstoffversorgungsstörungen des Myokards) nicht nur in einer Steigerung der Durchblutung, sonder auch der Durchtrittsräte der wichtigsten Substrate besteht"] (Kraupp

(1969), p. 153).

40. Articles of Raab appeared also in the German medical literature.

41. Mainzer (1958): ["Daß Coronarspasmen auch bei intakten Arterien vorkommen können, erweist neben vielen anderen Tatbeständen, die klassischen Beobachtung von Gruber und Lanz, die als Folge eines epileptischen Anfalles mit Herzbeklemmung Myokardnekrosen bei völlig einwandfreien Coronararterien feststellen konnten. Diese Sachlage wird auch durch hie wütigen Angriffe nicht geändert, die der englischen Kliniker Pickering undernommen hat, wobei er diese Anschauung verschiedentlich as 'grotesken Mythos von Idioten' bezeichnet hat"].

42. Payer (1988).

43. Charlier (1971).

44. The compound concerned is benziodarone; the successor of this compound was amiodarone but this drug was rapidly acknowledged as different from a 'coronary vasodilating agent'.

45. Charlier (1961).

46. This is an advantage since due to the dominance of Anglo-American medicine in the Post-Second-World-War period it is seldom the case that articles from different medical - including the German - contexts are covered. A clear disadvantage of Charlier's position, however, is that Charlier was also   director of the Labaz Laboratories, a Belgium-French pharmaceutical company that was involved in the development of coronary vasodilators (benziodarone, amiodarone). For this reason I checked Charlier's interpreted data; see also appendix III.

47. To understand the medical views about coronary vasodilators and beta blockers amongst general practitioners, particular in the United Kingdom, the journals J Coll Gen Pract and The Practitioner were screened using the key words "angina pectoris", "(coronary) vasodilators", "dipyridamole", "propranolol" and "ß-(adrenoreceptor)blockers/blockade" over the period 1958 - 1970. In the former journal one article, in the latter sixteen articles were retrieved. MacKinnon points out that "the majority of drugs in use at present are recommended because of their ability to increase coronary blood flow by producing coronary arterial dilatation in animal experiments" (MacKinnon (1960), p. 559). Amongst the short-acting coronary vasodilator drugs glyceryl trinitrate (trinitrin) was evaluated as the drug of first choice in relieving and aborting anginal attacks. Long-acting coronary vasodilator drugs amongst which dipyridamole, xanthines, khellin and derivatives, and derivatives of nitrites were disappointing. Thereafter only (long-acting) nitrites and beta blockers were the subject of discussion. Long-acting coronary vasodilators were evaluated negatively. In the early 1960s beta blockers were considered having a limited place in the treatment of angina pectoris; in the late 1960s with established value, though preserved for cases with a significant disability despite the use of glyceryl trinitrate.

48. The difference between the curve "clinical articles" and the curve of "positive clinical articles" concerns not negative clinical articles (there is merely one) but exploratory clinical articles the major part of which discussing beta blockade in relation to particularly cardiac insufficiency.

49. This example comes from Levine (1958), p. 349.

50. Parsons-Smith (1950): "He (MacKenzie, RV) regarded breathlessness, dropsy, engorgement of the liver, and renal congestion as indications of a deficient output into the systemic circulation, a smilar discrepancy in the lesser circulation being responsible for stasis and edema in the lungs" (Parsons-Smith (1950), p. 889).

51. Lawrence (1985).

52. Parsons-Smith (1950).

53. In America Harrison was among the first clinicians attempting to interpret Starling's observations clinically. He broke with the British tradition in heart failure by showing, as Pickering stated, "that the hypothesis of forward failure favored by the great masters MacKenzie and Lewis did not explain the phenomena of cardiac failure, which were more consistent with the alternative hypothesis of backward failure" (Pickering (1960).

54. Cf. Wood (1952); Pickering (1960) refers merely to the work of McMichael and Sharpey-Schaefer in the British context.

55. The controversy between the backward and forward failure theories was surpassed because the active role of the venous pressure in cardiac adjustment was stressed: "As opposed to the back-pressure and the forward-failure theories, in both of which a raised venous pressure was regarded as a passive development, the modern interpretation, based on Starling's law of the heart, is that the venous filling pressure plays an active part in regulating the range of the cardiac output, and that in a failing heart the rise of venous pressure is, for a time, a compensatory mechanism" (Parsons-Smith (1950), p. 890).

56. Wood (1952), p. 154.

57. Pickering (1950), p. 323.

58. Harrison (1977), Hurst (1966, 1970, 1974), Friedberg (1950,1956,1966).

59. See Friedberg (1966), p. 138.

60. For example, clinicians who assessed the role of the kidney in heart failure. Particularly in the United States the 'kidney' school has been very strong, paying attention to neurohumoral mechanisms of adaptation. However for some time the regulatory role of the kidney was shown with the help of hemodynamic studies. With so much emphasis laid upon the kidney, McMichael wondered whether heart failure was a failure of the kidney or of the heart (McMichael

(1962)).
61. This framework did more than redefining the language of everyday clinial practice; it added new subsets of heart failure too, e.g. "high-output" and "low-put" failure.
62. The issue is not whether Braunwald is right or wrong or even if Starling is right or wrong. The mere point is to show that medical and scientific perceptions in Anglo-American physiology and cardiology rely upon the applicability of Starling's Law of the Heart.
63. Braunwald, Ross and Sonnenblick (1967), p. 39. The authors use a nice analogy to explain the difference. Firstly, the number of horses for pulling a barrow: the more horses, the stronger the car is pulled; secondly, the strength of the (individual) horses: the stronger the horses the faster the car is pulled. The analogy is suitable to explain the contribution of the ultrastructural studies: the muscle filaments (the ultrastructural units) are the horses.
64. So influential was Starling's concept in cardiology that it was said that regulatory mechanisms **adjusted** the organism to the operation of the law. As Friedberg wrote: "Other collateral regulatory mechanisms as well as the sympathetic nervous system **add** their effects to the Starling relationship" (my emphasis, RV) (Friedberg (1966), p. 141). Or as Friedberg put it for the case of exercise: "..the Starling law is temporarily modified during exercise, not invalidated" (Friedberg (1966), p. 140); and: "The modifying autonomic and humoral regulatory factors which become notable with physiologic stress such as exericse are dominant **only for relatively brief periods of time**" (my emphasis, RV) (Friedberg (1966), p. 140).
65. Kaufmann (1926): ["In Wahrheit scheint mir die Sache so zu verhalten: Wenn wir älteren, in jüngster Zeit von W.R. Hess bereicherten Anschauungen folgend die Funktionen des Körpers in zwei Gruppen teilen, die animalischen, zu welchen die Funktionen der Sinnesorgane, der die Muskeln und Sinnesorgane versorgenden Nerven und vor allem die Funktionen der Körpermuskulatur gehören, und die vegetativen, zu welchen die Verdauung, die Ausscheidung und vor allem die Atmung gehören, so läßt sich das Verhältnis des Herzens zu diesen beiden Funktionen vielleicht zutreffend ausdrücken, wenn wir sagen: Das Herz ist ein Diener der animalischen, es ist ein Sklave der vegetativen Funktionen des Organismus"].
66. Wenckebach (1942), full quotation: "At this point the moment would have come for the Romantics among us to sit down by the side of the road and reflect on the transience of all great things. Harvey compared the heart to the outstanding character of his king (Charles I) to whom he was a loyal servant and to whom he dedicated his immortal opus "De motu cordis et sanguinis". In his dedication he ranked both heart and king with the sun, the centre of the world on which everything turns. (...) The "automation" of the heart muscle emerged as glorious victor from the long struggle of "neurogenic" against "myogenic". The laws of dynamics with regard to cardiac activity showed the exceptional adjustment of the heart to the demands required, no matter how great these demands were. Nevertheless, it was here that the term "slavery of the heart" was heard! Rudolf Kaufmann, our Viennese colleague, who died at too young an age, said in his last lecture for the Medical Society with all the emphasis of his serious manner: The heart is servant to the animal functions and slave to the vegetative functions of the organism". What would Harvey have said, had he lived to hear that statement? As an old, wise man he would have been comforted: He had already had to experience his king's head falling on the scaffold! For us it is an advance to have realised that the heart too must serve, not master, the well-being of the community"
["Hier wäre für den Romantiker unter uns der Augenblick gekommen, sich am Wegrand niederzulassen und über die Vergänglichkeit alles Großen nachzudenken. Harvey verglich das Herz mit der hervorragenden Figur seines Königs (Charles I.), dem er ein treuer Diener war und sein unsterbliches Werk "de motu cordis et sanguinis" widmete. In seiner Widmung stellte er beide auf eine Höhe mit der Sonne, dem Zentrum der Welt, um das sich alles dreht. (...) Die "Automatie" des Herzmuskels ging aus dem langen Kampfe "neurogen gegen myogen" in vollem Glanze als Sieger hervor. Die dynamischen Gesetze der Hertätigkeit zeigten die überragend autonome Anpassung des Herzens an jede Größe der ihm gestellten Anforderungen. Nichtsdestoweniger fiel hier das wort der "Knechtschaft des Herzens"! Rudolf Kaufmann, unser zu früh verstorbener Wiener Kollege, sagte in seinem letzten Vortrag in der Gesellschaft der Arzte mit dem ganzen Nachdruck seines ernsten Wesen: "Das Herzen ist ein Diener der animalischen, es ist der Sklave der vegetativen Funktionen des Organismus". Was hätte Harvey gesagt, wenn er diese Ausspruch erlebt hätte? Als alter, weiser Mann hätte er sich getröstet; er hat es ja auch erleben müssen, daß der Kopf seines Königs auf dem Schafott fiel! Für uns ist es ein Fortschritt, eingesehen zu haben, daß auch das Herz dem Wohl der Gemeinschaft zu dienen hat, sie nicht beherrscht"] (Wenckebach (1942), p. 95-96).
67. Quoted from Silber and Katz (1975); see also Katz (1960), (1966).
68. Florian was asked by the editorial board of the German medical journal to write a "state of the art" article about this subject.
69. Florian (1954), p. 1471.
70. It was extensively questioned whether a "sport heart" was normal or pathological.
71. The equivalent terms in German are: "Kontraktionsinsuffizienz" and "muskuläre Insuffizienz".
72. It is interesting to note that in order to achieve this beneficial state for the heart peripheral regulatory mechanisms were considered indispensable. Whereas Anglo-Saxon medicine declared these compensatory mechanisms to obscure

the operation of the Law of the Heart, German medicine appeals to them as necessary conditions for the operation of this Law. In the latter situation there is consequently no question of obscurity but actually the reverse, i.e. of clearness.

73. There were other terms in use (cf. Reindell et al. (1963), (1967).

74. Friedberg (1966), p. 152.

75. These observations were made in patients with heart failure on the basis of mitral stenosis, diphteria, multiple infarction, coronary insufficiency and a variety of other cardiovascular disorders (cf. Klepzig and Kaltenbach (1962), Klepzig (1964), (1968), (1972).

76. The pathologist Linzbach had quite some impact in Anglo-Saxon cardiology with the paper "Heart failure from the Point of View of Quantitative Anatomy" published in the American Journal of Cardiology (1960). Linzbach's findings contradicted the general view that hypertrophy is associated with an increase in diameter and volume of individual muscle fibres, not with an increase in number of fibres (cf Friedberg (1966), p. 151). Somewhat later his concept of "plastic dilatation" had impact too (cf. Hurst (1974), p. 420).

77. This concept was used by German clinicians to account for the observations made in mitral stenosis. This deviated clearly from Anglo-American views that the mechanical factor imposed on the (right) heart was more important to the development of heart failure in mitral stenosis than the pathological state of cardiac tissue. Friedberg, for example, acknowledged that heart failure of the (right) heart resulted in part from the mechanical disturbance, and in part from the pathological change which is generally of rheumatic origin. However, as he stated: "..as a rule the mechanical factor imposed....far exceeds any intrinsic myocardial disease in importance as a cause of right heart failure in mitral stenosis" (Friedberg (1966).

78. See for references Klepzig and Kaltenbach (1972), Klepzig (1964), Reindell et al. (1967).

79. Hegglin (1947); see further Florian (1954), p. 1470. See also "Fragen aus der Praxis" in the German medical journal on this issue and the answers provided by Delius (1953) implying that Hegglin's views had quite some impact.
It is interesting to note that Hegglin in fact takes a position relatively close to the Anglo-American position: he strongly distinguishes between the two forms of heart failure, one being dynamic (a la Starling), the other energetic requiring a biochemical-pathological approach.

80. The three major forms were "energetic insufficiency", "energetic-dynamic insufficiency" and "Hegglin's syndrome". The diagnosis could be made at the bedside. In the case of a prolongation of the QT-period, a normal ECG and the absence of congestion the diagnosis was energetic insufficiency; the same symptoms but including an untimely 2nd heart tone, energetic-dynamic insufficiency; and the symptoms as with the second syndrome but associated with AV-block or a positive reaction on a neurohumoral test, e.g. an adrenaline injection, the diagnosis was Hegglin's syndrome (Delius (1953)).

81. Cf. the spring and autumn meetings of the German Society of Cardiovascular Research (Tagungen) as well as the German Journal in the field (Zeitschrift für Kreislaufforschung.

82. This is not to deny their significance in Anglo-American medicine. The classification of the New York Heart Association dividing patients in four classes according to their symptoms with varying degrees of physical activity was very important. The classification has been used in the study of failure and pregnancy and of patients submitted to cardiac surgery for valvular heart disease. Cf. Friedberg (1966), p. 241.

83. Medical views in other countries were not investigated.

84. As Friedberg (1966, p. 336) wrote: "The various test of circulatory function or myocardial reserve are of very limited value. The responses of pulse and blood pressure to stress are too variable to be employed as a diagnostic test and there is considerable overlapping of the findings in normals and cardiac patients".

85. It is interesting to note that the varying perceptions of the major exception to Starling's conception, that of exercise, beautifully illustrates the marked differences between Anglo-Saxon and German views. Exercise diminishes cardiac volume yet is associated with increased stroke work.
According to Starling's law this is impossible since an increase in output originates from an increase in cardiac volume. The Anglo-American attitude to this exception consisted either in denying the relationship or by showing that despite this, the exercise was in accord with the applicability of Starling's law to man. Departing from exercise German and Scandinavian clinicians developed another view.

86. Naturally the methods were designed in such a way to discriminate between respiratory, circulatory and cardiac failure. In connection with the latter two categories, the test had to discriminate between nervous and organic states too.

87. Interview Kaltenbach: ["Ja, zur der Zeit in der fünfziger Jahren war die Schwedische Schule die Hoheschule der Kardiologie. Ja ich denke die waren auch wirklich gut damals"].

88. See Reindell, König and Roskamm (1967) for an extended list of references.

89. Engelhardt; Kaltenbach, personal communication.

90. Reindell et al (1967), particularly p. 82-83, and p. 86-87.

91. In fact, a continuous rise in pressure load; the hypertrophy that develops is essentially the same as in the case of training.

92. German terms are: "Bewegungsinsuffizienz", "Frühinsuffizienz" , "larvierten Formen der Insuffizienz", "latente Insuffizienz", and "Pre-insuffizienz".

93. Friedberg (1966), p. 726. There was however an important understream in Anglo-American cardiology which patronized the view that the angina patient was in a state of subliminal heart failure (c.f. Gorlin (1965)).

94. Dornhorst, interview.

95. The table is adapted from Friebel (1982).

96. Chamberlain, interview.

97. Cf. the different editions of Friedberg; and Braunwald in Harrison's textbook.

98. The most paradoxical and controversial therapeutic measure recently proposed and that is a direct consequence of this dynamic view, is the use of beta blockers in the treatment of heart failure.

99. German clinicians seemed to have had a rather primitive account of both Starling's experimental and the creative experiments performed during the 1940s and 1950s in the United Kingdom and America. The reverse, however, was also true.

100. It is difficult to retrieve from textbooks or scientific literature quantitative data with respect to the natural history of diseases. Under the heading of prognosis the course of the disease is discussed in qualitative terms: "some patients might develop...", "other patients...,"several patients...", etc. This enhances the difficulty in reconstructing contextual differences in patient profiles.

101. It is not stated whether these occurred simultaneously or not.

102. ["Aber alle auf dem Gebiete der Angina Pectoris erfahrenen Kliniker haben je und je **die Manigfaltigkeit ihrer Symptomatologie under ihres Verlaufes** betont"] Holzmann (1954), p. 1109.

103. The balance between these two major opposing views with respect to the nature and natural history of angina pectoris has been tipped in favour of either side throughout history. Cf. Monroe and Chung (1976).

104. Thus, a continuum existed ranging from little spots of necrosis, fibrosis and scars, "rudimentary" (anterior) infarction to myocardial infarction. The concept of "rudimentary" infarction encompassed all cases in which clinically and electrocardiographically an incomplete infarction pattern existed (cf. Holzmann (1954); Hauss (1954), (1958)).

105. At the therapeutic level contextual differences are more distinct. In Anglo-American medicine the treatment of angina pectoris was designed primarily to prevent or reduce the frequency of attacks, e.g. it was treatment of the pain. German medical literature focussed on the restoration of normal physiological conditions providing the heart with oxygen and nutrients in order to prevent damage of cardiac tissue.

106. This therapeutic view covers not only anginal treatment but also treatment of cerebral and peripheral disturbances. Vasodilators are a popular treatment in German medicine.

107. Levine (1958), p. 263. Admittedly, Levine also stresses prognostic and therapeutic aspects of this condition as the sentence which follows the quotation in the text expresses: "So often the physician errs and makes a 'cardiac cripple' out of one who is structurally sound" (ibidem).

108. Cf. Bargmann and Doerr (1963); Delius (1960), (1964), (1966); Grosse-Brockhoff (1964); Hauss (1954), (1966); Hoff (1948); Holzmann (1954); Klepzig (1968), (1972); Kottmaier and Schettler (1961); Parade and Bockel (1954); Reindel and Klepzig (1961); Reindel et al. (1967); Schimert et al. (1960); Schrenk (1967); Seitz (1966).

109. Cf. Hauss (1954), (1966); Keller (1960); Delius (1960), (1964), (1966); Parade and Bockel (1954).

110. This leads to another usage of the term "functional". For in Anglo-American medicine the term functional became synonymous with "from psychic origin". Hence, the distinction between organic and functional was overrided by that of "somatic" and "psychogenic".

111. The first meaning of the term "typical" is the relationship between the anginal attack and physical exercise. The second meaning denotes the clinical pattern that is so typical, once the anginal attack is manifest. This typicality ranges from anginal pain (e.g. typical nature and localization of the pain) to the full-blown picture (typical pain, typical electrocardiographic changes and other typical signs and symptoms).

112. See also the definition of angina pectoris and the lack of acceptance of exercise ECG tests in German medicine (section 7.2.1; notes 30 and 31).

113. Reindell en Klepzig (1961), p. 551: ["Das **klinische Bild** der Coronarinsuffizienz kann demnach durch ein vielfältiges Zusammenwirken von funktionellen und organischen Gefäßveränderungen ausgelöst werden"].

114. Since angina pectoris vera especially affected persons of sixty and seventy, and angina pectoris vasomotorica persons of thirty and forty, the group of persons of fifty was liable to both syndroms; furthermore, elderly people were characterized by vasovegetative lability.

115. Froment and Bruel, quoted from Mainzer: ["Wo immer bei Angina Pectoris die auslösende Faktoren, das zeitliche Verhalten, die Art der Ausstrahlung und die Reaktion des Angina Pectoris-Schmerz auf Nitrite vom typischen Verhalten abweichen, liegt Grund vor, die Ursache dafuer in der Mitwirkung modifizierender Einfluesse von gleichzeitig bestehenden anderweitigen Organerkrankungen zu suchen"] (Mainzer (1958), p. 750).

116. Particularly, the "vegetative chain of events" mediated these pain syndromes. This chain was considered as two-way-traffic. On the one hand these pain syndromes could be the result of genuine angina pectoris. On the other the

reverse situation was also held to be true.

117. Keller (1960), p. 1412: ["Besteht z.B. neben einer Erkrankung der Koronargefäße eine zweite, hiervon unabhängige Erkrankung, die außerhalb des Herzens lokalisiert ist, so erschöpt sich deren Vorhandensein keineswegs regelhaft in einer banalen 'Koexistenz'. Nicht selten kommt es vielmehr zu einer höchst komplizierten Verkettung oder Verflechtung der pathologischen Vorgänge, es entstehen neuartige pathogenetische Konditionenen, die das gewohnte klinische Bild des stenokardischen Anfalls in eigentümlicher Weise modifizieren. Daß atypische Angina pectoris-Anfälle in diesem Lichte zu deuten sind, daß sie unter dem Einfluß der Verkettung eine neuartige, doch wiederum typische Gestalt annehmen, war der klinischen Medizin lange verborgen und konnte erst in den letzten Jahren erhärtet werden"].

118. Engelhardt, interview: ["Dann wurde uns Ende der fünfziger Jahren bekannt daß ein Dichloorderivat des Aludrins bei Eli Lilly synthetisiert worden war, das hier bisher nicht hergestellt worden war und das wirkte so ein bischen wie ein elektrischer Schlag: 'Warum haben wir das nicht gemacht?', 'Ist das so schwer?' und so weiter. Also..und natürlich mit der Besonderheit das diese Verbindung ja auch nog blockierende Eigenschaften hatte. Also wir sind eigentlich durch's DCI auf dieses Thema gestoßen worden, durch die Findung des DCI's"].

119. Köppe (1977), (1986).

120. From the pharmacological and therapeutic point of view research in anorectic drugs unexpectedly branched into the realm of beta blockers. At the chemical level, however, this discontinuity seems to be less dramatic. The class of phenethanolamines was of considerable interest within the wider scope of research on sympathomimetic amines. By the end of the 1920s medicinal chemists had recognized four structural variants amongst sympathomimetic amines of therapeutic interest: adrenaline, tyramine, ephedrine and amfetamine. From these structures new drugs originated, particularly in view of indications as obesity, asthma, blood pressure disturbances, nasal congestion and the like. Manipulation of amfetamine, for example, led to derivatives as phenmetrazin, and several analogues of amfetamine were introduced as anorectic drugs (cf Sneader (1985).

121. Köppe (1986), p. 33; see also Engelhardt, Pharmacological Report, 19-5-1961.

122. Engelhardt, interview: ["Das war an sich mal zunächst vom rein pharmakologischen weil es ein neues Phenomenon war daß man den Sympathikus am Herzen blockieren konnte (...). Und da hab ich mir gesagt seiner Zeit das ist zunächst mal ein sehr interessanter und neuer pharmakologischen Befund aber habe noch kein Konzept gehabt, sagen wir mal, für eine therapeutische Ausnützung sondern habe mir nur gesagt das müsste eigentlich auch therapeutisch zu nutzen sein, im welchen Weise war...dazu konnte man theoretische Überlegungen anstellen. Die waren zu der Zeit von aller Ding, und das hat sich ja auch als wichtiges Prinzip für die Betablockern nachher ergeben, die Beeinflüssung der Herzfrequenz! Was daraus folgen würde jetzt für bestimmte Krankheiten und Indikationen. Dazu hätte Ich damals keine Ahnung"].

123. Engelhardt, interview: ["Natürlich. Also wenn wir was gefunden hätten, wäre das natürlich sofort eine Projekt geworden. Das ist klar!". For such a finding "hätte natürlich sehr nahegelegen beim den ganzen Konzept von Boehringer mit dem Aleudrin, nicht? Wir waren ja an die gleicher Zeit auch dabei ein Nachfolger des Aleudrins zu entwicklen. Das orciprenaline, ja"].

124. Engelhardt, interview.

125. The chemical and pharmacological reports of the compounds desribed in this section were provided by Boehringer.

126. In German: ["Zu untersuchen auf: Appetitzügelung"]. The form was signed by the chemist and the research director, i.e. Prof.Dr. Zeile who connived at the research into sympatholytic drugs (Dr. Köppe, pers. comm).

127. Engelhardt, interview: ["Na, wir haben zunächst mal natürlich, und da ging einige Zeit darüberhin, zusammen mit Herrn Dr. Köppe die Molekule optimiert, beziehungsweise untersucht. Was war jetzt maßgeblich für diese Wirkung? War das die Chlorsubstitution am Ring die wir zu anfangs postuliert hatten? Da merkten wir bald daß das gar nicht der Fall war. Und dann ein Preparat oder eine Substanz heraus zu suchen die optimal wirksam war und wenig toxisch"].

128. Kö 581 was synthesized on July 11, 1961.

129. The first pharmacological report referred to investigations of anorectic activity (February 28; March 13, 1962); the first report on isoprenaline antagonism in isolated guinea pig left atria appeared November 19, 1962.

130. The methods used were antagonism of adrenaline and isoprenaline induced bronchospasmolyse in quinea pigs (Konzett-Rössler system) in which bronchospasm was produced by acetylcholine and in isolated guinea pig left atrial preparations in which the effects of drugs on force of contraction and heart rate were expressed in terms of per cent of the post equilibration force as well as of the effects of isoprenaline.

131. That is, the LD-50 test.

132. Engelhardt, Pharmacological Report, June 14th 1962: ["Kö 592 ist unter die verwandten Verbindungen die bisher stärkste bradycardische Substanz, was evtl. auf eine Brauchbarkeit als Antiarrhythmikum hinweisen könnte, aber natürlich besonders geprüft werden muß"].

133. At this stage this was a general approach including effects on rhythmic and contractile function as well as general toxic effects on the cardiovascular system. A typical quotation of such a toxic effect with respect to Lg 32: "After 10 mg/

kg one animal died of strong bradycardia and the ECG-changes of a bundle branch heart block" ["Nach 10 mg/kg ging 1 Tier unter starker Bradykardie und den EKG-Veränderungen eines Schenkelblocks ein"]. (Engelhardt, Pharmacological Report May 27th 1963).

134. Lichterfeld, interview.

135. Engelhardt, interview: ["Nein. Es war an sich keine Überraschung. Es war nur ein stückchen weiter gedacht als wir selber hatten, nämlich jetzt nun auf eine besondere Krankheit ausgerichtet. Also auf der Angina Pectoris, auf die Koronarerkrankung was zunächst paradox erschien zu jener Zeit, denn die pharmakologische Koronartherapeutika beruhten ja auf Koronardilatation. Und das war nun bei den Betablockern überhaupt nicht der Fall. Die hatten keine Koronardilatierende Wirkung, unter Umstände sogar, unter bestimmten Konditionen sogar den Gegenteil im Effekt. Und trotzdem waren Sie einsetzbar für eine Koronarerkrankung. Das war überraschend"].

136. Köppe, interview: ["Wir wußten damals (1961/1962) überhaupt noch nicht daß einer sich Gedanken darüber hätten machen können was man damit anfangen kann, einfach therapeutisch. Wenn man das Herz ruhig stellt, was passiert dann? Ist das etwas günstiges? Kann man das Herz ökonomischer schlagen lassen? Hilft das? Heute ist es leicht zu sagen, es hilft ein Angina Pectoris Patient, nicht?"].

137. Letter (Engelhardt), October 31th 1962: ["Auf der Tabelle sind die wichtigsten Eigenschaften dieser Verbindungen der Bezugssubstanz Dichlorisoproterenol (DCI) gegenübergestellt. Alle Substanzen sind wesentlich weniger toxisch als DCI und hemmen die Herzwirkung des Aludrin 5 - 11 mal stärker. Sie unterscheiden sich hinsichtlich der bradycardischen Eigenwirkung, welche bei Th 293 fehlt, bei Kö 592 und 581 dagegen die Wirksamkeit des DCI um das 12- bzw. 23-fache übertrifft. Der bradycardische Eigeneffekt könnte Ausdruck einer zusätzlichen antiarrhythmischen Herzwirkung sein"].

138. The negative chronotropic activity ("Bradycardische Eigenwirkung") was distinguished from isoprenaline-antagonism in the sense that a potent "Bradycardische Eigenwirkung might express an anti-arrhythmic action in addition to the negative chronotropic effect of beta blockade. This differs from the ICI team who considered isoprenaline-antagonism as their prime criterium. To conclude this "cultural difference" on the basis of the use of two pharmacological parameters is far from convincing, but my impression is that such a letter would not have been written at ICI.

139. Engelhardt, interview.

140. Köppe, Engelhardt, interviews.

141. Engelhardt, interview: ["Also hier war sicherlich das Konzept der Koronardilatation in der praktischen Medizin sehr stark etabliert, nicht! (..) Und dies waren jetzt die Betablockern, Koronartherapeutika ohne koronardilatierende Wirkung und das war schwer verständlich"].

142. Lichterfeld, interview: ["Das Denken in Richtung des therapeutischen Prinzips "Koronardilatation" war ja auch bei Boehringer durch Persantin geprägt. Erst langsam kam durch die fehlenden klinischen Erfolge der reinen Koronardilatation ein Umdenken"].

143. Oxyfedrine (Ildamen) was a result of this idea (Lichterfeld, interview).

144. Lichterfeld, interview: ["Die Forschung der Firma richtete sich bisher auf die Agonisten der adrenergischen alpha- und beta-Rezeptoren. Neu und eine Wendung um 180° war die Entwicklung von Hemmstoffen des Sympathikus und das damit verbundene Denken"].

145. The most prominent German medical journals were: Arzneimittelforschung, Deutsche Medizinische Wochenschrift, Münchener Medizinische Wochenschrift, Medizinische Welt, Medizinische Monatschrift, Aertzliche Forschung, Therapie der Gegenwart, Aertzliche Praxis, Medizinische Klinik, Zeitschrift für Kreislaufforschung und Therapiewoche. Medical journals in other German speaking countries were most prominently: Wiener Medizinische Wochenschrift, Praktische Artzt (Wien), Wiener Zeitschrift für Innere Medizin, Wiener Klinische Wochenschrift, Schweizerische Medizinische Wochenschrift, Experientia (Basel) and Cardiologia (Basel). See also chapter 7, part 1.

146. Cf. the prospectus about Beta-Persantin, a combination preparation of Kö 592 and dipyridamole, published by Boehringer in August 1971.

147. Engelhardt, interview: ["Es fehlte hier bei Boehringer eigentlich der Impetus oder der gemeinsamen Entschluß jetzt mit der Substanzen voran zu gehen"].

148. Köppe, interview: ["Schon von Anfang an war man da erst mal vorsichtig als man diese neue Indikationsmöglichkeit sah, war das eine reine Angelegenheit von der Forschung. Wir haben es weiter betrieben aber es kannte keine Eingang in die Folgeabteilungen die danachkommen"].

149. Lichterfeld, interview.

150. The difference between Kö 581 and Kö 592 was explained as follows: "Kö 581 shows a moderate bradycardiac effect in non-anaesthesized animals and in itself it does not mobilize the non-esterified fatty acids. Therefore, the arresting effect on the tachycardiac and fatty acid mobilising effect of Aludrin is specifically and quantitatively of about the same strength as after Kö 592. However, since Kö 592 is somewhat less toxic and cheaper to produce, we recommend that further action be concentrated on this substance and that Kö 581 be put aside" ["Kö 581 zeigt an nicht narkotisierten Tieren eine mäßige bradykardische Eigenwirkung und mobilisiert selbst die unveresterten Fettsäuren

nicht. Der Hemmeffekt auf die tachykardische und fettsäuremobilisierende Aludrinwirkung ist daher spezifisch und quantitativ etwa ebenso stark wie nach Kö 592. Da Kö 592 aber etwas weniger toxisch und billiger herzustellen ist, empfehlen wir, die weiteren Arbeiten auf diese Substanz zu konzentrieren und Kö 581 zurückzustellen"] (Engelhardt, Pharmacological Report, September 11th, 1963).

151. Cf.: "Rather strong negative inotropic and to a lesser extent also negative chronotropic effects. 50% depression of the amplitude at the concetration 0.125 mg/50 ml." ["Ziemlich starke negativ inotrope und in geringerem Maße auch negativ chronotrope Eigenwirkung. 50% Amplitudendepression bei der Konzentration 0,125 mg/50 ml"] (Engelhardt, Pharmacological Report, November 29th, 1962).

152. Engelhardt, Pharmacological Report, August 28th, 1964: ["Lg 32 ist halb bis doppelt so wirksam wie Chinidin und wirkt damit am isolierten Herzvorhof stärker cardio-depressiv als Kö 592"].

153. Engelhardt, Pharmacological Report, April 11th, 1963: ["Zusammengefaßt ergaben die bisherigen Untersuchungen, daß Kö 592 ein spezifisches ß-Adrenolytikum ist und gegenüber bisher bekannte Substanzen dieser Art Vorteile bietet. Wir empfehlen eine vertieft pharmakologische Prüfung und bitten, ein Patent zu beantragen und die Trennung der optischen Isomeren in Angriff zu nehmen"].

154. Engelhardt, Pharmacological Report, October 15th 1963: "Tests on isolated heart preparations, on anaesthesized guinea pigs and on non-anaesthesized dogs have shown that, with regard to Aludrin-antagonism, Kö 592 has an effect on the heart that is at least twice as strong as Nethalide, and does not have any sympathomimetic characteristics of its own" ["Untersuchungen an isolierten Herzpräparaten, an narkotisierten Meerschweinchen und an nicht narkotisierten Hunden haben ergeben, daß Kö 592 am Herzen hinsichtlich Aludrinantagonismus mindestens doppelt so wirksam ist wie Nethalide, und selbst keine sympathomimetischen Eigenschaften besitzt"].

155. Lichterfeld, pers. comm.: ["Das Konzept der frühen klinischen Prüfung von Kö 592 war durch klinisch-pharmakologische Fragestellungen am gesunden Probanden bestimmt wie Ermittlung der dose-response und time-response für die aludrinantagonistische Wirkung und die "Eigenwirkungen", d.h. die Wirkungen per se. Die Parameter zielten auf adrenergisch vermittelte Funktionen von Herz und Kreislauf, Bronchien und Stoffwechsel, um Hinweise auf mögliche Indikationen und Kontraindikationen zu erhalten"].

156. Hähnel (1966); Kukovetz and Pöch (1965); Stock and Westermann (1965); Strubelt (1965); Levy and Richards (1966); Engelhardt (1964); Kuschinsky and Rahn (1965).

157. Lichterfeld, interview.

158. Lichterfeld, interview.

159. Kirchhoff (1965). This study on 50 human volunteers (age group: 18 - 35 year) was performed by Kirchhof while working at the medical department of the German Air Force. However, he had worked at the department of Reindell and the study of Kö 592 was in accordance with the functional-ergometric approach of Reindell; see Reindell and Kirchhoff (1956); Reindell et al. (1967).

160. Cf. Hähnel (1966).

161. Gebhardt et al. (1964); Gersmeyer (1965); see for references Hähnel (1966).

162. Lichterfeld, interview.

163. Lichterfeld, interview.

164. Kaltenbach, Bender, Pfennigsdorf, Haas and others (interviews); these reports also reached Boehringer. A German pharmacologist wrote October 18th, 1965 to Engelhardt after his visit to a symposium on beta blocking agents in Heidelberg: "From several sides we received warnings against possible side-effects, in particular cardiac depression" ["Von verschiedenen Seiten wurde vor den evtl. auftretenden Nebenwirkungen besonders der Herzdepression gewarnt"] (Letter to Dr. Engelhardt, October 18th 1965).

165. Cf. Patent application by G.H. Köppe, dated 23-4-1963, on behalf of the patent department of Boehringer. This letter contains information regarding reference substances for chemical and pharmacological screening, e.g. DCI and pronethalol, class exemplification and demarcation of patent rights. With regard to this latter aspect the various patents made by British Drug Houses which also patented a series of comparable compounds were included.

166. D.O.S. (Deutsches Offenlegungsschrift) 1493454.

167. Köppe and Engelhardt, interview.

168. On March 16, 1965 Boehringer received a letter from ICI claiming patent rights of this class of compounds. Priority dates referred to were 11-12-1962 and 19-7-1963; particularly with regard to Kö 592 ICI's patent application preceded that of Boehringer with less than 2 months. Cf. letter of patent department, 18-5-1988.

169. This was suggested by Köppe and Engelhardt, but was backed by the patent department of Boehringer.

170. Engelhardt, interview.

171. This is the case when considering the people who attended the meetings and received the relevant reports.

172. Engelhardt, interview.

173. Engelhardt, Pharmacological Report, March 8th, 1967: ["Sämtliche gemessenen Parameter wurden dosisabhängig im Sinne einer Cardiodepression verändert. Besonders und stärker betroffen als nach Kö 592 waren die Herzfrequenz und die Kontraktionskraft des rechten Ventrikels"].

174. Engelhardt, Pharmacological Report, March 31th 1967: ["Im Vergleich zu Chinidinsulfat war Propranolol hinsichtlich negativ inotroper Wirkung 5,9 (3,1 - 9,3) mal stärker, negativ chronotroper Wirkung 1,3 (0,9 - 1,5) mal stärker, negativ bathmotroper Wirkung 2,6 (1,8 - 3,7) mal stärker, Verlängerung der Refraktärzeit 2,1 (1,5 - 2,4) mal stärker. Unter den geprüften ß-Adrenolytika zeigte Propranolol am isolierten Meerschweinchen-Herzvorhof die stärkste cardiodepressive Wirkung"].

175. Letter Medical Department Boehringer, November 14th 1967: ["Es sieht so aus, als ob die Warnung der deutschen Kliniker, b-Rezeptorenblocker nicht für die ambulante Patienten freizugeben, auch für Kö 592 berechtigt sei und als ob auch Kö 592 kein 'Praxispräparat' werden kann"].

176. Letter Medical Department Boehringer November 14th 1967: ["Nach dem derzeitigen Stand des Wissens ist es nicht wahrscheinlich das b-Rezeptorenblocker gefunden werden, die Therapeutika für eine breite Praxisanwendung werden können"].

177. This was suggested several times when speaking with German clinicians. Due to the differences in health care system structure comparison is difficult. However, the following figures are impressive. The German Government (Daten des Gesundheitswesen (1977)) estimated the total number of specialists in internal medicine in 1960 on 7.550 of which 4.119 internists worked in private practice, 2641 in hospitals and 790 in administration and research (1970: 11.001, 5816, 3.977 and 1.208 respectively). In the United Kingdom the number of specialists working in private practice seemed to be considerable lower, i.e. under ten per cent of all specialists (Stevens (1966)).

178. Further research on cardiac insufficiency was recommended and the possibility of introducing another compound with a more marked intrinsic sympathomimetic activity, e.g. Kö 1313, was discussed Cf. letter Medical Department Boehringer Sohn, 14-11-1967. Compound Kö 1313 was valued for its similarity with alprenolol but it was argued that it was not certain at all that compounds with intrinsic activity were less riskfy and/or equally effective as propranolol.

179. Lichterfeld, interview: ["Aber ich glaube nicht, daß es daran lag, daß wir die falschen Konzepten hatten. Wir hatten die Konzepten die in der Luft lagen, inklusive der Angina pectoris und der labilen Hypertonie. Aber da war natürlich eine Bremswirkung, weil jeder representative wußte "irgendwo ist das Zeug gefährlich..". Und eigentlich kam dann kein Durchbruch und es trat eine Mutlosigkeit auf so daß man da nicht weiter durchgehalten hat und weitermachte"].

180. Interviews with the German industrial scientists and clinicians.

181. Letter Medical Department Boehringer, March 23rd 1970:
["Kö 592 besitzt pharmakologisch und toxikologisch größere therapeutische Breite. ß-adrenolytische Dosis und negativ inotrope Dosis sind weiter auseindergerückt als bei Propranolol"]
["Direkte und indirekte Hinweise sprechen für eine geringere kardiodepressive Wirkung von Kö 592 im pharmakologischen Experiment und in präliminären klinischen Befunden"].
This letter was send to marketing and foreign medical departments to provide information how to profile the drug. The addressed institutions were: "Pharma-Vertrieb CHBS Deutschland", "Marketing Information Ausland", "Region I", "Region II" and "Auslandsmedizin".

182. Letter Medical Department Boehringer, March 23rd 1970: ["Diese Ergebnisse dürfen nicht zu dem Fehlschluß verleiten, daß Kö 592 weniger sorgsam als Propranolol bei Herzinsuffizienz eingesetzt werden kann.
Die ß-Adrenolyse selbst, also die immanente Hauptwirkung, kann durch Hemmung des kompensatorisch verstärkten "sympathetic drive" bei Herzinsuffizienz zu einer Verschlechterung des Krankheitsbildes führen. Diese "Nebenwirkung" ist also dem therapeutischen Prinzip selbst und in klinisch-therapeutischen Dosierungen nicht den "kardiodepressiven" Eigenschaften anzulasten"].

183. This is a much more complex issue, particularly so from the theoretical point of view and related to the development of selectivity in the field of beta stimulating drugs. The question whether it was possible to dissociate these effects at the receptor level evolved during the 1960s.

184. Whether the parts of this preparation are administered separately or combined into one tablet is not important in this case. Neither would the association of these activities into one molecule make any difference, unless other demands are included into the wished functional profile: one tablet or one molecule, for example, might be preferred with regard to patient compliance.

185. The field of anti-arrhythmic drugs rapidly expanded during the 1960s not only because of the introduction of the beta blocking agents but also while cardiac dysrythm became a major clinical problem. In other words, the set of characteristics with respect to electrial function of the heart (with indirect consequences concerning mechanical activity) changed.

186. A non-empty intersection is a minimal condition in this respect.

187. Flörkenmeier (1980): ["Im Gespräch mit Kollegen aus der Praxis oder Klinik kommt es immer wieder vor, daß der eine oder andere Arzt seine Furcht vor einer Beta-Blocker-Anwendung zum Ausdruck bringt"].

188. The intermediate passage shows that there was a difference of acceptance between scientific and medical circles:

[RV: "Und sollte das bedeuten das diese Mediziner sehr stark an den Koronardilatatoren Konzept festhalteten?"
E: Das war ja damals eigentlich schon auch ein bischen an wackeln"
RV: "Ja, in pharmakologischen Kreisen und physiologischen Kreisen vielleicht"
E: "Ja, ja"
RV: "Aber wie war das in medizinische und therapeutische Kreisen?"
E: "Ja, hätte eigentlich nicht sein sollen, würde ich meinen aber ich weiss es nicht, also..."
RV: "Sie sagten: 'Das müsste nicht so sein'. Aber es war so?"].
(RV: "And would that mean that these physicians stuck to the coronary dilator concept very firmly?"
E: "In fact, at that time, that had also started to become somewhat wavering
RV:"Yes, perhaps in pharmacological circles and in physiological circles".
E: "Yes, yes".
RV: "But what was the situation in medical and therapeutical circles?"
E: "Well, it shouldn't have been like that, but, I don't know, anyway.."
RV: "You say: it shouldn't have been like that. But it was like that?").
189. E: "Wir haben den Mediziner den da seiner Zeit - der ist jetzt nicht mehr in der Firma (Dr. Graubner, RV) - sehr beknieen müssen und es war also sehr schwierig ihm zu überzeugen"
RV: "Aber bedeutet das daß man überhaupt das ganze Konzept bezweifelte?"
E: "Richtig, richtig! So ist es gewesen"
RV: "Und sollte das bedeuten das diese Mediziner sehr stark an den Koronardilatatoren Konzept festhalteten?"
E: Das war ja damals eigentlich schon auch ein bischen an wackeln"
RV: "Ja, in pharmakologischen Kreisen und physiologischen Kreisen vielleicht"
E: "Ja, ja"
RV: "Aber wie war das in medizinische und therapeutische Kreisen?"
E: "Ja, hätte eigentlich nicht sein sollen, würde ich meinen aber ich weiss es nicht, also..."
RV: "Sie sagten: 'Das müsste nicht so sein'. Aber es war so?".
E: "Ja, es war unbefriedigend letzes Endes und hat dann auch damit allem damit zugeführt daß wir mit unserem Doberol-Patent in der Priorität hinter der ICI standen"
K: "Obwohl wir ein, zwei Jahre hätten vorliegen können. Es gibt Situationen im Leben die man von sich aus nicht in der Griff bekommen kann von einem gewissen Position aus. Bedenken Sie bitte auch, wir waren 25 Jahre mindestens junger und da gibt es Älteren im höhere Positionen. Und da ist es nicht ganz so einfach eine neue, überraschende Erkenntnis um zu formen in ein verkäufliches Medikament. Das ist sehr schwierig vor allem Ding dann wenn da noch ein gewisses Risiko spricht, zum Beispiel die Kardiodepression vorhanden ist, und es bekannt war...eh..oder daß man davor Bange hatte. Sie wissen daß im Deutschland die Betablockern auch im nach hinein sehr viel später erst zu einem wirklich breiten Medikamentbereich geworden sind was in England, in den Skandinävischer Ländern schon Jahren vorher dann anerkannt war"] (Engelhardt, Köppe, interview).
190. Interview Lichterfeld: ["Aber mir ist auch bei der Rückblick eben klar geworden wie stark wir als Firma in das deutschen Umfeld eingebettet waren. (..) Das es nicht ein Versagen bestimmter Menschen war, sondern ein Umfeldproblem"].

Notes chapter 8.

1. These restrictions occur on the basis of the priority aspect which is omitted from the set-theoretical analysis. The results of these restrictions can still be registered with the help of the model. Actually, we assume implicitly in the text that in the context of wf^r/of^r and wf^{er}/of^{er} (see step 5) F is restricted to subsets F^r and F^{er}, respectively.
2. Without serious problems these steps can be described in terms of the set-theoretical model (see appendix IV). During step 3, for example, n times an introduction of a certain operational - functional and structural - profile occurs, while during step 4 it becomes clear that the extrinsic type of change, i.e. starting convergence with respect to the wished for profile, applies to compound x_1 and x_2, but not to the other synthesized substances.
3. There is no question of complete blindness. Even during a program of synthesizing and screening hundreds of thousands of substances, scientists make choices. The availability of raw material and equipment, the expertise of the chemist, the complexity of chemical synthesis, and the type of compounds already patented or studied by competitors influence the decisions made by the chemists. Further, one has to consider the wished for profile: compounds

containing chemical groups suspected of toxicity, for example, will be disregarded. Such considerations may also enter the search process later on.

4. Drews (1983), p. 49.

5. Drews (1983), p. 49.

6. Davey (1983), p. 47.

7. Austel and Kutter (1980), p. 39.

8. Austel and Kutter (1980); some papers of Austel and Kutter have been published since then which elaborate the principles discussed in the text and in appendix V in order to improve the activity of the medicinal chemist.

9. Three forms of structure-activity relationships are important to their analysis: 1) qualitative structure-activity relationships; 2) structure-activity classifications; and 3) quantitative structure-activity relationships cf Austel and Kutter (1980).

10. In chapter 2 this point has also been touched on when drawing attention to the controversy between "pictorial" and "sentential" imagery.

11. Cf. the Journal of Medicine and Philosophy, in particular Schaffner (1986) and Caplan (1986).

12. In medicine, as Schaffner argues, generalizations "fail to apply not only because they represent a stochastic process, i.e. are statistical generalizations, but also, and perhaps more often, because the generalizations represent only a partial fit due to individual or strain variation. The generalizations thus have a looser fit to their instances, which retain 'particularity' or their own individual differences more so than do (most) entities in the physicochemical sciences" (Schaffner, p. 77. 1986). As result, analogy or exemplar reasoning is prominent in medicine. An example of this is according to Schaffner, that biomedicine takes prototype-organisms such as the E. Coli bacterium as the exemplar, and "articulates a "mechanism" (more accurately an interlevel, idealized and usually temporal process) that explains some feature(s) of that organism. (A good example of such a 'mechanism' is the operon model for genetic regulation in the lac region of E. Coli K-12). The organism (or component part of the organism) is construed to be a prototype, and to have similarities with other organisms (or parts of organisms) - and ultimately and hopefully with humans - that license the extension of the 'mechanism' to a broader class of biological entities" (Schaffner (1986), p. 70). See also chapter 9 of this thesis for theory and concept forming at different levels in the organism.

13. Schaffner (1986), p. 71.

14. Collins (1987).

15. Collins (1987), p. 330.

16. Collins (1987), p. 336.

17. Cf. Collins (1987), p. 337.

18. Collins (1987), p. 335.

19. Collins (1987), p. 342.

20. Collins (1987), p. 345.

21. Notice the double sense of the term culture: the culture of the expert, i.e. the initiated, and of the end-user, i.e. the non-initiated.

22. Toulmin (1976).

23. Toulmin (1976), p. 36.

24. Toulmin (1976), p. 37.

25. Toulmin applies his map at a general level: medicine as a whole over a long period of time. My argument would be that we may seek lower levels of analysis and use the map for different purposes. In what way and to what extent depends on the issue at stake. We may focus on specific therapeutic fields or disease areas; or describe the contextual differences between British and German cardiology; we may do so for different groups or medical practices, e.g. the way cardiological problems are dealt with by cardiologists, gynaecologists, surgeons and general practitioners; and of course this can be done with respect to a department, a hospital, or a scientific discipline.

26. Toulmin (1976), p. 41.

27. In the diagram casual experience has an offshoot to the upper part of the map, i.e. general knowledge, indicating that the body of scientific therapeutic knowledge enters the realm of practical knowledge. In addition, it has an offshoot to collective knowledge, because physicians, e.g. general practitioners and occupational physicians, collect experiences about actual cases in taking care of particular groups of patients.

28. Cf. Stegmüller (1980); see also the discussion about the concept of application by Böhme in Starnberger Studien I, particularly p. 210-218 (reference by way of Hohlfeldt (1978). However, application is generally considerend in the context of the scientific theories. In this section the problem of application is interpreted by the author in terms of two-way-traffic between generalization and particularization with respect to a body of general knowledge composed of various threads of knowledge. This author's analysis results in the view of a circus movement of generalizing and particularizing medical knowledge. The basic idea is derived from Darden (1980) in which a general pattern of reasoning in theory construction (in genetics); and the figure (8.5) in the section of this thesis is adapted from Darden (1980, p. 155).

29. Toulmin (1976), p. 40.

30. Toulmin (1976), p. 43

31. Lasagna (1964), p.93-94.

32. The array of medical actions such as medical history taking, physical examination, laboratory measurements up to and including the prescription are left out of the analysis. The same applies to the activities of the patient and the pharmacist. Either these activities can be included into the stepwise reconstruction of the diagnostic-therapeutic process; or they are irrelevant for explaining the mechanisms of gathering new knowledge.

33. These changes can be described as transformation and differentiation (see appendix IV).

34. It might be the case that, though the drug was effective, the patient suffers anew from the same disease.

35. The drug might be effective or ineffective. In the case of a drug being effective: $CP'(i) = N \cup Q$, where Q is caused by that drug; in the case of a drug being ineffective: $CP'(i) = P \cup Q$ or $CP'(i) = P'' \cup Q$, where P'' is a change of P caused by that drug or through interference of Q with P.

36. In this case too the drug might be effective or ineffective.

37. This might concern a side-effect but this has been discussed under $BIIb_1$.

38. Bignami (1982) uses the term logic but does not define it in terms of logic. Since he treats ex juvantibus logic as a form of reductionist reasoning, the term form of reasoning is used in the text.

39. Bignami (1982), p. 96.

40. In this respect ex juvantibus logic comes close to the concept of retroduction/abduction of Peirce. However, because of the "distance" between theory and observation the term ex juvantibus logic is preferred by the author.

41. Van den Hoofdakker quoted from Termeer (1988), translation of quotation in Dutch: ["Iets nieuws ontdekken is in de praktijk niet de bedoeling. Er wordt juist verwacht dat je herkent wat je leermeesters al gezien hebben. Wat nieuw is, dat is lastig en gevaarlijk voor een jonge arts. Hij wil een oplossing, een diagnose. Het is voor hem heel moeilijk om te zeggen: ik weet het niet, dit heb ik nog nooit gezien, dit is nieuw. In het laboratorium moest ik op zoek naar wat nog nooit gezien was. Durven kijken, bij wijze van spreken. Dat was enorm boeiend...Natuurlijk kun je niet kijken met het ongewapende naieve oog. Basiskennis en een voorgeprogrammeerde blik heb je nodig. Maar de wetenschappelijke houding bestaat er nu juist uit, dat je die blik moet kunnen relativeren: oké, dit is onze huidige, diagnostische bril, die is niet eeuwig, die verandert. En hij verandert alleen doordat wij op een andere manier durven kijken. Dat is toch ook de motor van iedere vooruitgang, dat mensen anders durven kijken en niet langer denken dat ze het wel weten. Als je andere vragen stelt, komen er andere waarheden boven tafel"].

42. Cf. Howie (1972), Van Eijk (1979); and Gerritsma (1982). In this cycle the physician is guided by therapeutic objectives, i.e. restoring the normal condition of the patient, rather than correctly diagnosing the disease. However, the consequence (Bignami, type I) is clear.

43. Bignami (1982), p. 96.

44. The essence of the experiment lies in the fact that nature is being investigated under circumstances which do not normally exist. De Vries (1984, p. 15) writes [translation, RV]: "The experimenter has to change nature to a state in which it normally doesn't occur. Just as the geologist looks for fractures because there layers appear on the surface which otherwise lie hidden under the earth's surface, so, according to Bacon, should the physicist go to work. He has to produce "fractures"; because, after all, in experimental situations things appear which normally remain hidden under the surface".

In medicine it is repeatedly emphasized that disease is one of Nature's experiments. The analogy with the De Vries' geological fractures is perfect, since nature produces its own fractures which the experimenter makes use of. The second meaning, hidden in the above citation is that the experimenter creates these fractures. The medical practitioner is therefore involved in an experiment in two ways. On the one hand he acts and alters nature and on the other hand he treats disease as an experiment of nature.

45. Hacking (1989), p. 19; quotation translated: ["het uitzuiveren en stabiel houden van fenomenen die in pure toestand nergens in het universum bestaan"].

46. Hacking (1989), p. 20.

47. Wieland (1975).

48. The terminology which I use deviates from that normally used in ethical discussions. The diverse classifications of the therapeutic experiments in medical ethics will not be discussed further here. Generally speaking, the terms "therapeutic" and "experiment" are used in a broader sense than in medical ethics. Treatment given, for example, as part of a randomised clinical trial is considered therapeutic by the author but non-therapeutic in medical ethics. In relation to the term experiment, the prescription of an antibiotic for a woman with an urine bladder infection, is non-experimental according to the definition in medical ethics, while in this study it is regarded as an experiment.

Notes chapter 9.

1. Cf. Katz (1988).

2. Subsequent editions of the journal Trends in Pharmacological Sciences in recent years are evidence of this.

3. Hohlfeldt (1978); Zandvoort (1985), (1986).

4. This is also the case for studies of science looking at the relationship between social and cognitive aspects in the development of science (cf. the journal Social Studies of Science). In the above discipline concepts such as "style" or "heterogeneous network" illustrate the use of large analytical units.

5. Kuhn (1970).

6. Another model of the Starnberg group, i.e. the "alternatives" model, is left out from the analysis (cf. Zandvoort (1985); Boers (1981)).

7. In addition, the Starnberg group distinguishes between "functionalisation" and "finalisation". Functionalisation occurs in a situation where theories are lacking and trial-and-error strategies are important. Complex biological systems are considered as input-output systems, and manipulated accordingly. Pharmacology is considered pre-eminently as a scientific discipline in which functionalisation is central. Searching for medicines to treat headache, for example, pharmacologists proceed in a functional way by tracing causes of specific physiological effects, e.g. the dilation of blood vessels and hence, the search for vasoconstrictor agents. The theoretical explanation of underlying physiological mechanisms, then, is of minor importance.
The Starnberg group stresses that functionalisation as well as finalisation are important for the development of science. However, functionalisation is of primary importance in the pre-paradigmatic phase. Cf. Hohlfeldt et al. (1977); Rip and Groenewegen (1980); and Bodewitz and Stemerding (1979).

8. Cf. Rip and Groenewegen (1980).

9. Cf. Zandvoort (1985), (1986).

10. Kuipers (1989).

11. The more clinical medicine and general medical practice become the subject of philosophy, the development of medical knowledge cannot be described in terms of research programs.

12. Cf. the extensive discussion on the descriptive and normative nature of the concepts of health and disease in the Journal of Medicine and Philosophy; see also Vos and Willems (1987). Further, a philosophical justification for the claim that medical practice is a guide to medical science is not provided here. This claim can be justified, however, on the basis of Canguilhem's work. See particularly Hertogh (1987) who starts from Canguilhem in order to develop the concept of "clinical-therapeutical knowing".

13. Obviously, other classification levels can be found. In medicine "higher" levels including the social-cultural setting in which human beings live have to be considered.

14. Here the analysis is directed to the distinction between desired and undesired effects. However, the way of reasoning developed in the text also applies to the case of searching for more potent drugs in the sense of both inhibition or stimulation of specific physiological processes.

15. Moolenaar (1989).

16. Here we might consider reduction of phenomena (concepts) and relationships between phenomena (laws, theories). Standard examples of successful reductions, in physics, are the reduction of the law of Boyle/Gay-Lussac (or the ideal gas law) to the kinetic gas theory, and, in biology, of the two major laws of Mendel to the theory of molecular genetics. In the latter case the reduction of the concept of "gene" to the concept of "DNA-molecule" represents the reduction of concepts, in the sense of identification, i.e. "a gene is a piece of DNA-molecule" (Kuipers (1987a), (1987b)).

17. Hohlfeld (1978); Rip and Groenewegen (1980).

18. Other classifications are imaginable; a comprehensive overview is not provided here.

19. Due to the three-phase model the interaction between functionalisation and finalisation is not the subject of the analysis by the Starnberg group while this is especially so in this study. Specifically both processes are to be seen from the development of knowledge at different levels as distinguished in the text.

20. Carlsson (1983). In this article Carlsson mentions a number of important moments in the development of zimelidine, a medicine for depression. It is not important how truthful his discussion is, or how delighted clinicians should be with the drug, since it has already been withdrawn from the market because of its serious neurological side effects.

21. This does not mean that this knowledge always has to be published. The pharmaceutical industry maintains an extensive communication system with the medical profession via consultancies, symposia and congresses, panel review systems and market research. Usually this communication system is regarded as being uni-directional. The pharmaceutical industry provides information (to put it positively) to doctors or manipulates them (to put it negatively). This view fails to recognize that the communication system works in two directions - the "feelers" of the pharmaceutical industry.

22. Carlsson (1983), p. 38.

23. The term "case" (in Latin: casus = "declension" or "inflexion") is clarifying in this respect. By case is understood the declension of the nominative: in the (medical) case the disease as a general category is declined according to the situation of the patient, which is also declined in the process of diagnosis (Dillman and van Leeuwen (1989)).

24. In both cases the doctor will adjust his point of reference. Convergence and divergence here have a twofold relationship with each other. Because the theory (t) converges (c) to the orientation point as a general object (a): t + c + a. It diverges (d) however from this point as an particular object (i): t + d + i. Conversely, the practice (p) diverges: p + d + a; and converges: p + c + i. The result however forms a reciprocal convergence to the adjusted orientation point, i.e., to the object of the accumulated experience which forms a modification of the general object (a). Then the process begins again so that this interplay of movements can be viewed as a cycle.

25. Gross 1983, p. 64.

26. Barber (1979).

27. Veatch (1989).

28. Explicitly this view is held in radical circles; implicitly this view readily discussions on drug policy.

29. Payer (1988), p. 34.

References

Ablad B, Brogärd M, Ek L. Pharmacological properties of H56/28 - a ß-adrenergic receptor antagonist. Act Pharm Toxicol 1967a; 25(S2):9-40.

Ablad B, Johnsson G, Norrby A, Sölvell L. Potency and time-effect relationship in man of propranolol and H 56/28 - comparative studies after oral administration. Act Pharm Toxicol 1967b; 25(S2):85-94.

Ablad B, Brogard M, Carlsson E, Ek L. ß-Adrenergic receptor blocking properties of three alkyl-substituted phenoxypropanolamines. Eur J Pharm 1970; 13:59-64.

Ablad B. On the pharmacology of ß-adrenergic receptor blocking agents. In: Astra Chemical & Pharmaceuticals NV. Proceedings Swedish conference with Dutch specialists on hypertension. Gothenburg, May 17th-19th, 1972, Rijswijk: Astra, 1972: 75-103.

Ablad B, Carlsson E, Ek L. Pharmacological studies of two new cardioselective adrenergic beta-receptor antagonists. Life Sci 1973; 12:107-119.

Ahlquist RP. A Study of the adrenotropic receptors. Am J Phys 1948; 153:586-600.

Ahlquist RP. Adrenergic Drugs. In: Drill VA, ed. Pharmacology in Medicine, 2nd ed. New York: McGraw-Hill, 1958: 378-407.

Ahlquist RP. Adrenergic receptors: a personal and practical view. Persp Biol 1973; 17:119-122.

Ahlquist RP. Adrenoceptors: from figment to fact. In: Kalsner S, ed. Trends in Autonomic Pharmacology, vol. 2. Baltimore and Munich: Urban & Schwarzenberg, 1982.

Aisner M. Angina Pectoris 1768-1970. N Eng J Med 1970; 282:746-8.

Albert A. Selective Toxicity. 2nd ed. New York: Wiley, 1960.

Alleyne GAO et al. Effect of pronethalol in angina pectoris. Br Med J 1963; ii:1226-1229.

Ambrose AJ. Clinical impression against cold science [Points from letters]. Br Med J 1950; (ii):631.

Amsterdam EA, Mason DT. Coronary spasm: old problem, new questions. Am Heart J 1981; 101:242-3.

Anderson JL. Pharmacologic interventions in acute myocardial infarction. In: Maronde RF. Topics in Clinical Pharmacology & Pharmacotherapeutics. New York [etc.]: Springer-Verlag, 1986: 108-134.

Anonymous. Streptomycin in pulmonary tuberculosis. Br Med J 1948; ii:790-792.

Anonymous. Symposium on clinical trials. Br Med J 1958; i:1056-1057

Anonymous. The hemodynamic concept of atherosclerosis [editorial]. Am J Card 1960a; 5 (no. 3): 291-294.

Anonymous. The recognition of angina pectoris [editorial]. Circulation 1960b; 21 (6):1061-1064.

Anonymous. Effects of pronethalol. Br Med J 1963a; ii:1217.

Anonymous. To-days drugs. Coronary vasodilators. Br Med J 1963b (ii):103-105.

Anonymous. Discussion on side effects (Symposium on beta adrenergic receptor blockade - paper by Stephen. Directed by Prof. ML Rosenheim), Am J Card 1966; 18:438-472.

Anonymous. Claims for Cordilox. Drug Ther Bull 1967; 5:85-86.

Anonymous. To-days drugs. Verapamil. Br Med J 1968 (i):230.

Anonymous. Cordilox up to date. Drug Ther Bull 1969a;7:19-20.

Anonymous. Treatment of myocardial ischaemia. Br Med J 1969b; ii:249-50.

Anschütz F. Diagnose und Therapie der Angina Pectoris. Basel, Wiesbaden: Aesopus Verlag GmbH, 1982.

Anschütz F. Herzinsuffizienz. Erkennung und Behandlung in der Praxis, Basel, Wiesbaden: Aesopus Verlag GmbH, 1984.

Antman EM, Stone PH, Muller JE, Braunwald E. Calcium channel blocking agents in the treatment of cardiovascular disorders. Part 1: Basic and clinical electrophysiologic effects. Ann Int Med 1980;93:975-85.

Apthorp GH, Chamberlain DA, Hayward GW. The effects of sympathectomy on the electrocardiogram and effort tolerance in angina pectoris. Br Heart J 1964; 26:218-226.

Armstrong D. Clinical sense and clinical science. Soc Sci Med 1977; 11:599-601.

Aronow WS. Medical treatment of angina pectoris. VIII. Miscellaneous antianginal drugs. Am Heart J 1973a; 85:132-137.

Aronow WS. Management of stable angina. New Eng J Med 1973b; 289:516-20.

Austel V. and Kutter E. Practical Procedures in Drug Design. In: Ariëns EJ, ed. Drug Design. Medicinal Chemistry. A Series of Monographs. Volume X. New York [etc.]: Academic Press, 1980:1-69.

Barber B, Lally J, Loughlin Makarushka, Sullivan D. Research on human subjects. Problems of social control in medical experimentation. New Brunswick, New Jersey: Transaction Books, 1979.

Barger G, Dale HH. Chemical structure and sympathomimetic action of amines. J Physl Lon 1910; 41:19-59.

Bargmann W, Doerr W. Das Herzen des Menschen, Band I und II, Stuttgart: Georg Thieme Verlag, 1963.

Barrett AM, Crowther AF, Dunlop D, Shanks RG, Smith LH. Cardio-selective ß-blockade [Short communications/Kurzreferate, Teil 2]. N-S Arch Ph 1967/1968; 259:152-153.

Barrett AM Design of beta blocking drugs. Drug Design 1972; 3:205-228.

Bartholini G. Organization of Industrial Drug Research. In: Gross F, ed. Decision making in drug research. New York: Raven Press, 1983: 123-141.

Bassil GT. Treatment of angina pectoris. Br Med J 1969;ii:634

Bateman FJA. [Letter to the editor]. What is a ß-blocker? Lancet 1967 (ii):418.

Beamish RE, Sorrie VM. Impending myocardial infarction. Recognition and mangement. Circulation 1960; 21:1107-15.

Bender F, Kojima N. Reploh HD, Oelmann G. Behandlung tachykarder Rhythmusstörungen des Herzens durch Beta-Rezeptorenblockade desAtrioventrikulargewebes. Med Welt 1966; 17:1120-3.

Bender F, Schmidt E, Sieger W. Vergleichende Untersuchungen mit Beta-Receptorenblockern. Verh Dtsch Ges Inn Med 1968; 74:569-70.

Bender F, Schmidt E, Gradaus D. Medikamentöse Behandlung der Herzrhythmusstörungen. Schweiz Med Wschr 1969; 99:1539-42.

Bender F. Die Behandlung der tachycarden Arrhythmien und der arteriellen Hypertonie mit Verapamil. Arznei-For 1970; 20:1310-6.

Bender F. Medical treatment of cardiac arrythmias. N-S Arch Ph 1971; 269:272-82.

Biel JH, Lum BKB. The beta-adrenergic blocking agents: pharmacology and structure-activity relationships. Drug Res 1966; 10:46-87.

Biel JH, Martin YC. Organic synthesis as a source of new drugs. In: Gould RE, ed. Drug discovery. Science and development in a changing society. Advances in chemistry series 108, Washington: American Chemical Society, 1971.

Bignami, G. Disease models and reductionist thinking in the biomedical sciences. In: Rose S, ed. Against biological determinism. London: Allison & Busby, 1982.

Black JW. Electrocardiographic changes produced in rabbits by vasopressin (pitressin) and their alteration by prolonged treatment with a commercial heart extract. J Pharm Pharmacol 1959; 10:87-94.

Black JW, Stephenson JS, Pharmacology of a new adrenergic beta receptor blocking compound (Nethalide). Lancet 1962 (ii):311- 314.

Black JW, Crowther AF, Shanks RG, Dornhorst AC. A new adrenergic beta receptor antagonist. Lancet 1964 (ii):1080.

Black JW, Duncan WAM, Shanks RG. Comparison of some properties of pronethalol and propranolol. Brit J Pharmacol 1965; 25:577-591.

Black JW. The predictive value of animal tests in relation to drugs affecting the cardiovascular system in man (including discussion). In: Wolstenholme G, Porter R, eds. Drug responses in man. London: J&A Churchill Ltd., 1967: 111-124.

Black JW. Ahlquist and the development of beta-adrenoceptor antagonists. Postgrad Med J 1976; 52 (Suppl 4):11-13.

Bloom BM. Receptor theories. In: Burger A., ed. Medical Chemistry. 3d ed., New York: Wiley, 1970.

Blumberger Kj. Die Entwicklung der Strophanthinbehandlung seit Albert Fraenkel. In: Gädeke R, ed. Herztherapie in der Praxis, Stuttgart: Hippokrates-Verlag, 1964: 32-56.

Bodewitz H, Stemerding D. Wetenschap en samenleving en het werk van de Starnberg-groep. Kennis & Methode 1979; 3 (1):158-172.

Bodewitz H, Denig P. Dissenting views on the scientific base of drug regulation. Paper delivered at the 4th EASTT Conference, Strassbourg, 1986.

Bodewitz H, Bruins OB, Vos R. The strange case of metoprolol. One agent - two drugs. Paper delivered at 4th International Social Pharmacy Workshop, Stockholm, 1986.

Bodewitz H, De Vries G, Weeder P. Towards a cognitive model for technology-oriented R&D processes. Research Policy 1988; 17:213-224.

Boers CC. Wetenschap, techniek, en samenleving. Meppel [etc.]: Boom, 1981.

Böhm C, Schlepper M, Witzleb E. Eine neue koronar-gefäßerweiternde Substanz. Experimentelle und klinische Untersuchungen. Deut Med Wo 1960; 85:1405-8.

Bossert F, Vater W. Dihydropyridine, eine neue Gruppe stark wirksamer Coronartherapeutika. Naturwissenschaften 1971; 58:578.

Bousvaros GA, Campbell JE, McGregor M. Haemodynamic effects of dipyridamole at rest and during exercise in healthy subjects. Br Heart J 1966; 28:331-334.

Brändstrom A, Corrodi H, Junggren U, Jönsson T-E. Synthesis of some ß-adrenergic blocking agents. Acta Pharm Suecica 1966; 3:303-310.

Braunwald E. Symposium on beta adrenergic receptor blockade. an editorial introduction to the symposium. Am J Card 1966; 18:303-307.

Braunwald E, J. Ross and E.H. Sonnenblick, Mechanisms of contraction of the normal and failing heart [New England Journal of Medicine Medical Progress Series] London: J&A Churchill Ltd., 1968.

Braunwald E. Coronary spasm and acute myocardial infarction - new possibility for treatment and prevention. N Eng J Med 1978; 229:1301-1303.

Braunwald E. Coronary artery spasm as a cause of myocardial ischemia. J Lab Clin Med 1981; 97:299-312.

Braunwald E. Mechanism of action of calcium-channel-blocking agents. N Eng J Med 1982; 307:1618-27.

Braunwald E, ed. Heart Disease. A textbook of cardiovascular medicine. 2nd ed. Philadelphia: WB Saunders Company, 1984.

Bretschneider HJ. Pharmakotherapie coronarer Durchblutungsstörungen mit Kreislaufwirksamen Substanzen. Verh Dtsch Ges Inn Med 1963; 69:583-99.

Brick I, Glover WE, Hutchison KJ, Roddie IC. Effects of propranolol on peripheral vessels in man. Am J Card 1966; 18:329-332.

Brick I, Hutchison KJ, McDevitt DG, Roddie IC, Shanks RG. Comparison of the effects of I.C.I. 50172 and propranolol on the cardiovascular responses to adrenaline, isoprenaline and exercise. Br J Pharm 1968; 34:127-140.

Brick I, Hutchison KJ, Roddie IC, Shanks RG. Cardiac adrenergic blockade by 4-(2-hydroxy-3-isopropylaminopropoxy) acetanilide (I.C.I. 50172). [Short communications/Kurzreferate, Teil2]. N-S Arch Ph 1967/1968; 259:156-157.

Britchard G, Zimmermann PE. Treatment of arrhythmias with verapamil. Lancet 1970 (i):425.

Brittain RT, Dean CM, Jack D. Sympathomimetic bronchodilator drugs. Int Encyclopaedia of Pharmacology & Pharmacotherapeutics, Section 104 Respiratory Pharmacology (chapter 25), 1981: 613-655.

Bruce R. The treatment of angina pectoris with plaquenil. J Coll Gen Pract 1964; 7:290-294.

Brunner H, Hedwall PR, Meier M. Pharmakologische Untersuchungen mit 1-Isopropylamino-3-(o-allyloxyphenoxy)-2-propanol-hydrochlorid, einem adrenergischen ß-Receptorenblocker. Arznei-For 1968; 18:164-170.

Brunner H, Hedwall PR, Maier R, Meier M. Pharmacological aspects of oxprenolol. Postgrad Med J 1970; (suppl):5-14.

Brunner H, Hedwall PR, Meier M. General concepts in the use of ß-blockers: the relative roles of specific and unspecific effects. N Arch Pharmacol 1971; 269:219-231.

Büchner F. Die Koronarinsuffizienz. Dresden und Leipzig: Kreislaufbücherei 3, 1939.

Büchner F. Die Koronarinsuffizienz. In: Gebhardt W, ed., Koronarinsuffizienz, Freiburger Fortbildungskurse - Band 2, Stuttgart: Hippokrates - Verlag GmbH, 1967: 10-31.

Büchner F. Die Koronarinsuffizienz in alter und neuer Sicht, Sonderausgabe in der Reihe Forum Cariologicum. Mannheim: Boehringer Mannheim GmbH, 1970.

Bull JP. The historical development of clinical therapeutic trials. J Chron Dis 1959; 10:218-248.

Burch GE, DePasquale NP. A history of electrocardiography. Chicago: Year Book Medical Publishers, Inc., 1964.

Burkhardt R, Kienle G. Controlled clinical trials and medical ethics. Lancet 1978; (ii):1356-1359.

Burley DM, Binns TB, eds. Pharmaceutical medicine. London: Edward Arnold Publishers Ltd, 1985.

Burnett CF, Evans JA. Follow-up report on resection of the anginal pathway in thirty-three patients. JAMA 1956; 162:709-712.

Caplan AL. Exemplary reasoning? A comment on theory structure in biomedicine, The Journal of Medicine and Philosophy 1986; 11:93-105.

Carlsson A. The role of basic biomedical research in new drug development. In: Gross F, ed. Decision making in drug research. New York: Raven Press, 1983: 35-42.

Carlsson E, Ablad B, Brändström A, and Carlsson B. Differentiated blockade of the chronotropic effects of various adrenergic stimuli in the cat heart. Life Sciences 1972; 11 (part 1)953-958.

Carrier GO, Shlafer M. Raymond Ahlquist 26 July 1914 - 15 April 1983. Trends Pharmacol. Sci. 1984; 5 (2):41-44.

Casimir HBG. Toeval van de werkelijkheid. Een halve eeuw natuurkunde, (original title: Haphazard reality. Half a century of science). Amsterdam: Meulenhoff Informatief, 1983.

Cavallito CJ. Some relationships between chemical structure and pharmacological activities. Ann Rev Pharm 1968; 8:39-66.

Cavallito CJ. Some trends in the development of structure-activity relationships (SAR) and theory of receptors. In: Cavallito CJ, ed. Structure-Activity Relationships. Oxford: Pergamon, 1973.

Chamberlain DA, Howard J. The haemodynamic effects of ß-sympathetic blockade. Br Heart J 1964; 26:213-217.

Chamberlain DA, Howard J. Guanethidine and methyldopa: a hemodynamic study. Br Heart J 1964; 26:528-536.

Charlier R. Coronary vasodilators. Oxford: Pergamon Press, 1961.

Charlier R. Antianginal drugs. Berlin, Heidelberg, New York: Springer Verlag, 1971.

Christensen E, Juhl E, Tygstrup N. treatment of duodenal uler. randomized clinical trials of a decade (1964 to 1974). Gastroenterology 1977; 73:1170-1178.

Clark BJ. Pharmacology of beta-adrenoceptor blocking agents. In Saxena PR, Forsyth RP, eds. Beta Adrenoceptor Blocking Agents: The Pharmacological Base of Clinical Use. Amsterdam and Oxford: North Holland, 1976: 45-76.

Cochrane AL. Effectiveness and efficiency. Random reflections on health services. The Nuffield provincial hospitals trust, 1971.

Cohn PF, Braunwald E. Chronic ischemic heart disease. In: Braunwald E (ed). Heart Disease. A textbook of cardiovasculair medicine. 2nd ed. Philadelphia: WB Saunders Company, 1984: 1334-83.

Collins HM. Expert systems and the science of knowledge. In: Bijker WE, Hughes TP, and Pinch TJ, eds. The social construction of technological systems, The MIT Press, Cambridge [etc.] 1987: 329-348.

Comroe JH, Dripps RD. Scientific basis for the support of biomedical science. Science 1976; 192:105-111.

Comroe JH. Retrospectroscope: insights into medical discovery. California: Von Gehr Press, 1977.

Corrodi H, Persson H, Carlsson A, Roberts J. A new series of substances which block the adrenergic ß-receptors. J Med Chem 1963; 6:751-755.

Cotten M deV, Moran NC, Stopp PE. A comparison of the effectiveness of adrenergic blocking drugs in inhibiting the cardiac actions of sympathomimetic amines. J Pharm exp Ther 1957; 121:183-190.

Count DJ Le. Atenolol. In: Bindra JS, Lednicer D, eds. Chronicles of drug discovery, Vol 1. New York [etc.]: John Wiley & Sons, 1981:113-132.

Cozzens SE. Comparing the sciences: citation context analysis of papers from neuropharmacology and the sociology of science. Soc Stud Sci 1985; 15:127-53.

Craig PN. Guidelines for drug and analog design. In: De Wolff ME, ed. Burger's medicinal chemistry [part 1]. New York: A Wiley-Interscience Publication, 1980: 331-348.

D'Arcy hart P. Chemotherapy of tuberculosis. Research during the past 100 years. Br Med J 1946; (ii):805-810; 849-855.

Dale HH. On some physiological actions of ergot. J Physl Lon 1906; 34:163-206.

Darden L. Theory construction in genetics. In Nickles T, ed. Scientific discoveries: case studies. Dordrecht: D Reidel Publishing Company, 1980: 151-170.

Daten des Gesundheitswesens [Ausgabe 1977]. Der Bundesminister für Jugend, Familie und Gesundheit, Bonn-Bad Godesberg, 1977.

Davey DG. The validity of animal and other laboratory models. In: Gross F, ed. Decision Making in Drug Research. New York: Raven Press 1983: 45-47.

Daley R. The autonomic nervous system in its relation to some forms of heart and lung disease. Br Med J 1957; (ii):173-179.

Delius. in Rubrik "Fragen aus der Praxis" , einer Antwort auf eine Frage über die energetische Insuffizienz. Deut Med Wo 1953; 78:1118.

Delius L. Behandlung der Koronarleiden. Verh. Dtsch. Ges. Kreislaufforschung 26, 212, (Darmstadt) 1960.

Delius L. Das nervöse Herz und seine Behandlung. In: Gädeke R, ed. Herztherapie in der Praxis, Stuttgart: Hippokrates-Verlag, 1964: 156-169.

Delius L, Fahrenberg J. Psychovegetative Syndrome, Stuttgart: Georg Thieme Verlag, 1966.

Demany MA, Tambe A, Zimmerman HA. Coronary Arterial Spasm. Dis Chest 1968;53:714-21.

Demling L. Einführung in die Innere Medizin, 9th ed., Stuttgart: Georg Thieme Verlag, 1967.

Deutsch E. Comparison of German and American law concerning clinical trials. Contr Clin Trials 1981; 1:393-400.

Dexter L. A brief history of the clinical application of cardiac catheterization, 1929 - 1979. In: Snellen HA, Dunning AJ, Arntzenius AC, eds. History and Perspectives of Cardiology, Leiden University Press, The Hague/Boston/London 1981: 11-17.

Dhurandhar RW, DL Watt, MD Silver, AS Trimble and AG Adelman. Prinzmetal's variant form of angina with arteriographic evidence of coronary arterial spasm. Amer J Card 1972; 30: 902.

Dillman RJM, van Leeuwen E van. De redelijkheid van de ziekte. In: Parret H, ed. In alle redelijkheid. Meppel: Boom, 1989: 169-197.

Dollery CT, Paterson JW, Conolly ME. Clinical pharmacology of beta-adrenoceptor blocking drugs. Clin Pharm Ther 1969; 10:765-799.

Dolman H, Bolowitz H. Sedimentation of a scientific concept: the use of citation data. Soc Stud Sci 1985; 15:507-23.

Döring HJ, Kammermeier H, Fleckenstein A. Zur wechselseitigen Beeinflussung der Kontraktionskraft und der Frequenz des Herzens durch Proscillaridin und ‡-Isopropyl-‡-[(N-methyl-N-homoveratryl)-gamma-aminopropyl]-3,4-dimethoxyphenyl-acetonitril. Arznei-For 1966; 16:1197-1202.

Dornaus W. Zur Therapie pektanginöser Beschwerden. Therapiewoche 1967 (Heft 23):784-786.

Dornhorst AC, Laurence DR. Use of pronethalol in phaeochrome tumours. Br Med J 1963 (ii):1250-1251.

Dornhorst AC. Adrenergic blockade in cardiovascular disease. Pharm Rev 1966; 18(1):701-703.

Dresel PE. Blockade of some cardiac actions of adrenaline by dichloroisoproterenol. Can J Bioch Phys 1960; 38:375-381.

Drews J. Experimental models relevant for therapy. In: Gross F, ed. Decision Making in Drug Research. New York: Raven Press 1983: 49-55.

Dukes MNG. The effects of drug regulation. Falcon House: MTP Press, 1985.

Dungan KW, Lish PM. Bronchodilators: some qualitative and quantitative pharmacologic correlates in the guinea pig. J Allergy 1961; 32:139-151.

Dunlop D. The British system of drug regulation. In: Landau RL, ed. Regulating new drugs. Chicago: University of Chicago Press, 1973: 229-238.

Dunlop D, Shanks RG. Selective blockade of adrenoceptive beta receptors in the heart. Br J Pharm 1968; 32:201-218.

Engelhardt A. Methode zur Auswertung von ß-Adrenolytica am isolierten Herzvorhof. N-S Arch Ph 1965; 250:245-246.

Engelhardt A, Traunecker W. Pharmakologie einiger Phenoxy-propranolamin-Derivate mit ß-adrenolytischer Wirkung [Short communications/Kurzreferate]. N-S Arch Ph 1967; 256:203-204.

Engelhardt HT Jr. The concept of health and disease. In: Engelhardt HT, Jr. and Spicker SF, eds. Evaluation and explanation in the biomedical sciences. Dordrecht [etc.]: Reidel Publishing Company, 1975: 125-141.

Engelhardt HT Jr., Spicker SF, Towers B, eds. Clinical judgment: a critical appraisal. Dordrecht [etc.]: Reidel Publishing Company, 1979.

Feinstein AR. Clinical Judgment. Baltimore: Williams & Wilkins, 1967.

Feinstein AR, Koss N, Austin JHM. The changing emphasis in clinical research. Ann Int Med 1967; 66:397-419; 420-434.

Fildes P. A rational approach to chemotherapy. Lancet 1940; (i):955.

Fisher K. Beitrag zür medikamentösen Behandlung der Koronarinsuffizienz. Med Klin 1965; 60:847-51.

Fitgerald JD. Perspectives in adrenergic beta-receptor blockade. Clin Pharm Ther 1969; 10:292-306.

Fitzgerald JD, Barrett AM. [Letter to the editor]. What is a ß-blocker? Lancet 1967; (ii):310.

Fleck L. Über einige besondere Merkmale des ärztlichen Denkens. In: Schäfer L, Schnelle T. Ludwig Fleck - Erfahrung und Tatsache. Frankfurt am Main: Suhrkamp Taschenbuch Verlag, 1983: 37-45.

Fleckenstein A. Die Bedeutung der energiereichen Phosphate für Kontraktilität und Tonus des Myokards [The significance of energetic phosphates for the contractility and tone of the myocardium]. Verh Dtsch Ges Inn Med 1964; 70:81-99.

Fleckenstein A, Kammermeier H, Döring HJ, Freund HJ (in cooperation with Grün G, Kienle A). Zum Wirkungsmechanismus neuartiger Koronardilatatoren mit gleichzeitig Sauerstof-einsparenden Myokard-Effekten, Prenylamin und Iproveratril - Teil 1 [On the mechanism of action of novel coronary vasodilators with simultaneously oxygen saving myocardial effects, prenylamine and iproveratril - part 1]. Z Kreislaufforschung 1967a;56:716-744.

Fleckenstein A, Kammermeier H, Döring HJ, Freund HJ (in cooperation with Grün G, Kienle A). Zum Wirkungsmechanismus neuartiger Koronardilatatoren mit gleichzeitig Sauerstof-einsparenden Myokard-Effekten, Prenylamin und Iproveratril - Teil 2 [On the mechanism of action of novel coronary vasodilators with simultaneously oxygen saving myocardial effects, prenylamine and iproveratril - part 2]. Z Kreislaufforschung 1967b; 56:839-858.

Fleckenstein A, Döring J, Kammermeier H. Myokardstoffwechsel und Insuffizienz. Ärtzliche Forschung 1967c; 21:1-14.

Fleckenstein A, Döring HJ, Kammermeier H, Grün G. Influence of prenylamine on the utilization of high energy phosphates in cardiac muscle. Biochimica applicata 1968a; 14 (S1):323-344.

Fleckenstein A, Döring HJ, Kammermeier H. Einfluß von Beta-Rezeptorenblocker und verwandten Substanzen auf Erregung, Kontraktion und Energiestoffwechsel der Myokardfaser. Klin Woch 1968b;46:343-351.

Fleckenstein A, Tritthardt H, Fleckenstein B, Herbst A, Grün G. Selektive Hemmung der Myokard-Contractilität durch kompetitive Ca^{++}-Antagonisten (Iproveratril, D 600, Prenylamin). N-S Arch Ph 1969a; 264:227-228.

Fleckenstein A, Tritthart H, Fleckenstein B, Herbst A, Grün G. Eine neue Gruppe kompetitiver Ca^{++}-Antagonisten (Iproveratril, D 600, Prenylamin) mit starken Hemmeffekten auf die elektromechanische Koppeling im Warmblüter-Myokard. Pflügers Archiv 1969b; 307:R25.

Fleckenstein A. Die Zügelung des Myocardstoffwechsels durch Verapamil. Angriffspunkte und Anwendungsmöglichkeiten. Arznei-For 1970; 20(9a):1317-1322.

Fleckenstein A. Specific inhibitors and promotors of calcium action in the excitation-contraction coupling of heart muscle and their role in the prevention of production of myocardial lesions. In: Harris P, Opie LH, eds. Calcium and the heart. London, New York: Academic Press, 1971: 135-188.

Fleckenstein A. Physiologie und Pharmakologie der transmembranären Natrium-, Kalium- und Calcium-Bewegungen. Arznei-For 1972;22:2019-2028.

Fleckenstein A, Tritthart H, Döring HJ, Byron KY. Bay a 1040 - ein hochaktiver Ca^{++}-antagonistischer Inhibitor der elektro-mechanischen Koppelungsprocesse im Warmblüter-Myokard [Bay a 1040 - a very potent Ca^{++}-antagonistic inhibitor of excitation-coupling processes in the warm-blooded myocardium]. Arznei-For [Drug Res] 1972; 22:22-33.

Fleckenstein A. Specific pharmacology of calcium in myocardium, cardiac pacemakers and vascular smooth muscle. Ann Rev Pharm Tox 1977; 17:149-166.

Fleckenstein A. History of calcium antagonists. Circulation Res 1983a; 52(S1):I3-I16.

Fleckenstein A. Calcium antagonism in heart and smooth muscle. Experimental facts and therapeutic prospects. New York: John Wiley & Sons, 1983b.
Fletcher SW, Fletcher RH, Greganti MA. Clinical research trends in general medical journals, 1946 - 1976. In: Roberts E, et al., eds. Biomedical innovation. Massachuchets: The MIT Press, 1980: 284-300.

Florian HJ. Über die Formen der Herzinsuffizienz. Deut Med Wo 1951; 46:1466-1471.

Flörkenmeier V. Keine Angst vorm Beta-Block. Ein Lernprogramm für Klinik und Praxis, Programmierte Arztinformationen IV, Deutscher Ärzte/Verlag GmbH, Köln-Lövenich, 1980.

Folkow B. Impulse frequency in sympathetic vasomotor fibres correlated to the release and elimination of the transmitter. Act Phys S 1952; 25:49-76.

Folkow B. Nervous control of blood vessels. Physiol Rev 1955; 35:639-663.

Folkow B, Hamberger C-A. Characteristics of sympathetic neuroeffectors in man. J appl Physiol 1956; 9:268-270.

Folkow B, Löfving B, Mellander S. Quantitative aspects of the sympathetic neuro-humoral control of the heart rate. Acta Physiol Scand 1956; 37:363-369.

Folkow B, Häggendal J, Lisander B. Extent of release and elimination of noradrenaline at peripheral adrenergic nerve terminals. Act Phys S 1967 (Suppl. 307):5-38.

Follansbee WP, Shaver JA. Pharmacologic interventions in angina. In: Maronde RF, ed. Topics in Clinical Pharmacology & Pharmacotherapeutics. New York [etc.]: Springer-Verlag, 1986: 83-107.

Forsberg S-A, Johnsson G. Hemodynamic effects of propranolol and H56/28 in man - a comparative study of two ß-adrenergic receptor antagonists. Life Sci 1967; 6:1147-1154.

Fowler NO. "Preinfarctional" Angina. A need for an objective definition and for a controlled clinical trial of its management. Circulation 1971; 44:755-8.

Friebel H. Arzneimittelverbrauch. Ein Vergleich der Verbrauchsituation in einigen europäischen Ländern, Deutsche Apotheker Zeitung 1982; 122:815-819.

Friedberg CK. Diseases of the heart, 1st ed 1949 (reprint 1950); 2nd ed. 1956; 3rd ed. Philadelphia & London: WB Saunders Company, 1966.

Friedberg CK. Some comments and reflections on changing interesets and new developments in angina pectoris. Circulation 1972; 46:1037-47.

Fuchs RM, Becker LC. Pathogenesis of angina pectoris. Arch Int Med 1982; 142:1685-92.

Furchgott RF. The receptors for epinephrine and norepinephrine (adrenergic receptors). Pharm Rev 1959; 11:429-441.

Furchgott RF. The pharmacological differentiation of adrenergic receptors. Ann NY Acad Sci 1967; 139: 139:553.

Gau DW. Use of beta-blockers in general practice in the United Kingdom. In: Schweizer W, ed. Beta-blockers - present status and future prospects. Bern [etc]: Hans Huber Publishers, 1974: 135-137.

Gazes PC, Mobley Jr. EM, Fairs Jr. HM, Duncan RC, Humphries GB. Pre-infarctional (Unstable) Angina - a prospective study - ten year follow-up. New Eng J Med 1973; 48: 331 -338.

Gebhardt W, Büchner F. Zur medikamentösen Behandlung der koronaren Herzkrankheiten. In: Gebhardt W, ed. Koronarinsuffizienz. Freiburger Fortbildungskurse (Nov. 1965) - Band 2, Stuttgart: Hippokrates - Verlag GmbH, 1967: 151-168.

Gerritsma JGM. De werkwijze van huisarts en internist [Dissertation]. Utrecht: Wetenschappelijke Uitgeverij Bunge, 1982.

Gersmeyer EF. 6. Frühjahrstagung Dtsch. Pharmakol. Gesellschaft, Mainz 1965.

Gill EW, Vaughan Williams EM. Local anaesthetic activity of the ß-receptor antagonist, pronethalol. Nature 1964 (January 11):199.

Gillam PMS, Prichard BNC. Use op propranolol in angina pectoris. Br Med J 1965; (ii):337.

Gillespie JS, ed. Summary of discussion and commentary, 2nd symposium on catecholamines. Pharm Rev 1966; 18(1):537-540.

Glover WE, Greenfield ADM, Shanks RG. Effect of dichloroisoprenaline on the peripheral vascular response to adrenaline in man. Brit J Pharmacol 1962; 19:235-244.

Godfraind T, Kaba A. Inhibition by cinnarizine and chlorpromazine of the contraction induced by calcium and adrenaline in vascular smooth muscle. Br J Pharmacol 1969; 35:P354-5.

Goodman LS, Gilman A, eds. The pharmacological basis of therapeutics, 1st ed. 1941; 2nd ed. 1955, [etc.], 6th ed. New York: The MacMillan Company, 1975.

Goodman Gilman A, Goodman LS, Gilman A, eds. Goodman and Gilman's The Pharmacological Basis of Therapeutics, 6th ed. 1980, 7th ed. New York: The MacMillan Company, 1985.

Goodman LS. The problem of efficacy: an exercise in dissection. In: Talalay P, ed. Drugs in our society. Baltimore: The Johns Hopkins Press, 1964: 49-68.

Gorlin R. et al. Effect of nitroglycerin on the coronary circulation in patients with coronary artery disease or increased left ventricular work. Circulation 1959; 19:705-718.

Gorlin R. Pathophysiology of cardiac pain. Circulation 1965; 32:138-148.

Grandjean T, Rivier JL. Schweiz. Med. Wschr. 1963; 93:1101.

Grant RHE, McDevitt DG, Shanks RG. Is verapamil a ß-blocker? Lancet 1968; (i):362-3.

Green FHK. The clinical evaluation of remedies. Lancet 1954; (ii):1085-1090.

Gregg DE, Sabiston DC. Current research and problems of the coronary circulation. Circulation 1956; 13:916-27.

Griffith GC. Coronary Artery Disease: Looking Back. In: Russek HI, Zollman BI. Coronary Heart Disease. A medical surgical symposium. Philadelphia, Toronto: JB Lippincott Co, 1971: 3-5.

Gross F. Drug utilization - Theory and practice. The present situation in the Federal Republic of Germany. Eur J Clin Pharm 1981; 19:387-394.

Gross F, ed. Descision Making in Drug Research. New York: Raven Press, 1983.

Grosse-Brockhoff Fr, Effert S. Herz- und Gefäßkrankheiten. In H. Dennig H, ed. Lehrbuch der Inneren Medizin, erster band, 6. Auflage. Stuttgart: Georg Thieme Verlag, 1964: 732-884.

Haas H, Fink H, Härtfelder G. Das placeboproblem. In: Beckett AH, Büchi J, Chen KK, et al. Progress in Drug Research, Vol 1. Basel/Stuttgart: Birkhäuser Verlag, 1959: 279-454.

Haas H, Härtfelder G. ‡-Isopropyl-‡-[(N-methyl-N-homoveratryl)-gamma-aminopropyl]-3,4-dimethoxyphenylacetonitril, eine Substanz mit coronargefäßerweiternden Eigenschaften. Arznei-For 1962; 12:549-58.

Haas H. Zum Wirkungsmechanismus des ‡-Isopropyl-‡-[(N-methyl-N-homoveratryl)-gamma-aminopropyl]-3,4-dimethoxyphenylacetonitrils, einer Substanz mit coronargefäßerweiternden Eigenschaften. Arznei-For 1964a; 14:461-8.

Haas H. Coronarwirksame Substanzen. Pharmazeutische Zeitung 1964b; 109:1855-62.

Haas H. Selektive Sympathikolyse und Myokardfunktion. Deut Med Wo 1964c; 89:2117-21.

Haas H, Busch E. Vergleichende Untersuchungen der Wirkung von ‡-Isopropyl-‡-[(N-methyl-N-homoveratryl)-gamma-amino-propyl]-3,4-dimethoxyphenylacetonitril, seiner Derivate sowie einiger andere Coronardilatatoren und ß-Receptor-affiner Substanzen. Arznei-For 1967; 17:257-72.

Haas H. Vergleichende Untersuchungen zum Wirkungsmechanismus von ‡-Isopropyl-‡-[(N-methyl-N-homoveratryl)-gamma-amino-propyl]-3,4-dimethoxyphenylacetonitril und seiner Derivate. Arznei-For 1968; 18:89-105.

Haas H, Igarashi T. Vergleichende Untersuchungen am Herz-Lungen-Präparat des Hundes Über das Wirkungsspektrum von Verapamil, Chinidin und einigen ‡- und ß- Sympathicolytica sowie ihre Beeinflussung durch Adrenalin. Arznei-For 1968; 18:1373-80.

Haas H. Veränderungen des Mechanograms und anderer Kreislaufparameter durch Isoprenalin und Adrenalin unter der Einwirkung von Verapamil, Chinidin und antiadrenerg werksamen Substanzen. Arznei-For 1970; 20:501-9.

Haas H. Studien mit coronarwirksamen Substanzen. Arznei-For 1970; 20:1299-1304.

Haas H, Gokel M. Der Einfluß von Verapamil auf den Myocardstoffwechsel. Arznei-For 1970; 20:647-55.

Hacking I. Representing and intervening. Introductory topics in the philosophy of natural science. Cambridge [etc.]: Cambridge University Press, 1983.

Hacking I. Filosofen van het experiment (translated) [Philosophers of the experiment]. Kennis & Methode 1989; 13:11-27.

Haferkamp H. Das Altersherz. Die Medizinische 1956; 11 (17. März 1956):389-391.

Hahn FE. Strategy and tactics of chemotherapeutic drug development. Die Naturwissenschaften 1975; 62:449-458.

Hähnel J. Wirkungsnachweis einer Beta-Rezeptoren blockierenden Substanz am Verhalten einiger Kreislaufwerte. Z für Kreislaufforschung 1966; 55:1023-1035.

Hamner CE. Drug development. Boca Raton: CRC Press, 1982.

Hanna C, Schmid JR. Antiarrhythmic actions of coronary vasodilator agents Papaverine, Dioxyline and Verapamil. Arch Int Pharmacodyn 1970; 185:228-233.

Hansen EH, Launso/ L. Development, use and evaluation of drugs: the dominating technology in the health care system. Soc Sci Med 1987; 25:65-73.

Hanson NR. Perception and discovery. San Francisco: Freeman, Cooper & Company, 1969.

Hanson NR. Patterns of discovery. [1st print 1958], Cambridge: Cambridge University Press, 1972.

Harris P, Opie Lh (eds). Calcium and the heart. London, New York: Academic Press, 1971: 1-24.

Thorn GW, Adams RD, Braunwald E, Isselbacher KJ, Petersdorf RG. Harrison's Principles of Internal Medicine. 8th ed. A Blakiston Publication, McGraw-Hill Kogakusha Ltd., 1977.

Hashimoto K. Opening Address. In: Hashimoto K, Kimura, E, Kobayashi T (eds). First International Nifedipine >> Adalat[R] << Symposium. New Therapy of Ischemic Heart Disease. Tokyo: University of Tokyo Press, 1975: xv-xvi.

Hasskarl HW. Legal problems of controlled clinical trials. Contr Clin Trials 1981; 1:401-409.

Hauss WH. Angina Pectoris, Stuttgart: Georg Thieme Verlag, 1954.

Hauss WH. Lehrbuch der Inneren Medizin. München: J.F Lehmans Verlag , 1966.

Hegglin R. Klinik der energetisch-dynamischen Herzinsuffizienz, Basel: Karger, 1947.

Helms RB, ed. Drug development and marketing. Washington DC: American Enterprise Institute for Public Policy Research, 1975.

Hemminki E. Study of information submitted by drug companies to licensing authorities. Br Med J 1980 (i):833-838.

Hemminki E, Falkum E. Psychotropic drug registration in the scandinavian countries: the role of clinical trials. Soc Sci Med 1980; 14(A):547-559.

Hertogh PM. De medische rede in de wetenschapsfilosofie van Canguilhem. Scripta Medico-Philosophica 1987 (schrift 4):22-39.

Hilger HH. Experimental tests of the action of coronary dilators in humans/Probleme der Klinische Pharmakologie der Coronardilatatoren. N-S. Arch Ph 1969; 263:168-183.

Hill GB. Controlled clinical trials - the emergence of a paradigm. Clin Inv Med 1983; 6:25-32.

Hillis LD, Braunwald E. Coronary-artery spasm. N Eng J Med 1978; 299:695-702.

Hills EA, Downes EM. Verapamil and cardiac pain. Lancet 1967; ii:1149-50.

Hirsch W. und G. Woschée. Klinische Beobachtungen zur Behandlung des Symptoms Angina Pectoris. Therapie der Gegenwart 1967: 809-817.

Hofbauer K. Zur Behandlung stenokardischer Beschwerden mit Iproveratril. Wien Med Wschr 1966; 116:1155-6.

Hoff F. Medizinische Klinik. Ein Fortbildungskurs für Aerzte, Stuttgart: Georg Thieme Verlag, 1948.

Hoffmann P. Behandlung koronarer Durchblutungsstörungen mit Isoptin[R] in der Praxis. Med Klin 1964; 59:1387-91.

Hohlfeld R. Praxisbezüge wissenschaftlicher Disziplinen. Das Beispiel der Krebsforschung. In: Böhme G, van den Daele W, Hohlfeld R et al. Starnberger Studien I. Die Gesellschaftliche Orientierung des wissenschaftlichen Fortschritts. Suhrkamp Verlag, Frankfurt am Main 1978: 131-194.

Holtz P. Introduction. Probleme der Klinische Pharmakologie der Coronardilatatoren. N-S Arch Ph 1969; 263:121-127.

Holzmann M. Differenzierungsmöglichkeiten bei der Angina Pectoris, Deut Med Wo 1954; 79:1109-1115.

Horwitz RI. The experimental paradigm and observational studies of cause-effect relationships in clinical medicine. J Chron Dis 1987; 40:91-99.

Howe R, Rao BS, Chodnekar MS. ß-Adrenergic blocking agents - VII. J Med Chem 1970; 13:169-176.

Howie JGR. Diagnosis. J R Coll Gen Pract 1972; 22:310-315.

Hucklenbroich P. Action theory as a source for philosophy of medicine. Metamedicine 1981; 2:55-74.

Hunter KM. A science of individuals: medicine and casuistry. The Journal of Medicine and Philosophy 1989; 14:193-212.

Hurst JW (ed), Logue RB, Schlant RC, Kass WN (co-eds). The heart. Arteries and veins, 1st ed. 1966; 2nd ed. 1970; 3rd ed. New York: McGraw Hill Book Co, 1974.

Huxley HE. The mechanism of muscular contraction. Science 1969; 164:1356-66.

Idänpään-Heikillä JE. Adverse reactions and post-marketing-surveillance (1985) In: Burley DM, Binns TB, eds. Pharmaceutical Medicine. London: Edward Arnold (Publishers) Ltd, 1985: 126-148.

Imai S, Tadeka K. Calcium and contraction of heart and smooth muscle. Nature 1967; 213:1044-5.

Imhof PR. Characterization of beta-blockers as antihypertensive agents in the light of human-pharmacology studies. In: Schweizer W, ed. Beta-blockers - present status and future prospects. Bern [etc]: Hans Huber Publishers, 1974: 40-46.

James TN. Angina without coronary disease (sic). Circulation 1970; 42:189-191.

Jölndal B. Regulation for need - the Norwegian experience. J Soc Adm Pharmacy 1984; 2(2):81-84.

Jolles G, Wooldrigde KRH, eds. Drug design: fact or fantasy? London [etc.]: Academic Press, Inc., 1984.

Jong FJ de. Boven en onder het mes. Een bijdrage tot de filosofie van de geneeskunde. Delft: Eburon, 1988.

Juhl E, Christen E, Tygstrup N. The epidemiology of the gastrointestinal randomized clinical trial. New Engl J Med 1977; 296:20-22.

Julian DG, ed. Angina pectoris. London and New York: Churchil Livingstone, 1977.

Kadatz R, Diederen W. Contribution to the discussion - Effects of coronary dilators on the oxygen tension in the myocardium/ Probleme der Klinische Pharmakologie der Coronardilatatoren. N-S Arch Ph 1969; 263:156-167.

Kalsbeek F. Alfa- en beta-adrenerge receptoren. De merkwaardige geschiedenis van een curieus concept. Ned T Geneesk 1969; 113:383-390.

Kaltenbach M, Klepzig H. Das EKG während Belastung und seine Bedeutung für die Erkennung der Koronarinsuffizienz. Z Kreislaufforschung 1963; 63:486-97.

Kaltenbach M, Zimmermann D. Zur Wirkung von Iproveratril auf die Angina pectoris und die adrenergischen ß-Rezeptoren des Menschen. Deut Med Wo 1968; 93:25-8.

Kaltenbach M. Medikamentösen Therapie der Angina pectoris. Prüfung verschiedener Medikamente mit Hilfe von Arbeitsversuchen. Arznei-For 1970; 20:1304-10.

Kaltenbach M, Becker H-J, Kollath J, Spitz E, Kober G. Exercise electrocardiogram and selective coronary arteriography. In: Kaltenbach M, Lichtlen P (eds.). Coronary heart disease. Stuttgart: Georg Thieme Verlag, 1971: 66-78.

Kaltenbach M, Hopf R, Keller M. Calciumantagonistische Therapie bei hypertroph-obstruktiven Kardiomyopathie. Deut Med Wo 1976; 101:1284-7.

Katz, A.M. Molecular biology in cardiology, a paradigmatic shift. J Mol Cell Cardiol 1988; 20:355-366.

Katz LN, Feinberg H, Shaffer AB. Hemodynamic aspects of congestive heart failure. Circulation 1960; 21:95-111.

Keller CH. Leitsymptom: "Herzschmerzen" und ihre Deutung. Münch med Wschr 1960; 30:1409-1415.

Kernohan RJ. What is a ß-blocker? [letter to the editor]. Lancet 1967; (ii):716.

Kienle G. Arzneimittelsicherheit und Gesellschaft. Eine kritische Untersuchung. Stuttgart-New York: FK Schattauer Verlag, 1974.

Kirchhoff HW. Zur Wirkung einer ß-adrenolytische Substanz in Belastungs- und Kipptisch-Untersuchungen. Z für Kreislaufforschung 1965; 55:583-593.

Klaes L, Seeback R, Lex C, Feich J, Mayntz R. Regulative Politik und politisch-administrative Kultur. Ein Vergleich von fünf Ländern und vier Interventionsprogrammen, Köln: Universität zu Köln, 1982.

Klaus W, LÜllmann H. Calcium als intracelluläre Überträgersubstanz und die mögliche Bedeutung dieses Mechanismus fÜr pharmakologische Wirkungen. Klin Woch 1964; 42:254-257.

Klepzig H, Kaltenbach M. Die Belastungsinsuffizienz des Herzens und ihre Erkennung. Deut Med Wo 1962; 87:35-38.

Klepzig H. Die Behandlung der Herzinsuffizienz in der Praxis. In: Gädeke R, ed. Herztherapie in der Praxis, Stuttgart: Hippokrates-Verlag, 1964: 56-66.

Klepzig H. Herz- und Gefäßkrankheiten, 1. Auflage 1968. 3e Auflage. Stuttgart: Georg Thieme Verlag, 1972.

Klever R. Die Behandlung pektanginöser Beschwerden in der Allgemeinpraxis. Therapiewoche 1968 (Heft 19):5-6.

Kochsiek K, Bretschneider HJ, Scheler F. Vergleichende experimentelle Untersuchungen über die coronargefäßerweiternde Wirkungen von Phenyl-propyl-diphenyl-propyl-amin. Arznei-For 1960; 10:576-583.

Köhler U. Aktuelle Probleme der Herzinsuffizienz. Deut Med Wo 1956; 81:1892-1896.

Kolodzig S. Klinische Erfahrungen in der Behandlung der Koronarinsuffizienz und des Herzinfarktes mit Persantin forte. Therapiewoche 1966 (Heft 43):1479-1481.

König K, Reindell H. Die Altersinsuffizienz des Herzens. In: Gädeke R, ed. Herztherapie in der Praxis, Stuttgart: Hippokrates-Verlag, 1964: 79-96.

Köppe HG. Recent chemical developments in the field of beta adrenoceptor blocking drugs. Progr Clin Biochem Med 1986; 3:31-72.

Köppe HG. The development of mexiletine. Postgr Med J 1977; 53 (Suppl):22-25.

Kottmaier J, Schettler G. Taschenbuch der praktischen Medizin, 5th ed., Stuttgart: Georg Thieme Verlag, 1961.

Krantz JC, Carr CJ. The pharmacological principles of medical practice, 2nd ed. 1951; 3rd ed. 1954; 6th. ed. Baltimore: The Williams & Wilkins Company, 1965.

Krauß J. Die Behandlung des chronischen Herzversagens. Deut Med Wo 1961; 86:2385-2395.

Kraupp O. Zum Wirkungsmechanismus der Coronardilatatoren/On the mechanism of action of coronary dilators. N-S Arch Ph 1969; 263:144-155.

Kreuzer H. Klinische Beurteilung von Coronardilatatoren/The Clinical Evaluation of Coronary Dilators. NS Arch Pharmakol Exp Path 1969; 263:186-194.

Kroneberg G. Pharmacology of nifedipine (Adalat). In: Hashimoto K, Kimura E, Kobayashi T, eds. 1st International Nifedipine - Adalat - Symposium. New therapy of ischemic heart disease. Tokyo: University of Tokyo Press, 1975: 3-10.

Kübler W, Tillmans H. Management of coronary vasometric angina. Eur Heart J 1985; 6 (Suppl F):27-31.

Kuhn T.S. The structure of scientific revolutions, 2nd ed. (enlarged). Chicago: The University of Chicago Press, 1970.

Kuipers TAF. Approaching descriptive and theoretical truth. Erkenntnis 1982; 18(3):343-378.

Kuipers TAF. Reductie van wetten: een decompositiemodel. Kennis & Methode 1987a; 11 (1):125-135.

Kuipers TAF. Reductie van Begrippen. Kennis & Methode 1987b; 11 (4):330-342.

Kuipers TAF. Cognitive patterns in the empirical sciences: examples of cognitive studies of science. Communication & Cognition 1988;21:319-341.

Kuipers TAF. Onderzoeksprogramma's gebaseerd op een idee. Impressies van een wetenschapsfilosofische praktijk. Assen: Van Gorcum, 1989.

Kukovetz WR, Pöch G. Die Hemmung mechanischer und metabolischer Katecholaminwirkungen durch Isopropylmethoxamine und Kö 592 am Herzen. N-S Arch Ph 1967; 256:310-318.

Kuschinsky G, Rahn KH. Untersuchungen über die Beziehungen zwischen chinidinartigen und ß-adrenolytischen Wirkungen von 1-(3-Methylphenoxy)-2-hydroxy-3-isopropylaminopropan (Kö 592). NS Arch Exp Path Pharmakol. 1965; 252:50-62.

Kuschinsky G, Lüllman H. Kurzes Lehrbuch der Pharmakologie, 1st ed. 1964; 3rd ed. 1967; 5th ed. 1972, 9th ed. Stuttgart: Georg Thieme Verlag, 1981.

Kvam DC, Riggilo DA, Lish PM. Effect of some new ß-adrenergic blocking agents on certain metabolic responses to catecholamines. J Pharm exp Ther 1965; 149:183-192.

Landau RL, ed. Regulating new drugs. Chicago: University of Chicago Press, 1973.

Lands AM, Arnold A, McAuliff JP, Luduena FP, Brown, Jr., TG. Differentiation of receptor systems activated by sympathomimetic amines. Nature 1967; 214:597-598.

Langley P, Simon HA, Bradshaw GL, Zytkow JM. Scientific discovery. Computational explorations of the creative processes. Cambridge [etc.]: The MIT Press, 1987.

Larsen AA, Lish PM. A new bio-isostere: alkylsulphonamidophenethanolamines. Nature 1964; 203:1283-1284.

Larsen AA, Gould WA, Roth HR, Comer WT, Uloth RH. Sulfonamides - II. Analogs of catecholamines. J Med Chem 1967; 10:462-472.

Lasagna L. On evaluating drug therapy: the nature of the evidence. In: Talalay P, ed. Drugs in our society. Baltimore: The Johns Hopkins Press, 1964: 91-106.

Lawrence C. Moderns and ancients: the 'new cardiology' in Britain 1880 - 1930. Medical History 1985; 29 (Suppl, No. 5):1-33.

Leibowitz JO. The history of coronary heart disease, London: Wellcome Institute of the History of Medicine, 1970.

Leufkens HGM. Farmacie en Samenleving [unpublished educational document]. Pharmacy & Society Department, University Leiden, 1982.

Levine SA. Clinical Heart Disease. 5th ed. Philadelphia, London: WB Saunders Co, 1958: 89-163.

Levy B. Alterations of adrenergic responses by N-iso-propyl methoxamine. J Pharm exp Ther 1964; 146:129-138.

Levy B. The adrenergic blocking activity of N-tert.-butylmethoxamine (butoxamine). J Pharm exp Ther 1966a; 151:413-422.

Levy B. Dimethyl isopropylmethoxamine: a selective ß-receptor blocking agent. Brit J Pharmac Chemother 1966b; 27:277-285.

Levy B. A comparison of the adrenergic receptor blocking properties of 1-(4'-methylphenyl)-2-isopropylamino-propranol HCL and propranolol. J Pharm exp Ther 1967; 156:452.

Levy B, Wilkenfield BE. An analysis of selective beta receptor blockade. Eur J Pharm 1969; 5:227-234.

Levy JV, Richards V. Inotropic and chronotropic effects of a series of ß-adrenergic blocking drugs: some structure-activity relationships. Proc Soc Exp Biol Med 1966; 122:373-379.

Lewis T. Research in medicine: its position and its needs. Br Med J 1930; (i):479-483.

Lichtlen PR. Zur Therapie der Angina pectoris in heutiger sicht. Z Kreislaufforschung 1972; 61:193-223.

Lichtlen PR, Ebner F. Nifedipine - Historical Aspects. In: Lichtlen PR, ed. New therapy of ischaemic heart disease and hypertension. Proceedings 6th International Adalat Symposium, Geneva 18 -20 April 1985, Amsterdam [etc]: Excerpta Medica, 1986: 3-19.

Lie RK. Theory change in cardiovascular research [Dissertation]. Minnesota: University of Minnesota, 1987.

Likoff W. Coronary arterial spasm: reexamination of an old concept. In: Russek HI (ed). Cardiovascular Problems. Baltimore: University Park Press, 1976: 241-245.

Lilienfeld AM. Ceteris paribus: the evolution of the clinical trial. Bull Hist Med 1982; 56:1-18.

Lindner E. Phenyl-propyl-diphenyl-propyl-amin, eine neue Substanz mit koronargefäßerweiternder Wirkung. 1. Mitteilung: Wirkung auf den Kreislauf. Arznei-For 1960a; 10:569-573.

Lindner E. Phenyl-propyl-diphenyl-propyl-amin, eine neue Substanz mit koronargefäßerweiternder Wirkung. 2. Mitteilung: Weitere pharmakologische Wirkungen. Arznei-For 1960b; 10:573-576.

Linzbach . Heart failure from the point of view of quantitative anatomy. Am J Card 1960; 5:370-382.

Lish PM, Dungan KW, Peters EL. A study of the effects of isoxsuprine on nonvascular smooth muscle. J Pharm exp Ther 1960; 129:191-199.

Lish PM, Weikel JH, Dungan KW. Pharmacological and toxicological properties of two new ß-adrenergic receptor antagonists. J Pharm exp Ther 1965; 149:161-173.

Livesley B, Catley PF, Campbell RC Oram S. Double-blind avaluation of verpamil, propranolol and isosorbide dinitrate against a placebo in the treatment of angina pectoris. Br Med J 1973; (i):375-8.

Lochner W. The physiology of the coronary circulation as a basis for evaluation of coronary vasodilators/ Probleme der Klinische Pharmakologie der Coronardilatatoren. N-S Arch Ph 1969; 263:127-144.

Lucchesi BR, Hardman RF. The influence of dichloroisoproterenol (DCI) and related compounds upon oubain and acetylstrophanthidin induced cardiac arrhythmias. J Pharm exp Ther 1961; 132:372-381.

Luebs ED, Cohen A, Zaleski EJ, Bing RJ. Effect of nitroglycerin, intensain, isoptin and papaverine on coronary blood flow in man. Measured by the coincidence counting technic and rubidium. Am J Card 1966; 17:535-541.

MacAlpin RN. Coronary spasm as a cause of angina. N Eng J Med 1973a; 288:788-9.

MacAlpin RN, Kattus AA, Alvaro AB. Angina pectoris at rest with preservation of exercise capacity. Prinzmetal's variant angina. Circulation 1973b; 47:946-58.

MacAlpin RN. Provoking variant angina. N Eng J Med 1976; 294:277-9.

MacAlpin RN. Coronary Arterial Spasm: A historical perspective. J Hist Med 1980; :288-311.

MacKinnon J. Current therapeutics - CLIV. Drugs in the treatment of angina pectoris. The Practitioner 1960; 185:557-563.

Mainzer F. Atypische Angina Pectoris. Der Zusammenhang zwischen Angina Pectoris und Wirbelsäulenerkrankung: Verkettungsangina und pseudo-anginöses Wurzelsyndrom. Klin Woch 1958; 36:749-760.

Martin GJ. Biological antagonism. Philadelphia: Blakiston, 1951.

Martini P. Methodenlehre der therapeutischen Untersuchung. Berlin: Verlag von Julius Springer, 1932.

Maseri A, L'Abbate A, Chierchia S et al. Significance of spasm in the pathogenesis of ischemic heart disease. Am J Card 1979; 44:788-92.

Maseri A. Pathogenetic mechanisms of angina pectoris: expanding views. Br Heart J 1980; 43:648-60.

Maseri A. The changing face of angina pectoris: practical implications. Lancet 1983; ii:746-9.

Maseri A, Chierchia S, Kaski JC. Mixed Angina Pectoris. Am J Card 1985; 56:30E-33E.

Mason DT, Spann JF, Zelis R, Amsterdam EA. Physiologic approach to the treatment of angina pectoris. N Eng J Med 1969; 281:1225-8.

Matoren GM, ed. The clinical research process in the pharmaceutical industry. New York and Basel: Marcel Dekker, Inc., 1984.

Matthews MB. Historical background. In: Julian DG, ed. Angina pectoris. Churchill Livingstone, 1977: 1-13.

Matthews MB, Turck WPG. Drugs in the management of angina pectoris. The Practitioner 1969; 202:230-7.

Maxwell RA. The state of the art of the science of drug discovery - an opinion. Drug Dev Res 1984; 4:375-389.

McMichael J. Changing views on heart failure. Ann Int Med 1959; 51:635-640.

McNeill RS, Ingram CG. Effect of propranolol on ventilatory function. Am J Card 1966; 18:473-475.

Mechelke K. Korrelation von Herz und Kreislauf zur Psyche und Konstitution. Münch Med Wschr 1962; 104:1361-5.

Medical Research Council (Streptomycine in Tuberculosis Trials Committee). Streptomycin treatment of pulmonary tuberculosis. Br Med J 1948; (ii):769-783.

Meier M. Effects of oxprenolol on cardiac contractile force, heart rate and coronary circulation. Postgrad Med J 1970 (suppl):15-21.

Meller J, Pichard A, Dack S. Coronary arterial spasm in Prinzmetal's angina: a proved hypothesis. Am J Card 1976; 37:938-40.

Melville KI, Shister HE, Huq S. Iproveratril: experimental data on coronary dilatation and antiarrythmic action. Can Med Ass J 1964; 90:761-70.

Melville KI, Benfey BG. Coronary vasodilatory and cardiac adrenergic blocking effects of iproveratril. Can J Phys Pharm 1965; 43:339-42.

Mignault de LJ. Coronary cineangiographic study of intravenously administered Isoptin. Can Med Ass J 1966; 95:1252-1253.

Mol A, Lieshout P van. Ziek is het woord niet. Medicalisering, normalisering en veranderende taal in huisartsgeneeskunde en geestelijke gezondheidszorg, 1945-1985. Nijmegen: SUN, 1989.

Monroe MT, Chung EK. Antianginal agents for coronary heart disease. In: Chung EK, ed. Controversy in cardiology. The practical clinical approach. Springer-Verlag, New York Heidelberg Berlin 1976: 115-126.

Moolenaar WH. Trends in research on oncogens and growth factors [Lecture delivered at the congress Drug design and development in perspective, Groningen Centre for Drug Research, Groningen 9 mei, 1980.

Moore JI, Swain HH. Sensitization to ventricular fibrillation. I. Sensitization by a substituted propiophenone, U-0882. J Pharm exp Ther 1960; 128:243-252.

Moran NC, Perkins ME. Adrenergic blockade of the mammalian heart by a dichloro analogue of isoproterenol. J Pharm exp Ther 1958; 124:223-237.

Moran NC, Moore JJ, Holcomb AK, Musket G. Antagonism of adrenergically-induced cardiac arrhythmias by dichloroisoproterenol. J Pharm exp Ther 1962; 136:327-335.

Moran NC. Pharmacological characterization of adrenergic receptors. Pharm Rev 1966; 18(1):503-512.

Moravcsik MJ, Murugesan P. Citation patterns in scientific revolutions. Scientometrics 1979; 1:161-9.

Morris JN. Uses of epidemiology. 3rd ed. Edinburgh London and New York: Churchill Livingstone, 1975.

Mulkay M. Patterns of scientific growth. Curr Soc 1980; 28(3):15-22.

Mulrow CD, Feussner JR, Velez R. Reevaluation of digitalis efficacy. New light or old leaf. Ann Int Med 1984; 101:113-117.

Nägle S. Die Bedeutung von Kreatinphosphat und Adenosintriphosphat im Hinblick auf Energiebereitstellung, -transport und -verwertung im normalen und insuffizienten Herzmuskel. Klin Woch 1970; 48:332-41.

Nayler WG. Calcium exchange in cardiac muscle: A basic mechanism of drug action. Am Heart J 1967; 73:379-94.

Nayler WG, McInnes I, Swann JB et al. Some effects of iproveratril (Isoptin) on the cardiovascular system. J Pharm exp Ther 1968; 161:247-61.

Neiss ES, Boyd TA. Pharmacogenology: The Industrial New Drug Development Process. In: Matoren GM, ed. The Clinical Research Process in the Pharmaceutical Industry. New York and Basel: Marcel Dekker, Inc., 1984: 1-33.

Neumann M, Luisada AA. Effect of rapid- and slow-acting "coronary" drugs on precordial pain of the aged. Am J Med Sci 1964; 247:156-63.

Neumann M, Luisada AA. Double blind evaluation of orally administered iproveratril in patients with angina pectoris. Am J Med Sci 1966; 25:552-556.

Newman RK, Bishop VS, Peterson DF, Leroux EJ, Horwitz LD. Effect of verapamil on left ventricular performance in conscious dogs. J Pharm Exp Ther 1977; 201:723-730.

Nickerson M. The pharmacology of adrenergic blockade. Pharm Rev 1949; 1:27-101.

Nickerson M. Blockade of the actions of adrenaline and noradrenaline. Pharm Rev 1959; 11:443-461.

Oates JA. Clinical investigation: a pathway to discovery [presidential address]. Trans Ass Am Phys 1982; 95:lxxviii-xc.

Östholm I. Presentation of Hässle's research and development work. In: Astra Chemical & Pharmaceuticals NV. Proceedings Swedish conference with Dutch specialists on hypertension. Gothenburg, May 17th-19th, 1972, Rijswijk: Astra, 1972: 15-24.

Paget GE. Carcinogenic action of pronethalol. Br Med J 1963; ii:

Papp C, Smith KS. Status anginosus. Br Heart J 1960; 22:259-73.

Parade GW, Bockel P. Angina Pectoris und Herzinfarkt. Stuttgart: Ferdinand Enke Verlag, 1954.

Parodi O, Maseri A, Simonetti I. Management of unstable angina at rest by verapamil. Br Heart J 1979; 41:167-174.

Parsons-Smith BT. Cardiac failure. The Lancet 1950; (i): 889-894;943-947.

Payer L. Medicine & culture. Varieties of treatment in the United States, England, West Germany, and France. New York: Henry Holt and Company, 1988.

Pellegrino ED. The identity crisis of an ideal. In: Ingelfinger FJ, Ebert RV, Finland M, Relman AS, eds. Controversy in internal medicine - II. Philadelphia: WB Saunders Company, 1974: 41-50.

Peltzman S. The benefits and costs of new drug regulation. In: Landau RL, ed. Regulating new drugs. Chicago: University of Chicago Press, 1973: 113-212.

Phear DN. Verapamil in angina: a double-blind trial. Br Med J 1968 (ii):740-741.

Pickering GW. Starling and the concept of heart failure. Circulation 1960; 21:323-331.

Pickering GW. Vascular spasm. The Lancet 1951 (ii):845-850.

Powell CE, Slater IH. Some aspects of blockade of inhibitory adrenergic receptors by a dichloro analogue of isoproterenol. J Pharm exp Ther 1958; 122:480-488.

Powell CE, Slater IH. Some aspects of blockade of inhibitory adrenergic receptors or adrenoceptive sites [Symposium on Catecholamines, Oct. 1958]. Pharm Rev 1959; 11:462-463.

Preston TA. Coronary artery surgery. New York: Raven Press, 1977.

Prichard BNC. Hypotensive action of pronethalol. Br Med J 1964; (i):1227-1228.

Prinzmetal M, Kennamer M, Merliss R, Wada T, Bor N. Angina pectoris: 1. Variant from angina pectoris: preliminary report. Am J Med 1959; 27:375-388.

Prinzmetal M, Goldman A, Shubin H, Bor N, Wada T. Angina pectoris: 2. Observations on classic form of angina pectoris (preliminary report). Am Heart J 1959; 57:530-543.

Prinzmetal M, Ekmekci A, Toyoshima H, Kwoczynski JK. Angina pectoris: 3. Demonstration of chemical origin of ST deviation in classic angina pectoris, its variant form, early myocardial infarction, and some noncardiac conditions. Am J Card 1959; 3:276-293.

Prinzmetal M, Ekmeckci A, Kennamer R. Kwoczynski JK, Shubin H, Toyoshima H. Variant form of angina pectoris. Previously undelineated syndrome. JAMA 1960; 174:1794-1800.

Prinzmetal M, Toyoshima H, Ekmekci A, Mizuno Y, Nagaya T. Myocardial ischemia. Nature of ischemic electrocardiographic patterns in the mammalian ventricles as determined by intracellular electrographic and metabolic chanes. Am J Card 1961; 8:493-503.

Proger S, Naimi S. Acute and chronic coronary heart disease. In: Friedberg CK (ed). Modern trends in disease of coronary arteries and ischemic heart disease. New York, London: Grune & Stratton, 1964: 1-13.

Proudfit WL, Hogdman JR. Physical signs during angina pectoris. Progr Card Dis 1968; 10:283-286.

Raab W. Roentgen treatment of the adrenal glands in angina pectoris (one hundred cases). Ann Int Med 1940; 14:688-710.

Raab W. Myocardial metabolism in the pathogenesis and treatment of angina pectoris. Cardiologia 1953; 22:291-303.

Raab W. The sympathogenic biochemical trigger mechanism of angina pectoris - Its therapeutic suppression and long-range prevention. Am J Cardiol 1962; 9:576-590.

Raab W. The complex pathogenesis of so-called "coronary" heart disease. In: Russek HI, Zohmann BL. Coronary Heart Disease. A medical-surgical symposium. Philadelphia, Toronto: JB Lippincott Co, 1971: 85-96.

Refsum H, Landmark K. The effect of a calcium-antagonistic drug, nifedipine, on the mechanical and electrical activity of the isolated rat atrium. Act Pharm Toxic 1975; 37:369-376.

Reindell H, Klepzig H. Krankheiten des Herzens und der Gefäße. In: Heilmeyer LN, ed. Lehrburch der Inneren Medizin, 2e Auflage, Berlin Göttingen Heidelberg: Springer Verlag, 1961: 450-516.

Reindell H. Ueber Albert Fraenkels Wirken. In: Gädeke R, ed. Herztherapie in der Praxis, Stuttgart: Hippokrates-Verlag, 1964: 11-19.

Reindell H, König K, Roskamm H. Funktionsdiagnostik des gesunden und kranken Herzens. Stuttgart: Georg Thieme Verlag, 1967.

Reindell H, Keul J, Doll E. Herzinsuffizienz. Pathophysiologie und Klinik. Stuttgart: Georg Thieme Verlag, 1968.

Reiser SJ. Medicine and the reign of techology. Cambridge [etc.]: Cambridge University Press, 1978.

Reploh HD, Bender F, Schürmeyer E. Gesichtspunkte bei der modernen Behandlung tachykarder Herzrythmusstörungen. Verh Dtsch Ges Inn Med 1967; 73:570-571.

Reuter H. Ion channels in cardiac cell membranes. Ann Rev Physiol 1984; 46:473-84.

Rip A, Groenewegen P, eds. Macht over kennis. Mogelijkheden van wetenschapsbeleid, Alphen aan den Rijn/Brussel: Samsom Uitgeverij, 1980.

Roberts J, Baer R. A method for the evaluation of depressants of subatrial rhythmic function in the heart of the intact animal. J Pharm exp Ther 1960; 129:36-41.

Roskamm H. Zur Bewegungstherapie der Koronarinsuffizienz. In: Gebhardt W, ed., Koronarinsuffizienz, Freiburger Fortbildungskurse - Band 2, Stuttgart: Hippokrates - Verlag GmbH, 1967: 168-181.

Ross G, Jorgensen CR. Cardiovascular actions of iproveratril. J Pharm exp Ther 1967; 158:504-9.

Ross OB, Charlotte NC. Use of controls in medical research. JAMA 1951; 145:72-75.

Ruesch J. Declining clinical tradition. JAMA 1962; 182:110-115.

Russek HI, Urbach KF, Doerner AA. Choice of a coronary vasodilator drug in clinical practice. Evaluation of effects by electrocardiographic tests. JAMA 1953; 153:207-211.

Sackett DL, Haynes RB, Tugwel P, eds. Clinical epidemiology. A basic science for clinical medicine. Boston/Toronto: Little, Brown and Company, 1985.

Sandler G. Verapamil bei der Behandlung der Angina pectoris. Arznei-For 1970; 20:1323-5.

Sandler G, Clayton GA, Thornicroft SG. Clinical evaluation of verapamil in angina pectoris. Br Med J 1968 (iii):224-227.

Saren MA. Classification and review of models of the intra-firm innovation process. R&D Management 1984; 14(1):11-24.

Sato M, Nagao T, Yamaguchi I, Nakajima H, Kiyomoto, A. Pharmalogical studies on a new 1,5-benzothiazepine derivative (CRD-401). 1. Cardiovascular actions. Arznei-For 1971; 21:1338-43.

Saviotti PP, Metcalfe JS. A theoretical approach to the construction of technological output indicators. Research Policy 1984; 13:141-151.

Schaefer J. The case against coronary artery surgery. A paradigm for studying the nature of a so-called scientific controversy in the field of cardiology. Metamedicine 1980; 1:155-176.

Schaffner KF. Discovery in the Biomedical Sciences: Logic or Irrational Intuition? In: Nickles T, ed. Scientific Discovery: Case Studies. Dordrecht [etc]: D. Reidel Publishing Company, 1980: 171-205.

Schaffner KF. Logic of Discovery and Diagnosis in Medicine. Berkeley [etc.]: University of California Press, 1985.

Schaffner KF. Exemplar reasoning about biological models and diseases: a relation between the philosophy of medicine and philosophy of science. The Journal of Medicine and Philosophy 1986; 11:63-80.

Schamroth L, Krikler DM, Garrett C. Immediate effects of intravenous verapamil in cardiac arrhythmias. Br Med J 1972; i:660-2.

Scherf D, Cohen J. "Variant" Angina Pectoris. Circulation 1974; 49:787-9.

Schimert G. et al. Die Koronarerkrankungen, Koronarinsuffizienz, Angina Pectoris und Herzinfarkt. In: Handbuch der Inneren Medizin, 4. Aufl., IX/3, Berlin-Göttingen-Heidelberg 1960.

Schlant RC. Altered cardiovascular physiology of coronary atherosclerotic heart disease. In: Hurst JW (ed.). The Heart. Arteries and veins. 3rd ed. New York, etc.: McGraw-Hill, 1974: 1021-33.

Schlepper M, Witzleb E. Tierexperimentelle Untersuchungen Über die Veränderungen von Coronardurchblutung und Sauerstoffverbrauch des Herzens nach ‡-Isopropy-‡[(N-methyl-N-homoveratryl)-gamma-animo-propyl]-3,4-dimethoxyphenylacetonitril. Arznei-For 1962; 12:559-61.

Schmid JR, Hanna C. A comparison of the anti-arrhythmic actions of two new synthetic components, iproveratril and MJ 1999, with quinidine and pronethalol. J Pharm exp Ther 1967; 156:331-8.

Schmidt AM. The politics of drug research and development. In: Wechsler H, Lamont-Havers RW, Cahill, Jr. GF. The social context of medical research. Cambridge [etc]: Ballinger Pubishing Company, 1981: 233-262.

Schmidt HD, Schmier J. Die kontraktilitätsmindernde Eigenwirkung verschiedener ß-Adrenolytika am Herz-Lungen-Präparat des Hundes. Z Kreislaufforschung 1967; 56:1137-1150.

Schmidt L. Pharmakologische Grundlagen der Digitalis- und Strophanthintherapie. In: Gädeke R, ed. Herztherapie in der Praxis, Stuttgart: Hippokrates-Verlag, 1964: 19-31.

Schöne H-H, Lindner E. Die Wirkung des N-[3'-Phenyl-propyl-(2')]-1,1-diphenyl-propyl-(3)-amins auf den Stoffwechsel von Serotonin und Noradrenalin. Arznei-For 1960; 10:583-5.

Schrenk M. Die Angina Pectoris. Südhoffs Archiv 1967; 51:165-83.

Schwartz A, Taira N. Introduction. Circul Res 1983; 52(S1):I1-2

Schwartz A. Studies on mechanisms of calcium channel modulators. J Mol Cell Cardiol 1987; 19 (suppl. II:
The Calcium-Antagonists. The Fleckenstein Symposium. XIIth Congress of the International Society for
Heart Research, Melbourne, Australia, 9 - 13 February 1986):49-62.

Schwartzmann D. Innovation in the pharmaceutical industry. Baltimore: The John Hopkins University
Press, 1976.

Segall HN. Drugs for anginal pain. Can Med Ass J 1964; 90:491.

Seitz W. Taschenbuch der inneren Medizin, 7th ed., Stuttgart: Wissenschaftliche Verlagsgesellschaft
MBH, 1966.

Selzer A, Langston M, Ruggeroli C, Cohn K. Clinical syndrome of variant angina with normal coronary
arteriogram. N Eng J Med 1976; 295:1343-7.

Shanks RG. Methods for the evaluation of adrenergic beta-receptor antagonists. In: Mantegazza P,
Piccinini F, eds. Methods in drug evaluation, Proceedings of the International Symposium held in Milano,
20-23 September 1965, Amsterdam: North-Holland Publishing Company, 1966a: 183-198.

Shanks RG. The effect of propranolol on the cardiovascular responses to isoprenaline, adrenaline and
noradrenaline in the anesthetized dog. Br J Pharm 1966b; 26:322-333.

Shanks RG. The pharmacology of beta sympathetic blockade. Am J Card 1966c; 18:308-316.

Shanks RG. [Letter to the editor]. What is a ß-blocker? Lancet 1967a (ii):560-561.

Shanks RG. The peripheral vascular effects of propranolol and related compounds. Br J Pharm 1967b;
29:204-217.

Shanks RG. The discovery of beta adrenergic blocking drugs. In: Parnham MJ, Bruinvel J, eds. Discoveries
in pharmacology, vol2: haemodynamics, hormones and inflammation. Amsterdam: Elseviers Science
Publishers BV, 1984: 37-72.

Shanks RG, Wood TM, Dornhorst AC, Clark ML. Some pharmacological properties of a new adrenergic
ß-receptor antagonist. Nature 1966; 212:88-90.

Silber EN, Katz LN. Clinical impression and clinical investigation [editorial]. JAMA 1953; 151 (1):44.

Silber EN, Katz LN. Coronary dilators and angina. Reappraisal. JAMA 1953; 153 (2):1075-1076.

Silber EN, Katz LN (eds). Heart disease. New York: Macmillan Publishing Co, Inc, 1975.

Silverman KJ, Grossman W. Angina Pectoris. National History and Strategies for Evaluation and
Management. N Eng J Med 1984; 310:1712-7.

Silvertssen E, Bay G, Grendahl H. The effect of propranolol and verapamil on atrial and atrioventricular
refractory periods in man. Angiology 1975; 26:605.

Singh BN, Vaughan Williams EM. A third class of anti-arrhythmic action. Effects on atrial and ventricular intracellular potentials, and other pharmacological action on cardiac muscle, of MJ 1999 and AH 3474. Br J Pharmac 1970; 39:675-687.

Singh BN, Vaughan Williams EM. A fourth class of anti-dysrhythmic action? Effect of verapamil on ouabain toxicity, on atrial and ventriculair intracellular potentials, and on other features of cardiac function. Cardiovasc Res 1972; 6:109-19.

Singh BN, Ellrodt G, Peter CT. Verapamil: a review of its pharmacological properties and therapeutic uses. Drugs 1978;15:169-97.

Singh BN. Verapamil (Isoptin^R): Historical perspective and general pharmacological profile of a prototype slow-channel inhibitor. In: Singh BN, Zipes DP, Sung RJ et al. The role of calcium ion antagonists in the management of supraventricular arrythmias — Isoptin^R. Proceedings of a symposium, Key Biscayne, Florida, january 14, 1980. Amsterdam: Excerpta Medica, 1980:1-26.

Smith RB. The development of a medicine. New York: M Stockton Press, 1985.

Sneader W. Drug discovery: the evolution of modern medicines. Chichester [etc]: John Wiley & Sons, 1985.

Sneader W. Drug Development: from laboratory to clinic. Chichester [etc]: John Wiley & Sons Ltd., 1986.

Somani P, Lum BKB. The antiarrhythmic actions of beta adrenergic blocking agents. J Pharm exp Ther 1965; 147:194-204.

Spang K. Die primär-pulmonale Rechtsinsuffizienz. Deut Med Wo 1954; 79:9-15.

Spilker B. Multinational drug companies. Issues in drug discovery and development. New York: Raven Press, 1989.

Stanton HC, Kirchgessner T, Parmenter K. Cardiovascular pharmacology of two new ß-andrenergic receptor antagonists. J Pharm exp Ther 1965; 149:174-182.

Stauch M, Schairer K. Hämodynamik nach Beta-Rezeptoren-Blockade. Z Kreislaufforschung 1968; 58:586-592.

Stegmüller W. Neue Wege der Wissenschaftsphilosophie. Berlin [etc.]: Springer-Verlag, 1980.

Stephen SA. Unwanted effects of propranolol. Am J Card 1966; 18:463-468.

Stevens R. Medical practice in modern England. The impact of specialization and state medicine. New Haven and London: Yale University Press, 1966.

Stock JPP, Dale N. Beta-adrenergic receptor blockade in cardiac arrhythmias. Br Med J 1963; (ii):1230-1233.

Stock K, Westermann E. Hemmung der Lipolyse durch ‡- und ß-Sympatholytica, Nicotinsäure und Prostaglandin E$_1$. N-S Arch Ph 1966; 254:334-354.

Stone PH, Antman EM, Muller JE, Braunwald E. Calcium channel blocking agents in the treatment of cardiovascular disorders. Part 2: Hemodynamic effects and clinical applications. Ann Int Med 1980; 93:886-904.

Strässle B, Burckhardt D. Isoptin (D-365), klinische Untersuchungen zur Behändlung coronarer Herzkrankheit. Schweiz Med Wschr 1965; 95:667-72.

Swales JD. Platt versus Pickering. An episode in recent medical history, The Keynes Press, British Medical Association, 1985.

Talalay P, ed. Drugs in our society. Baltimore: The Johns Hopkins Press, 1964.

Temin P. Taking your medicine: drug regulation in the United States. Cambridge [etc]: Harvard University Press, 1980.

Termeer G. De onmogelijke scheiding tussen poëzie en wetenschap [interview with R. van den Hoofdakker]. Universiteitskrant RU Groningen, 5-29 september 1988.

Thompson RH, Letley E. What is a ß-blocker? Lancet 1967;ii: 1149.

Toulmin S. On the nature of the physician's understanding. J Medicine Philosophy 1976; 1:32-50.

Traks E, Hackel DB, Sancetta SM. Effects of a 'new coronary vasodilator' on the general and coronary hemodynamic and myocardial metabolism of man. Ann Int Med 1959; 51 (1):31.

Tschirdewahn B, Klepzig H. Klinische Untersuchung Über die Wirkung von Isoptin und Isoptin S bei Patienten mit Koronarinsuffizienz. Deut Med Wo 1963; 88:1702-7.

Uloth RH, Kirk JR, Gould WA, Larsen AA. Sulfonaminedes - I. Monoalkyl- and arylsulfonamidophenethanolamines. J Med Chem 1966; 9:88-97.

Vakil RJ. Intermediate Coronary Syndrome. Circulation 1961; 24:557-71.

Van Eijk JThM. Verschillen in praktijkvoering van huisartsen. Een methode om van te leren. Medisch Contact 1979; 34:987-991.

VanDeripe DR, Ablad B, Moran NC. ß-Adrenergic receptor blockade by four methyl substituted N-isopropylphenylethanolamines. Federation Proc 1964; 23:124.

VanDeripe DR, Moran NC. Comparison of cardiac and vasodilator adrenergic blocking activity of DCI and four analogs. Federation Proc 1965; 24:712.

Varley KG, Dhalla NS. Excitation-contraction coupling in heart. XII. Subcellular calcium transport in isoproterenol-induced myocardial necrosis. Exp Mol Path 1973; [rest].

Vater W, Kroneberg G, Hoffmeister F et al. Zur Pharmakologie von 4-(2'-Nitrophenyl)-2,6-dimethyl-1,4-dihydropyridin-3,5-dicarbonsäuredimethylester (Nifedipine, Bay a 1040). Arznei-For 1972; 22:1-14.

Veatch RM. Drug research in humans: the ethics of nonrandomized access. Clin Pharm 1989; 8:366-370.

Veer R van der, Miedema S, Ijzendoorn MH. Simons inductivistische benadering van de ontdekking. Kennis & Methode 1983; 7:35-46.

Vereiniging der Bad Neuheimer Ärzte. Angina Pectoris, pp. 1-188, 27. Fortbildungslehrgang (29 Sept. - 1 Oct. 1961). Darmstadt: Dr. Dietrich Steinkopff Verlag, 1962.

Vos R, Bodewitz H. The dynamics of clinical-therapeutic objectives and the role of medical professional groups in drug innovation. In: Callebaut W, Cozzens SE, Lecuyer B-P, Rip A, Van Bendegem JP, eds. George Sarton Centennial. Ghent: Communication and cognition, 1984, 343-346.

Vos R, Willems D. Semiotiek als wijsgerige bezinning op de geneeskunde. Het wijsgerig denken over feiten en waarden in de geneeskunde. Scripta Medico-Philosophica 1987 (Schrift 4):40-54.

Vos R, Bodewitz H. Experimental and therapeutic profiling in drug innovation - the early history of the beta blockers. Persp Biol 1988; 469-479.

Vos R, Willems D. Hoe besmettelijk is wetenschap? Een semiotische beschouwing van de verspreiding en receptie van wetenschappelijke kennis. Kennis & Methode 1989; 13:206-224.

Vries GH de. De ontwikkeling van wetenschap. Een inleiding in de wetenschapsfilosofie. Groningen: Wolters-Noordhoff, 1984.

Wardell WM. Are these requirements enough of too much. In: De Schaepdrijver et al. The scientific basis of drug research and development. Ghent: Heymans Foundations Ghent 1978a.

Wardell WM. Controlling the use of therapeutic drugs - an international comparison. Washington DC: American Enterprise Institute for Public Policy Research, 1978b.

Wardell WM, Velo G. Drug development, regulatory assessment and post-marketing-surveillance. New York-London: Plenum Press, 1981.

Warner JH. The therapeutic perspective in medical practice. Knowledge and identity in America, 1820 - 1885. Cambridge: Harvard University Press, 1986.

Wartak J, Fenna D, Callaghan JC. Numerical approach to classification of angina. Am Heart J 1984; 107:402-404.

Wehrmacher WH. Pain in the Chest. Springfield, Illinois: Charles C Thomas, Publisher, 1964.

Wenckebach KF. Herz- und Kreislaufinsuffizienz, (Series: Medizinische Praxis. Sammlung fuer Aerztliche Fortbildung, L.R. Grote et al. (Hrsgg.)) 1. Auflage 1934; 4. Auflage, Dresden und Leipzig: Verlag von Theodor Steinkopff, 1942.

Wette K, Heimsoth V, Jansen FK. Einfluß von Iproveratril auf EKG-Veränderungen bei Hochdruck-patienten mit Angina Pectoris. MÜn Med Wschr 1966; 108:1238-42.

White PD. The psyche and the soma: the spiritual and physical attributes of the heart. Ann Int Med 1951; 35:1291.

White PO. The historical background of angina pectoris. Mod Conc Cardiovasc Dis 1974; 43:109.

Whiting RB, Klein MD, Vander Veer J, Lown B. Variant angina pectoris. N Eng J Med 1970; 282:709-12.

Wieland W. Diagnose: Überlegungen zur Medizintheorie. Berlin: Walter de Gruyter, 1975.

Wilkinson JCM. [Letter to the editor]. What is a ß-blocker? Lancet 1967 (ii):617.

Willems D, Vos R. Hoe besmettelijk is wetenschap? Een semiotische beschouwing van de verspreiding en receptie van wetenschappelijke kennis. Kennis & Methode 1989; 13:206-224.

Winbury MM. Angianginal drugs. In: Parnham MJ, Bruinvel J, eds. Discoveries in pharmacology, vol2: haemodynamics, hormones and inflammation. Amsterdam: Elseviers Science Publishers BV, 1984: 141-162.

Winbury MM. Experimental approaches to the development of antianginal drugs. In: Garattini S, Shore PA, eds. Advances in Pharmacology. vol. 3. New York and London: Academic Press, 1964: 2-82.

Wood P. Diseases of the heart and circulation. 2nd impr, 1st ed. Eyre & Spottiswoode, 1952.

Woodbridge JA. Social aspects of pharmaceutical innovation: heart disease [dissertation]. Birmingham: University of Aston, 1981.

Wulff HR, Pedersen SA, Rosenberg R. Philosophy of Medicine. Oxford [etc.]: Blackwell Scientific Publications, 1986.

Wulff HR. Rational diagnosis and treatment. Oxford [etc.]: Blackwell Scientific Publications, 1976.

Wyngaarden JB. The clinical investigator as an endangered species. N Engl J Med 1979, 301;1254-1259

Zandvoort H. Models of scientific development and the case of NMR [dissertation] Groningen, 1985.

Zandvoort H. Milieukunde en interdisciplinariteit. Kennis & Methode 1986; 10 (3):230-251.

Zimmer V. Ein Beitrag zur Behandlung von Herzinsuffizienz mit Koronarinsuffizienz. Med Welt 1966; 17:2806-2808.

Zipes DP, Besch HR, Watanabe AM. Role of the slow current in cardiac electrophysiology. Circulation 1975; 51:76-86.

Zipes DP, Troup PJ. New antiarrhythmic agents amiodarone, aprindine, disopyramide, ethmocin, mexiletine, tocainide, verapamil. Am J Card 1978; 41:1005-1014.

Zsotér TT, Church JG. Calcium antagonists. Pharmacodynamic effects and mechanism of action. Drugs 1983; 25:93-112.

Zwieten PA van. Calcium antagonists - terminology, classification, and comparison. Arznei-For 1985; 25:298-301.

Appendix I. The ranking order aspect of the concept of profile

In this appendix the ranking aspect of the concept of profile will be briefly elaborated. This ranking aspect has many forms in medical practice but here emphasis is on the pathognomonic sign, that is: a feature which is so typical for a certain disease that the physician will diagnose a patient with that feature, immediately and without doubt as suffering from that disease. Examples are (Levine (1958):

. The typical feature that when in case of a young adult who is suddenly afflicted with painful joints which are tender, warm, swollen and red, the symptoms are jumping from one joint to another in rapid succession, is pathognomonic for rheumatic fever.
. A continuous machinery murmur at the second left interspace of the chest is pathognomonic of patent ductus arteriosus, an abnormal connection in the heart.

In both cases a disease characteristic is considered **more important** than any other characteristic of the disease concerned. Henceforth, such a disease characteristic will be called a **dominant** characteristic.
Firstly, the concept of dominance and the comparison of profiles will be defined. Then, the concept of pathognomonic sign will be elaborated.

General definitions: dominance and comparison

If:

C: the set of disease characteristics
M: the set of human beings
$P: M \rightarrow \mathbf{P}(C)$, that is: P is a function from M to the power set of C, i.e. the set of all subsets of C;

Then: $P(i) \subseteq C$, where $P(i)$ denotes the disease profile of patient i.

Let E be an **elementary disease profile**, where E is a subset of C but we do not assume that all subsets need to be an elementary disease profile. Hence, if EDP represents the set of elementary disease profiles, then:

  i) $EDP \subseteq \mathbf{P}(C)$
  ii) $E \in EDP$
  iii) $E \subseteq C$

Further, Z is a **complex disease profile**, that is: a set of elementary disease profiles: $Z \subseteq EDP$

Definition I.1:

$c \in C$ is a dominant characteristic of $Z := \{c\} \in Z$

Definition I.2:

$P(i)$ looks **qualitatively** more like E_2 dan $E_1 :=$

$$E_2 \, \Delta \, P(i) \subset E_1 \, \Delta \, P(i)$$

On the basis of definition I.2 it is possible to compare at the level of elementary disease profiles. Further, we should be able to compare at the level of complex disease profiles.

Definition I.3: P(i) looks **qualitatively** more like Z_2 than Z_1:=

there is an E_2 in Z_2 such that for all E_1 in Z_1:

$$E_2 \Delta P(i) \subset E_1 \Delta P(i)$$

Proposition I.a. If $Z_2 = \{E_2\}$ and $Z_1 = \{E_1\}$, then definition I.3 corresponds with I.2.

Proof:

From I.3 it follows by substituting $Z_2 = \{E_2\}$ and $Z_1 = \{E_1\}$ that:

P(i) looks qualitatively more like $\{E_2\}$ than $\{E_1\}$ is equivalent to $E_2 \Delta P(i) \subset E_1 \Delta P(i)$,

because Z_2 and Z_1 contain merely one element. This is precisely the condition of I.2.

The preceding analysis has been restricted to the qualitative definitions; quantitative definitions can be similarly treated.

The pathognomonic disease characteristic

The following interpretation of the pathognomonic disease characteristic will be proposed. A disease characteristic will be called pathognomonic when a certain feature suggests the diagnosis more accurately than any other symptom or sign of the disease concerned. This proposal should include also the situation that a clinical picture composed of a pathognomonic sign is more suggestive for the diagnosis than any other combination of disease characteristics which does not encompass a pathognomonic sign.

Definition I.4: c is called pathognomonic with respect to $Z := c \in P(i) \cdot P(i) \in Z$.

This definition expresses that patient i has complex disease profile Z if and only if the disease profile of patient i belongs to Z.
When assuming that:
(1) c is pathognomonic with respect to Z;
(2) $c \in P(1)$;
(3) $c \notin P(2)$, it follows that:

(4) $P(1) \in Z$ (on the basis of definition I.4 and assumption (1) and (2));
(5) $P(2) \notin Z$ (on the basis of definition I.4 and assumption (1) and (3)).

Now P(1) looks more like Z than P(2) does, because from (4) and (5) it follows that

$$\{P(1)\} \Delta Z \subset \{P(2)\} \Delta Z.$$

Typical pattern of disease characteristics

The above proposal does not take into account the possibility that a certain number of clues, none of them characteristic enough to be pathognomonic, but when considered in their combination suggests a disease as much as the presence of a pathognomonic feature.

An example is provided by Levine (1958, p. 10-11): "It is well known that nosebleeds occur in many normal individuals and in a variety of diseases, but I know of no group of individuals who have repeated epistaxis (nosebleed, RV) as frequently as rheumatic children. (..) At any rate, a history of repeated nosebleeds, together with other features, which may be of doubtful significance in themselves, should make one strongly suspect that the patient is rheumatic".

Thus, a combination of disease features might be as suggestive for the disease as a single pathognomonic sign. Henceforth, such a combination will be called a **typical pattern**. This possibility will be briefly elaborated in this section.

When T represents a particular set of disease characteristics ($T \subseteq C$; $T \subseteq E$), and further when the pathognomonic sign $c \notin T$, then:

Definition I.5: T will be called a typical pattern with respect to $Z := T \subseteq P(i) \rightarrow P(i) \in Z$.

This definition expresses that patient i has complex disease profile Z if and only if the disease profile of patient i belongs to Z.

When assuming that:
(1) T is a typical pattern with respect to Z;
(2) $T \subseteq P(1)$;
(3) $T \not\subseteq P(2)$;
(4) $c \notin P(1), P(2)$, it follows that:

(5) $P(1) \in Z$ (on the basis of definition I.5 and assumptions (1) , (2) and (4));
(6) $P(2) \notin Z$ (on the basis of definition I.5 and assumption (1), (3) and (4)).

Now P(1) looks more like Z than P(2) does, because from (4) and (5) it follows that

$\{P(1)\} \Delta Z \subsetneq \{P(2)\} \Delta Z$.

Combining the definitions I.4 and I.5 it follows that a clinical picture containing a pathognomonic feature suggests the diagnosis **as much as** a picture containing the typical pattern:

If:

c is pathognomonic with respect to Z
T is a typical pattern with respect to Z
$c \in P(1)$
$T \subset P(2)$
$c \notin P(2)$
$T \not\subseteq P(1)$,

Then:

$|\{P(1)\} \Delta Z| = |\{P(2)\} \Delta Z|$.

Appendix II. Bibliometrical analysis of the impact of Fleckenstein's concept of calcium antagonism

A bibliometrical analysis was performed in order to gain insight in the extent to and the mechanism through which the concept of calcium antagonism elaborated by Fleckenstein was accepted by the scientific and medical community.

The assumption is that Fleckenstein developed the concept of calcium antagonism: "Major credit must be given to Fleckenstein for first pointing out the possibility of selective calcium inhibition".[1]

However, various scientists examined the role of calcium ions in the human organism. Moreover, the concept of "antagonism" is a well-known pharmacological and physiological notion. Thus, the combination of the term calcium and antagonism is not revolutionary in itself. Furthermore, the issue of excitation-contraction coupling, described in the text, was a rapidly developing subject in cardiac physiology in the late 1950s and 1960s.

From the **Five year Cumulation 1965-1969**' edition of the Science Citation Index it becomes clear that various articles were published with titles which linked calcium and drug therapy. In 1969 the term "Antagonists & Inhibitors" is for the first time used in The Cumulated Index Medicus as a subheading to the category "Calcium", and encompasses five articles. Two papers are published by Fleckenstein and co-workers, two other papers concern sodium-calcium- and calcium-magnesium-antagonism respectively, and the fifth concerns the inhibition by cinnarizine and chlorpromazine of the contraction induced by calcium. While the other authors discuss antagonism of calcium for describing pharmacological and physiological processes, Fleckenstein uses it to clarify a new pharmacodynamic principle. In this sense Fleckenstein can be credited with the discovery of this concept.

The bibliometrical analysis comprises two methods:
1. Counting the number of citations;
2. Citation-context analysis.

Counting the number of citations

A simple computerized search in the data base Scisearch (SCI = Science Citation Index) in the period 01/01/1974 - 23/02/1986 - using the key-word "Fleckenstein A" - yielded 118 (cited) papers published by Fleckenstein (as first author) in the period 1942 - 1985. Subsequently, the number of citations of each paper was calculated by computer. Seven papers were quoted more than 100 times; another eight more than 50 times.

Next, the counting of the number of citations of the seven most cited papers was repeated but now by hand on the basis of an analysis of the SCI-handbooks - the analysis stretched from 1961 being the first year of publication of the SCI, up till and including 1985. Some changes in the ranking according to the number of citations occurred, particularly so because of mistakes of the SCI-database (spelling-mistakes, wrongly given references, etc.) which were eliminated by the hand-made analysis. Therefore, a count by hand of the number of citations of the additional set of papers - being cited more than 50 times in the original set - was performed as well. As a result, a list of 10 most-cited papers of Fleckenstein and co-workers was retrieved (table A-II.1), the criterium being "cited more than 100 times in the period 1961-1985".

	I	II	III	IV	V	Total
1) F(1977)	-	-	-	140	1071	1211
2) F(1971a)	-	-	71	264	305	640
3) F(1972)	-	-	32	87	126	245
4) F(1969)	-	-	5	90	80	175
5) F(1971b)	-	2	23	47	96	168
6) F(1967a)	-	-	47	69	46	162
7) F(1983)	-	-	-	-	162	162
8) F(1968)	-	22	40	27	46	135
9) F(1974)	-	18	48	29	15	110
10) F(1964)	1	43	11	11	39	105
11) F(1967b)	-	13	27	14	17	71
Total	1	98	304	778	2003	3184

Table A-II.1
Citation score of most-cited papers of Fleckenstein

F = Fleckenstein; I: 1961-1965;

II: 1966-1970; III: 1971-1975;

IV: 1976-1980; V: 1981-1985.

One article, i.e. 11), was added because it formed the second part of a paper of which the first part, i.e. 6), belonged to the "top 10".[2] Citations by Fleckenstein or his co-workers (called "in house" citations) are excluded. Though absolute criteria for what counts as a high number of citations do not exist, a total number of more than 1000 citations of one paper (F(1977)), is extraordinarily high; this paper has been discussed as a "citation-classic" in the SCI (1988). Most striking is the difference in the total number of citations of the papers 1) and 2) compared with that of the other papers. This indicates that the first two papers had the greatest impact in the scientific community. Since plan and contents of both papers are rather similar, the 1977' paper may be considered as the 'mature' version of the 1971' paper.
The curves A, B, C, and D of figure 5.2 are based on this hand-made analysis (numbers of citations counted per year).

Citation-context analysis

A major problem with counting the number of citations is the lack of insight into the nature of the citation: what component of the paper is cited, and how is it cited. To gain deeper understanding of the way scientists referred to Fleckenstein's work, a citation-context analysis was performed in the following way.[3]
The SCI gives the title of the citing paper, the author(s), the affiliation and the periodical in which the citing paper appeared. Thus, articles citing Fleckenstein's papers can be listed and retrieved from the library. Subsequently, that part of the citing paper which specifically refers to Fleckenstein's paper can be found and studied. The context of the citation was defined as the sentence immediately preceding and following the citation. In doubtful cases the wider context, i.e. the paragraph, of the citation was used.
First, to restrict the large set of cited papers published by Fleckenstein a smaller set of papers was defined meeting two conditions. One condition was that the papers were acknowledged by the scientific community as important contributions to the field, i.e. being frequently cited papers. The other was that they represented Fleckenstein's work in an adequate way.
The set of cited papers was restricted to those papers published during the period 1964 - 1971 because the analysis comprised the period 1973 - 1977 (to be explained below). Therefore, the papers 1), 3), 7), and 9) of the "top 11"-cited papers of Fleckenstein were excluded. Further, paper 5) of the top-11 list was left out because it concerned calcium antagonism with regard to uterus-relaxation, not to cardiovascular applications. Hence, six articles (2), 4), 5), 6), 8), 10) and 11) were included. Further, two papers (Fleckenstein (1967c), (1970)) were added because they represented essential components of Fleckenstein's research on phosphates and cardiac metabolism.[4] As a result, eight papers were selected: Fleckenstein (1964), 1967a), (1967b), (1967c), (1968), (1969), (1970) and (1971). This set contains the article published in 1971 which because of its high number of citations may be considered important in its relation to neighboring fields, such as clinical medicine.

The years 1973, 1975 and 1977 were selected as "mark year" for the following reasons. Firstly, the middle 1970s were considered particularly interesting to see whether clinicians connect basic concepts with therapeutic developments in their own field at an early stage. This phase is the second stage which is covered fairly well by the period 1973 - 1977 taking 1975 as the turning-point of the S-shaped curve D. The first stage is deliberately left out because based on literature analysis and interviews, the impression was that Fleckenstein's work was known to few clinicians.[5] Secondly, 1973 was in any case still an early stage as suggested by curves A and D (figure 5.2), and the impact of the 1971 paper can be measured here. Thirdly, 1977 was taken as the final mark year because the qualitative results from literature-analysis and interviews suggested that late 1970s and during the 1980s medical opinion leaders formed the mediators between experimental research and clinical medicine. Moreover, taking 1977 as the final mark year was practically useful in order to keep the sample of articles to be analyzed within reasonable limits.

All articles citing the sample of Fleckenstein's articles in 1973, 1975 and 1977 were retrieved from Medlar's database by computerized SCI-search. Excluding the in-house citations the total set retrieved contains 138 articles (with 169 references) published in 64 different journals amongst which 22 journals (33 articles) were not available (table A-II.2).

Table A-II.2

Number of references to the defined sample of Fleckenstein's
articles, number of articles and journals in which
the references and the articles appeared.

	References	Articles	Journals
Total	191	150	67
In house	22	12	8 (a)
Relevant of which:	169	138	64
outside	48	33	20
in Groningen.	121	105	44 (b)

(a) Three of these eight journals, i.e. "Annual Review of Pharmacology and Toxicology", "Klinische Wochen-schrift", "Medizinische Klinik", merely contained articles of Fleckenstein and/or co-workers.
(b) One article (published in "Albrecht von Graefes Archiv für klinische und experimentelle Ophthalmologie") referred to an article of Fleckenstein in the list of references but not in the text.

The decision was made to include the articles available in the library of the University of Groningen into the sample of the analysis. Thus, the total number of articles of the sample amounted to 104, namely 105-1 (table A-II.2 and note (b)). These articles were published in 43 different journals and with 120 references according to SCI).

Table A-II.3 shows the journals (un)available in the library of the University of Groningen and the number of citing articles per journal. From the table it follows that renowned journals are included in the sample and that the journals are equally distributed over the set of articles available in Groningen and the set of articles not available as far as the disciplinary origin is concerned.

Table A-II.3

List of journals containing the papers citing Fleckenstein's papers categorized according to availability in Groningen and the number of the citing articles that appeared in the journals listed

	Available in Groningen	Number of Articles
Acta Pharmacologica et Toxicologica	yes	5
Advances in Cyclic Nucleotid Research	yes	1
Agressologie. Revue internationale de physio-biologie et de pharmaco-logie appliqués aux effets de l'agression	no	1

Angiology	yes	1
Annals of the New York Academy of Sciences	yes	2
American Heart Journal	yes	1
American Journal of Physiology	yes	1
Archives internationales de pharma-codynamie et de thérapie	yes	3
Arzneimittel Forschung/Drug Research	yes	16 (2 I.H.) Basic
Research in Cardiology	no	5 (2 I.H.)
Biochemical Pharmacology	yes	2
Biochemical Society Transactions	yes	1
Biochimica et Biophysica Acta	yes	2
Brain Research	yes	1
British Journal of Pharmacology	yes	6
British Medical Journal	yes	1
Canadian Journal of Physiology and Pharmacology	yes	1
Cardiovascular Research	yes	3
Circulation	yes	3
Circulation Research	yes	2
Comparative Biochemistry and Physiology c.comparative pharmacology	no	1
Cryobiology. Journal of the Society for Cryobiology	no	1
Deutsche Medizinische Wochenschrift	yes	1
Diabetes. The Journal of the American Diabetes Association	yes	1
Endocrinology (Los Angeles)	yes	1
European Journal of Clinical Pharmacology	yes	1
European Journal of Pharmacology	yes	9
Experientia	yes	2
Experimental and molecular Pathology	yes	1
Gastroenterology	yes	1
General Pharmacology	no	1
Herz-Kreislauf	no	5 (1 I.H.)
Internist	yes	1
Japanese Heart Journal	no	3
Japanese Journal of Pharmacology	no	5
Japanese Journal of Physiology	no	1
Journal of the American Veterinary Medical Association	no	1
Journal of Endocrinology	yes	1
Journal of Molecular and Cellular Cardiology	no	4
Journal of Pharmacology and Experimental Therapeutics	yes	8
Journal of Physiology	yes	3
Lancet	yes	1
Life Sciences	yes	1
Lyon Médical	no	1
Metabolism. Clinical and Experimental	yes	1
Monatschrift für Kinderheilkunde	yes	1

Naunyn-Schmiedebergs Archiv für experimentelle Pathologie und Pharmakologie	yes	11 (2 I.H.)
Pfluegers Archiv für die gesammte Physiologie	yes	7 (3 I.H.)
Pharmazie	yes	1
Pharmacology and Therapeutics. b. general and systematic pharmacology	no	1
Pharmacology and Therapeutics. c. clinical pharmacology and therapeutics	no	1
Physiologia Bohemoslavaca	yes	1
Postgraduate Medical Journal (London)	no	1
Proceedings of the Society for experimental Biology and Medicine (New York)	yes	1
Progress in Cardiovascular Diseases	yes	1
Research Communications in Chemical Pathology and Pharmacology	no	1
Sbornik Lekarsky (Praag)	no	1
Scandinavian Journal of Clinical and Laboratory Investigation	yes	2
South African Medical Journal	no	1
Surgical Forum	yes	1
Tohoku Journal of Experimental Medicine	no	1
Virchows Archiv für pathologische Anatomie und klinische Medizin	yes	1
Zeitschrift für Gastroenterologie	no	1

* I.H. = "in house" citations.

In order to check that the decision to include only articles available in Groningen did not affect the sets of articles distributed over the mark years unequally, table A-II.4 may be constructed.

Table A-II.4 The distribution of the number of articles citing Fleckenstein's papers included in the sample over the sets of articles available respectively non-available in Groningen

	Availability in Groningen		
	Yes	No	Total
1973	18	6	24
1975	45	12	57
1977	41	15	56
	- - -	- -	- - -
	104	33	137

From table A-II.4 it follows that the references to both categories of articles, i.e. available and non-available, are distributed reasonably well.

Finally, the articles referring to Fleckenstein were classified as "(animal) experimental", "human-experimental" and "clinical-therapeutic". The second category, i.e. "human-experimental", designated the exploration of mechanisms of actions or pathogenetic mechanisms in human subjects; the third, i.e. "clinical-therapeutic", the assessment of therapeutic efficacy in patients.

The passages in the articles in which Fleckenstein's work was referred to, that is, the "citation-contexts"[6], were also classified into three categories: 'experimental', 'conceptual' and 'therapeutic' as illustrated by the following examples:

a. **experimental**: specific experimental results or conditions are referred to, for example:

"Fleckenstein (1971) has demonstrated an increase in calcium influx into the isoproterenol-induced necrotic heart.."[7];

b. **conceptual**: the concept of calcium antagonism is quoted from a pharmacological, biochemical or physiological perspective, for example:

"(..) nifedipine, which inhibits the transmembrane calcium influx during excitation without affecting the simultaneous sodium movements (Fleckenstein 1971; Fleckenstein et al. 1972)(..)"[8]

c. **therapeutic**: the concept of calcium antagonism is quoted with respect to therapeutic applications, for example:

"The antiarrhythmic properties of verapamil have been explained by interference with calcium conductance (Fleckenstein, 1968)."[9]

In this way table 5.2 is obtained.

The difference between the numbers of references in the table presented in the text and table A-II.2 is due to the fact that during the analysis articles containing two or more references in the text were found - this was the case for 46 articles of the set (= 104 articles).

Notes appendix II.

1. Singh (1980).
2. One article published in 1953 with 116 citations was excluded from the analysis. It concerns an article about the classification of sympathomimetic amines based on experimental research by Fleckenstein carried out as a British Council Exchange Lecturer at the Department of Pharmacology at the University of Oxford. This article has no (direct) influence on Fleckenstein's research on calcium antagonists and calcium antagonism.
3. Cozzens (1985); Dolman and Bodewitz (1985).
4. Both papers being full articles were selected from a total number of 42 papers published by Fleckenstein and co-workers in the period 1964-1971 (and cited). The other papers being abstracts, monographs and/or dealing with other subject, and not available in the library of the University of Groningen were excluded.
5. In addition, Fleckenstein charged the medical world with the deplorable lack of acquaintance with his work; furthermore, the first series of Adalat-symposia which was attended by pharmacologists, physiologists and clinicians Fleckenstein was actually the "only one" who used the word calcium antagonism (Fleckenstein, pers. comm.).
6. The citation-context was defined as the sentence in the article referring to Fleckenstein, and the sentence before and after this sentence. In doubtful cases the passage was taken as the citation-context.
7. Varley and Dhalla (1973), p. 103.
8. Refsum and Landmark (1975), p. 374.
9. Silvertssen et al. (1975), p. 605.

Appendix III. Bibliometrical analysis of Charlier's "Antianginal Drugs"

In this book Charlier reviews the state of affairs regarding anti-anginal drugs. After a general overview of basic concepts, pathophysiology, hemodynamics and pharmacological and clinical methods for investigating and evaluating anti-anginal drugs (117 pp.) he discusses the pharmacological and clinical features of antianginal drugs. In his review of each group of preparations - subdivided in individual members - he discusses experimental and clinical observations hereby referring to articles in the relevant fields. Propranolol was chosen being the representative of the beta-adrenoceptor blocking agents, the five compounds mentioned in the text being the representatives of the coronary vasodilators. Since the book appeared in 1971, Charlier's review of the literature in 1970 and 1971 was considered to be incomplete and 1969 was chosen as the final mark year. Since dipyridamole was marketed in 1959 and the other four coronary vasodilators selected were developed during the 1960s, the period of 1959 - 1969 was chosen.
The analysis comprises a text-analysis while selecting and investigating the references made by Charlier in the text.

The following procedure was followed.
1. The sample of articles was formed by selecting those articles Charlier referred to in passages dealing with angina pectoris, and excluding those dealing with myocardial infarction, cardiac arrhythmias, etc. For example: articles referred to by Charlier when stating "Although its antianginal effect has been..."; and "As regards the effect of....on angina pectoris subjects..." were included. Doubtful cases such as "...in the treatment of cardiac pain in particularly painful cases of acute infarction" were excluded.
2. The retrieved articles were classified as experimental or clinical. By definition, an article was categorized as clinical whenever Charlier **explicitly** referred in the text to a clinical situation: "According to ..., the beneficial effect of ... on the angina subject.."; "...of favorable results to be achieved (102 patients)"; "With 41 patients..."; "Eight clinical tests have been carried out double-blind..."; and so on. Otherwise, articles were classified as experimental.
3. The journals in which the articles were published were headed according to origin: "Anglo-American", "German" and "Other". The placement of articles matched fairly well the location of the laboratory or clinic of the authors concerned meaning that Anglo-Saxon doctors published in Anglo-Saxon journals and German doctors in German journals.
4. Clinical articles were classified as positive or negative whenever Charlier explicitly referred to them as yielding beneficial or negative clinical results with the concerned drug in antianginal treatment: "The efficacy of....is likewise beyond doubt in the opinion of other clinicians"; "Although its antianginal effect has been denied by certain...authors, especially under double-blind conditions...other clinicians....claim that this drug is effective as preventive treatment against anginal attacks". Doubtful cases as "...led its authors to consider the antianginal effect...as being very relative" or articles referred to by Charlier as positive at one place but negative at another were labeled as 'exploratory'; the same applies to articles discussing specific aspects or pathogenetic mechanisms.

This bibliometrical procedure was checked by analyzing the articles about dipyridamole as reviewed by Charlier by performing an independent evaluation of the articles about dipyridamole using the same categories (angina pectoris, positive, negative, etc.). Charlier reviewed 39 articles about dipyridamole which were retrieved from the library: 33 articles concerned dipyridamole whereas 6 concerned dipyridamole in combination with a sedative. These six articles were excluded from analysis. Moreover, from the set of 33 articles another four articles were excluded: one article could not be located in the journal referred to by Charlier; the other three were published in journals not available in the Netherlands. The results obtained by the author's analysis matched the results of the bibliometrical analysis of Charlier's textbook.
Charlier's sample of verapamil (see 5.3.) was also checked and with the same result. Verapamil was left out from the analysis being discussed as a coronary vasodilator and as a beta blocker.
Further, through a computerized search in MEDLARS database using the name of the drugs respectively and angina pectoris as key words, the articles published during 1966-1975 were retrieved. The cross-check between Charlier's and the computer's sample has been conducted for the years 1966-69.

Charlier's review is reasonably complete, considering that his sample covers about 65% of the sample retrieved by computer, and even about 85% if articles in East-European, Spanish or Italian language are excluded. Charlier's sample can be considered as well representing the Anglo-American and German medical world.

NAME INDEX

Ablad 101, 109, 115, 120
Ahlquist 71–73, 75–77, 83, 97–98, 100, 104, 119
Albert 74
Ambrose 6
Aphthorp 91
Ariens 74
Aristotle 251
Austel 243–244
Bacon 33
Barber 276
Barger 73
Barrett 87, 89–90, 93, 95, 101, 103, 110, 121, 126–127
Bateman 127–129
Bayes 49
Beecher 5, 162
Bender 138, 191
Berntsson 110
Bignami 260, 263
Black 72, 77–78, 81–85, 87, 89, 91, 97, 101, 106, 119–120
Bradshaw 29
Brauer 202
Braunwald 99, 103, 169, 198
Bricks 95
Brittain 95
Bruel 213
Brunner 118
Brunton 186–187
Büchner 126, 207–208, 210
Burley 118
Cannon 83, 111
Carlsson 100–101, 108, 110, 274
Carrier 75
Chamberlain 91–92, 164–165, 206
Charlier 125, 193, 195
Church 35, 38
Clark 74
Clymer 10
Cochrane 4
Cohen 178
Collins 248, 250
Corrodi 108
Cournand 198
Crowther 84–86
Dale 71–73, 91–92
Davey 103, 242
Delius 214

Dengel 135
Dexter 159
Dollery 91, 165, 184
Dornhorst 84–85, 89, 205
Dresel 104
Drews 241–242
Drill 83
Dunlop 95, 98
Engelhardt 46, 99–100, 216–218, 220–222, 225, 237
Favorolo 161
Feinstein 6, 46–47
Fildes 74
Fisch 190
Fitzgerald 89, 92, 101, 103, 121, 126–127
Fleck 47
Fleckenstein 123, 126, 129–136, 138, 140, 150, 152–154, 201
Fletcher 3–5, 17
Florian 199
Folkow 107, 111, 113
Forsberg 114
Fourneau 84, 110
Friebel 205
Friedberg 158–159, 163, 167–168, 176, 198
Froment 213–214
Furchgott 74, 76
Gaddum 74
Gazes 174
Gebhardt 126
Gill 86
Gillam 91, 93
Gilman 187
Gonin 213
Goodman 187
Goodwin 92
Gorlin 177
Grandjean 118
Graubner 218, 221–222
Gregg 82, 189
Greiner 5
Gross 118, 276
Gruber 193
Haas 124
Hacking 33–34, 264
Hamilton 75
Harrison 91, 198
Harvey 188, 196, 199
Haynes 16

SUBJECT INDEX

Developments in Cardiovascular Medicine

1. Ch.T. Lancée (ed.): *Echocardiology*. 1979   ISBN 90-247-2209-8
2. J. Baan, A.C. Arntzenius and E.L. Yellin (eds.): *Cardiac Dynamics*. 1980
                                                   ISBN 90-247-2212-8
3. H.J.Th. Thalen and C.C. Meere (eds.): *Fundamentals of Cardiac Pacing*. 1979
                                                   ISBN 90-247-2245-4
4. H.E. Kulbertus and H.J.J. Wellens (eds.): *Sudden Death*. 1980   ISBN 90-247-2290-X
5. L.S. Dreifus and A.N. Brest (eds.): *Clinical Applications of Cardiovascular Drugs*.
   1980   ISBN 90-247-2295-0
6. M.P. Spencer and J.M. Reid: *Cerebrovascular Evaluation with Doppler Ultrasound*.
   With contributions by E.C. Brockenbrough, R.S. Reneman, G.I. Thomas and D.L.
   Davis. 1981   ISBN 90-247-2384-1
7. D.P. Zipes, J.C. Bailey and V. Elharrar (eds.): *The Slow Inward Current and Cardiac
   Arrhythmias*. 1980   ISBN 90-247-2380-9
8. H. Kesteloot and J.V. Joossens (eds.): *Epidemiology of Arterial Blood Pressure*. 1980
                                                   ISBN 90-247-2386-8
9. F.J.Th. Wackers (ed.): *Thallium-201 and Technetium-99m-Pyrophosphate. Myocardial Imaging in the Coronary Care Unit*. 1980   ISBN 90-247-2396-5
10. A. Maseri, C. Marchesi, S. Chierchia and M.G. Trivella (eds.): *Coronary Care Units*.
    Proceedings of a European Seminar, held in Pisa, Italy (1978). 1981
                                                   ISBN 90-247-2456-2
11. J. Morganroth, E.N. Moore, L.S. Dreifus and E.L. Michelson (eds.): *The Evaluation of
    New Antiarrhythmic Drugs*. Proceedings of the First Symposium on New Drugs and
    Devices, held in Philadelphia, Pa., U.S.A. (1980). 1981   ISBN 90-247-2474-0
12. P. Alboni: *Intraventricular Conduction Disturbances*. 1981   ISBN 90-247-2483-X
13. H. Rijsterborgh (ed.): *Echocardiology*. 1981   ISBN 90-247-2491-0
14. G.S. Wagner (ed.): *Myocardial Infarction*. Measurement and Intervention. 1982
                                                   ISBN 90-247-2513-5
15. R.S. Meltzer and J. Roelandt (eds.): *Contrast Echocardiography*. 1982
                                                   ISBN 90-247-2531-3
16. A. Amery, R. Fagard, P. Lijnen and J. Staessen (eds.): *Hypertensive Cardiovascular
    Disease*. Pathophysiology and Treatment. 1982   IBSN 90-247-2534-8
17. L.N. Bouman and H.J. Jongsma (eds.): *Cardiac Rate and Rhythm*. Physiological,
    Morphological and Developmental Aspects. 1982   ISBN 90-247-2626-3
18. J. Morganroth and E.N. Moore (eds.): *The Evaluation of Beta Blocker and Calcium
    Antagonist Drugs*. Proceedings of the 2nd Symposium on New Drugs and Devices,
    held in Philadelphia, Pa., U.S.A. (1981). 1982 ISBN 90-247-2642-5
19. M.B. Rosenbaum and M.V. Elizari (eds.): *Frontiers of Cardiac Electrophysiology*.
    1983   ISBN 90-247-2663-8
20. J. Roelandt and P.G. Hugenholtz (eds.): *Long-term Ambulatory Electrocardiography*.
    1982   ISBN 90-247-2664-6
21. A.A.J. Adgey (ed.): *Acute Phase of Ischemic Heart Disease and Myocardial
    Infarction*. 1982   ISBN 90-247-2675-1
22. P. Hanrath, W. Bleifeld and J. Souquet (eds.): *Cardiovascular Diagnosis by
    Ultrasound*. Transesophageal, Computerized, Contrast, Doppler Echocardiography.
    1982   ISBN 90-247-2692-1

Developments in Cardiovascular Medicine

Developments in Cardiovascular Medicine

43. S. Sideman and R. Beyar (eds.): [3-D] *Simulation and Imaging of the Cardiac System.* State of the Heart. Proceedings of the International Henry Goldberg Workshop, held in Haifa, Israel (1984). 1985   ISBN 0-89838-687-X

44. E. van der Wall and K.I. Lie (eds.): *Recent Views on Hypertrophic Cardiomyopathy.* Proceedings of a Symposium, held in Groningen, The Netherlands (1984). 1985
                                                                ISBN 0-89838-694-2

45. R.E. Beamish, P.K. Singal and N.S. Dhalla (eds.), *Stress and Heart Disease.* Proceedings of a International Symposium, held in Winnipeg, Canada, 1984 (Vol. 1). 1985   ISBN 0-89838-709-4

46. R.E. Beamish, V. Panagia and N.S. Dhalla (eds.): *Pathogenesis of Stress-induced Heart Disease.* Proceedings of a International Symposium, held in Winnipeg, Canada, 1984 (Vol. 2). 1985   ISBN 0-89838-710-8

47. J. Morganroth and E.N. Moore (eds.): *Cardiac Arrhythmias.* New Therapeutic Drugs and Devices. Proceedings of the 5th Symposium on New Drugs and Devices, held in Philadelphia, Pa., U.S.A. (1984). 1985   ISBN 0-89838-716-7

48. P. Mathes (ed.): *Secondary Prevention in Coronary Artery Disease and Myocardial Infarction.* 1985   ISBN 0-89838-736-1

49. H.L. Stone and W.B. Weglicki (eds.): *Pathobiology of Cardiovascular Injury.* Proceedings of the 6th Annual Meeting of the American Section of the I.S.H.R., held in Oklahoma City, Okla., U.S.A. (1984). 1985   ISBN 0-89838-743-4

50. J. Meyer, R. Erbel and H.J. Rupprecht (eds.): *Improvement of Myocardial Perfusion.* Thrombolysis, Angioplasty, Bypass Surgery. Proceedings of a Symposium, held in Mainz, F.R.G. (1984). 1985   ISBN 0-89838-748-5

51. J.H.C. Reiber, P.W. Serruys and C.J. Slager (eds.): *Quantitative Coronary and Left Ventricular Cineangiography.* Methodology and Clinical Applications. 1986
                                                                ISBN 0-89838-760-4

52. R.H. Fagard and I.E. Bekaert (eds.): *Sports Cardiology.* Exercise in Health and Cardiovascular Disease. Proceedings from an International Conference, held in Knokke, Belgium (1985). 1986   ISBN 0-89838-782-5

53. J.H.C. Reiber and P.W. Serruys (eds.): *State of the Art in Quantitative Cornary Arteriography.* 1986   ISBN 0-89838-804-X

54. J. Roelandt (ed.): *Color Doppler Flow Imaging and Other Advances in Doppler Echocardiography.* 1986   ISBN 0-89838-806-6

55. E.E. van der Wall (ed.): *Noninvasive Imaging of Cardiac Metabolism.* Single Photon Scintigraphy, Positron Emission Tomography and Nuclear Magnetic Resonance. 1987
                                                                ISBN 0-89838-812-0

56. J. Liebman, R. Plonsey and Y. Rudy (eds.): *Pediatric and Fundamental Electrocardiography.* 1987   ISBN 0-89838-815-5

57. H.H. Hilger, V. Hombach and W.J. Rashkind (eds.), *Invasive Cardiovascular Therapy.* Proceedings of an International Symposium, held in Cologne, F.R.G. (1985). 1987   ISBN 0-89838-818-X

58. P.W. Serruys and G.T. Meester (eds.): *Coronary Angioplasty.* A Controlled Model for Ischemia. 1986   ISBN 0-89838-819-8

59. J.E. Tooke and L.H. Smaje (eds.): *Clinical Investigation of the Microcirculation.* Proceedings of an International Meeting, held in London, U.K. (1985). 1987
                                                                ISBN 0-89838-833-3

Developments in Cardiovascular Medicine

Developments in Cardiovascular Medicine

78. M.M. Scheinman (ed.): *Catheter Ablation of Cardiac Arrhythmias*. Basic Bioelectrical Effects and Clinical Indications. 1988   ISBN 0-89838-967-4
79. J.A.E. Spaan, A.V.G. Bruschke and A.C. Gittenberger-De Groot (eds.): *Coronary Circulation*. From Basic Mechanisms to Clinical Implications. 1987
ISBN 0-89838-978-X
80. C. Visser, G. Kan and R.S. Meltzer (eds.): *Echocardiography in Coronary Artery Disease*. 1988   ISBN 0-89838-979-8
81. A. Bayés de Luna, A. Betriu and G. Permanyer (eds.): *Therapeutics in Cardiology*. 1988   ISBN 0-89838-981-X
82. D.M. Mirvis (ed.): *Body Surface Electrocardiographic Mapping*. 1988
ISBN 0-89838-983-6
83. M.A. Konstam and J.M. Isner (eds.): *The Right Ventricle*. 1988   ISBN 0-89838-987-9
84. C.T. Kappagoda and P.V. Greenwood (eds.): *Long-term Management of Patients after Myocardial Infarction*. 1988   ISBN 0-89838-352-8
85. W.H. Gaasch and H.J. Levine (eds.): *Chronic Aortic Regurgitation*. 1988
ISBN 0-89838-364-1
86. P.K. Singal (ed.): *Oxygen Radicals in the Pathophysiology of Heart Disease*. 1988
ISBN 0-89838-375-7
87. J.H.C. Reiber and P.W. Serruys (eds.): *New Developments in Quantitative Coronary Arteriography*. 1988   ISBN 0-89838-377-3
88. J. Morganroth and E.N. Moore (eds.): *Silent Myocardial Ischemia*. Proceedings of the 8th Annual Symposium on New Drugs and Devices (1987). 1988
ISBN 0-89838-380-3
89. H.E.D.J. ter Keurs and M.I.M. Noble (eds.): *Starling's Law of the Heart Revisted*. 1988   ISBN 0-89838-382-X
90. N. Sperelakis (ed.): *Physiology and Pathophysiology of the Heart*. (Rev. ed.) 1988
ISBN 0-89838-388-9
91. J.W. de Jong (ed.): *Myocardial Energy Metabolism*. 1988   ISBN 0-89838-394-3
92. V. Hombach, H.H. Hilger and H.L. Kennedy (eds.): *Electrocardiography and Cardiac Drug Therapy*. Proceedings of an International Symposium, held in Cologne, F.R.G. (1987). 1988   ISBN 0-89838-395-1
93. H. Iwata, J.B. Lombardini and T. Segawa (eds.): *Taurine and the Heart*. 1988
ISBN 0-89838-396-X
94. M.R. Rosen and Y. Palti (eds.): *Lethal Arrhythmias Resulting from Myocardial Ischemia and Infarction*. Proceedings of the 2nd Rappaport Symposium, held in Haifa, Israel (1988). 1988   ISBN 0-89838-401-X
95. M. Iwase and I. Sotobata: *Clinical Echocardiography*. With a Foreword by M.P. Spencer. 1989   ISBN 0-7923-0004-1
96. I. Cikes (ed.): *Echocardiography in Cardiac Interventions*. 1989
ISBN 0-7923-0088-2
97. E. Rapaport (ed.): *Early Interventions in Acute Myocardial Infarction*. 1989
ISBN 0-7923-0175-7
98. M.E. Safar and F. Fouad-Tarazi (eds.): *The Heart in Hypertension*. A Tribute to Robert C. Tarazi (1925-1986). 1989   ISBN 0-7923-0197-8
99. S. Meerbaum and R. Meltzer (eds.): *Myocardial Contrast Two-dimensional Echocardiography*. 1989   ISBN 0-7923-0205-2

Developments in Cardiovascular Medicine

Developments in Cardiovascular Medicine

Previous volumes are still available

KLUWER ACADEMIC PUBLISHERS – DORDRECHT / BOSTON / LONDON